Books should be returned to the SDH Library on or before
the date stamped above unless a renewal has been arranged

Salisbury District Hospital Library

Telephone: Salisbury (01722) 336262 extn. 4432 / 33
Out of hours answer machine in operation

Michigan Manual of Plastic Surgery

David L. Brown, MD
Assistant Professor of Plastic Surgery
Former Fellow, Section of Plastic Surgery
University of Michigan Medical Center

Gregory H. Borschel, MD
Resident, Section of Plastic Surgery
University of Michigan Medical Center

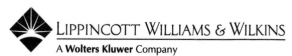
LIPPINCOTT WILLIAMS & WILKINS
A **Wolters Kluwer** Company
Philadelphia · Baltimore · New York · London
Buenos Aires · Hong Kong · Sydney · Tokyo

Acquisitions Editor: Craig Percy
Developmental Editor: Scott Scheidt
Supervising Editor: Erica Woods
Production Editor: Richard Rothschild, Print Matters, Inc.
Manufacturing Manager: Colin J. Warnock
Cover Designer: Christine Jenny
Compositor: Compset, Inc.
Printer: R.R. Donnelley-Crawfordsville
Illustrator: Holly R. Fischer, MFA

© 2004 by LIPPINCOTT WILLIAMS & WILKINS
530 Walnut Street
Philadelphia, PA 19106 USA
LWW.com

Printed in the USA

Library of Congress Cataloging-in-Publication Data

Michigan manual of plastic surgery / [edited by] David L. Brown, Gregory H. Borschel.
    p. ; cm.
  Includes bibliographical references and index.
  ISBN 0-7817-5189-6
    1. Surgery, Plastic—Handbooks, manuals, etc. I. Title: Manual of plastic surgery. II. Brown, David L., MD. III. Borschel, Gregory H.
    [DNLM: 1. Reconstructive Surgical Procedures—Outlines. WO 18.2 M624 2004]
  RD118.M456 2004
  617.9'5—dc22

                                                              2004046580

ISBN 13: 978-0-7817-5189-6
ISBN 10: 0-7817-5189-6
10 9 8 7 6 5 4 3 2

This work is dedicated to our wives, Andrea Brown and Tina Mullick Borschel, for their inspiration, example, and encouragement.

Also, to our families, for without their undying support, this would not have been possible:

Matthew and Andrew Brown, Lyn Brown, David A. Brown, PhD, Chad Brown, and Dorothy and Lawrence Brown; Anjali Borschel, Audrey and Michael Borschel, Amanda Borschel-Dan, David Borschel and Jacqueline Rankin.

Contents

Foreword

The Michigan Manual of Plastic Surgery is a book that we need. I can't think of any better way to state the import and utility of this book to nurses, to physician's assistants, to medical students, to residents, to physicians outside the specialty of plastic surgery, and to all of us in plastic surgery. Drs. Borschel, Brown and their co-authors have assembled a practical and concise reference manual that is remarkably comprehensive in its coverage of the broad field of plastic and reconstructive surgery. The result is a book that will serve anyone involved in the care of a plastic surgery patient. The book is an excellent reference for busy medical students, residents, emergency room physicians, and others who are not plastic surgeons. Because many of the book chapters have been written by residents, medical students and residents will find that the level of the material included is just right for their needs, making this book an outstanding tool for a first-pass survey of plastic surgery. The practical and concise information in this book will provide a handy reference for the nonplastic surgeon to provide appropriate initial treatment and subsequent referral of patients with the broad array of diagnoses that are treated by plastic surgeons. For the plastic surgeon, this book will serve as a practical, up-to-date reference for those areas of plastic surgery that are outside our own practices. It will also serve as a tool when preparing for re-certification and as a pocket manual during our day-to-day work. I predict that there will be many thumb-worn copies of this smart little manual in our clinics and hospitals, and that the improved care of our patients will be testament to its ultimate value.

William M. Kuzon, Jr., M.D., Ph.D.
Professor and Section Head,
Plastic Surgery
University of Michigan

Preface

The Michigan Manual of Plastic Surgery was originally conceived in response to our search for a concise, pocket-sized, comprehensive manual of plastic surgery. To our surprise we found that no such manual existed. The goal of this manual is to present the entire scope of plastic surgery in a format that is easy to read and is able to fit into a coat pocket. It is primarily aimed at providing medical students and surgical residents with core information useful for seeing patients in consultation, in the clinic, and in preparing for the operating room. Our hope is that residents will also find the information useful in preparing for the plastic surgery inservice examination and as an adjunct for study for the written boards. As plastic surgery has interaction with many other disciplines, this book will also be a valuable resource for residents, attendings, and nurses in many related fields.

This book was written by residents at the University of Michigan. Although the book is centered around the plastic surgery training program, the contributors were drawn from the many disciplines with whom we interact on a daily basis, including dermatology, general surgery, neurosurgery, oral and maxillofacial surgery, orthopedics, otolaryngology, and urology. We wish to thank our section editors, Christi Cavaliere, Steve Haase, Richard Klein, Anil Mungara, and Andrew Rosenthal for their authorship and other editorial contributions to this work. We also are indebted to our illustrator, Holly Fisher, for her fine artwork.

We hope that you enjoy this book and the material presented herein. It is our privilege to be able to contribute to the education that is so vital to the practice of plastic surgery.

David L. Brown, MD
Gregory H. Borschel, MD

About the Authors

David L. Brown, MD, FACS is an Assistant Professor of Plastic Surgery at the University of Michigan in Ann Arbor. He attended Wittenberg University in Springfield, Ohio and went to medical school at Vanderbilt University in Nashville, Tennessee. He performed his training in general surgery at the University of Cincinnati under the tutelage of Josef Fischer, in plastic surgery training at the University of Michigan with David Smith, Jr. and in microsurgery at St. Vincent's Hospital and the University of Melbourne in Australia with Wayne Morrison.

Gregory H. Borschel, MD will complete his plastic surgery residency training at the University of Michigan in June 2005, under William M. Kuzon, Jr. He attended medical school at the Johns Hopkins University School of Medicine in Baltimore, Maryland, and went to Emory University in Atlanta, Georgia for his undergraduate education.

Contributing Authors

Amy Alderman, MD, MPH	Resident, Section of Plastic Surgery University of Michigan Medical Center
John C. Austin, MD	Resident, Department of Orthopaedic Surgery University of Michigan Medical Center
Gregory H. Borschel, MD	Resident, Section of Plastic Surgery University of Michigan Medical Center
David L. Brown, MD	Assistant Professor of Plastic Surgery Former Fellow, Division of Plastic Surgery University of Michigan Medical Center
Michelle S. Caird, MD	Resident, Department of Orthopaedic Surgery University of Michigan Medical Center
Marlene S. Calderon, MD, PhD	Resident, Section of Plastic Surgery University of Michigan Medical Center
Christi M. Cavaliere, MD	Resident, Section of Plastic Surgery University of Michigan Medical Center
Edwin Y. Chang, MD	Resident, Section of Plastic Surgery University of Michigan Medical Center
Joon Y. Choi, MD	Resident, Section of Plastic Surgery University of Michigan Medical Center
Catherine Curtin, MD	Resident, Section of Plastic Surgery University of Michigan Medical Center
Sean P. Edwards, MD, DDS	Resident, Section of Oral and Maxillofacial Surgery University of Michigan Medical Center
Steven C. Haase, MD	Resident, Section of Plastic Surgery University of Michigan Medical Center
Jafar S. Hasan, MD	Resident, Section of Plastic Surgery University of Michigan Medical Center

Adam S. Hassan, MD

Fellow, Eye Plastic and Orbital Surgery
Department of Ophthalmology
University of Michigan Medical Center

Brent K. Hollenbeck, MD

Resident, Department of Urology
University of Michigan Medical Center

Emily Hu, MD

Resident, Section of Plastic Surgery
University of Michigan Medical Center

Timothy A. Janiga, MD

Resident, Section of Plastic Surgery
University of Michigan Medical Center

Lynn C. Jeffers, MD

Former Resident
Section of Plastic Surgery
University of Michigan Medical Center

Sameer S. Jejurikar, MD

Resident, Section of Plastic Surgery
University of Michigan Medical Center

Richard D. Klein, MD, MPH

Resident, Section of Plastic Surgery
University of Michigan Medical Center

Jenny B. Lynch, MB, BCh BAO

Research Fellow, Section of Plastic Surgery
University of Michigan Medical Center
Registrar, Cork University Hospital
Cork, Ireland

Keith Lodhia, MD, MS

Resident, Department of Neurosurgery
University of Michigan Medical Center

Anil Mungara, MD

Research Fellow, Section of Plastic Surgery
University of Michigan Medical Center

Caleb P. Nelson, MD

Resident, Department of Urology
University of Michigan Medical Center

Salvatore Pacella, MD

Resident, Section of Plastic Surgery
University of Michigan Medical Center

Anastasia Petro, MD

Resident, Department of Dermatology
University of Michigan Medical Center

Andrew H. Rosenthal, MD

Resident, Section of Plastic Surgery
University of Michigan Medical Center

Douglas Sammer, MD

Resident, Section of Plastic Surgery
University of Michigan Medical Center

Cecelia E. Schmalbach, MD

Resident, Department of Otolaryngology—
Head and Neck Surgery
University of Michigan Medical Center

Andrew P. Trussler, MD

Resident, Section of General Surgery
University of Michigan Medical Center

Brent B. Ward, MD, DDS

Oncology Fellow
Division of Oral and Maxillofacial Surgery
University of Michigan Medical Center

Nicholas C. Watson, MD

Resident, Section of Plastic Surgery
University of Michigan Medical Center

J. Jason Wendel, MD

Assistant Professor of Plastic Surgery
Vanderbilt University;
Former Resident, Section of Plastic Surgery
University of Michigan Medical Center

Jonathan S. Wilensky, MD

Resident, Section of Plastic Surgery
University of Michigan Medical Center

Keith G. Wolter, MD

Resident, Section of Plastic Surgery
University of Michigan Medical Center

Andrew S. Youkilis, MD

Resident, Department of Neurosurgery
University of Michigan Medical Center

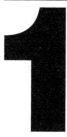

Tissue Injury and Repair

Douglas Sammer

Skin Structure

I. **Anatomy** (Fig. 1-1)
  A. **Epidermis**
   1. Stratified, keratinized.
   2. Avascular.
   3. **Stratum germinativum** (basal layer)
    a. Hemidesmosomes connect basal cells to basement membrane.
    b. Melanocytes produce melanin, which is phagocytized by surrounding keratinocytes.
   4. **Stratum spinosum:** Desmosomes connect cells, creating a spiny appearance.
   5. **Stratum granulosum:** Cytoplasm contains granules that later contribute to keratin.
   6. **Stratum lucidum:** Layer of dead cells without nuclei.
   7. **Stratum corneum:** Nearly acellular layer of keratin.
  B. **Dermis**
   1. **Papillary dermis:** Superficial thin layer of loose vascular tissue.
   2. **Reticular dermis:** Deeper layer of denser tissue, less vascular.
   3. Fibroblasts, adipocytes, macrophages, collagen, and ground substance are present.
   4. Contains sweat glands, hair follicles, sebaceous glands, nerve endings, and blood vessels.
   5. Blood vessels enter the dermis from the subcutaneous tissue and branch into subdermal and subepidermal plexuses.
II. **Adnexa**
  A. **Hair follicle**
   1. Ingrowth of epidermis into dermis and subcutaneous tissue.
   2. Associated sebaceous glands secrete into the hair follicle.
   3. Retained in thick split-thickness skin grafts.
  B. **Eccrine sweat gland**
   1. Coiled secretory structure in subcutaneous tissue with a single duct passing to the surface.
   2. Decreased or absent in skin grafts, leading to dryness.
  C. **Apocrine sweat gland**
   1. Found in the axilla and inguinal regions.
   2. Secrete into hair follicles.
   3. Become active at puberty.
  D. All adnexal structures are sources of epithelialization in partial-thickness wounds.
III. **Collagen**
  A. **Thirteen types:** The predominant types are as follows.
   1. **Type I:** Skin, tendon, and mature scar (4:1 type I–type III).
   2. **Type II:** Cartilage.
   3. **Type III:** Blood vessels and immature scar.
   4. **Type IV:** Basement membrane.

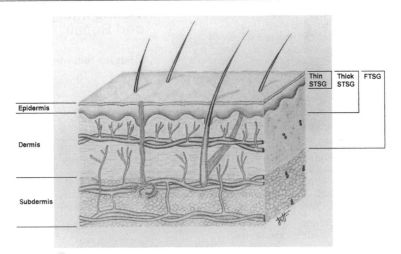

Fig. 1-1. Anatomy of the skin and levels of skin grafts.

    B. Procollagen: A single chain of amino acids.
    C. Tropocollagen: Three procollagen chains bound by disulfide bonds, forming a triple helix.
        1. Secreted by cells, and combines to form filaments.
        2. Filaments combine to form fibrils, which combine to form fibers.
    D. Vitamin C (ascorbic acid): Coenzyme involved in hydroxylation of proline and lysine, the amino acids involved in cross-linking collagen.

Normal Wound Healing

I. Wound closure
    A. Primary closure: Wound closed surgically soon after creation.
    B. Delayed primary closure
        1. Wound remains open for a few days before surgical closure.
        2. Decreases the risk of infection in contaminated wounds.
    C. Secondary closure
        1. Wound closes over time by contraction.
        2. Appropriate for infected or contaminated wounds.
        3. Allows drainage of fluid.
        4. Allows debridement with dressing changes.
        5. Prolonged inflammatory phase, leading to increased scarring and wound contracture.
II. Phases of wound healing
    A. Three phases: Inflammatory, proliferative, and remodeling.
    B. Inflammatory phase
        1. Begins at the time of injury; lasts 2 to 3 days.
        2. Begins with **vasoconstriction** to achieve hemostasis (epinephrine and thromboxane).
        3. Platelet plug forms and clotting cascade is activated, resulting in fibrin deposition.
        4. Platelets release platelet-derived growth factor (PDGF) and transforming growth factor β (TGF-β) from their alpha granules, attracting **inflammatory cells, particularly macrophages.**
        5. After hemostasis is achieved, **vasodilation** occurs and vascular permeability increases (due to histamine, platelet-activating factor, bradykinin,

prostaglandin I_2, prostaglandin E_2, and nitric oxide), aiding the infiltration of inflammatory cells into the wound.

6. **Neutrophils peak at 24 hours** and help with débridement.
7. **Monocytes** enter the wound, becoming macrophages, and peak within 2 to 3 days.
8. Limited numbers of **lymphocytes** arrive later, but their significance is unknown.
9. Macrophages produce PDGF and TGF-β, attracting fibroblasts and stimulating **collagen production.**

C. **Proliferative phase**
   1. **Begins around day 3, as fibroblasts arrive; lasts through week 3.**
   2. **Fibroblasts:** Attracted and activated by PDGF and TGF-β; arrive day 3, reach peak numbers by day 7.
   3. **Collagen synthesis (mainly type III), angiogenesis, and epithelialization occur.**
   4. **Total collagen content increases for 3 weeks,** until collagen production and breakdown become equal and the remodeling phase begins.

D. **Remodeling phase**
   1. Increased collagen production and breakdown continue for 6 months to 1 year.
   2. **Type I collagen replaces type III until it reaches a 4:1 ratio** of type I to type III (that of normal skin and mature scar tissue).
   3. Wound strength increases as collagen reorganizes along lines of tension and is cross-linked.
   4. Vascularity decreases.
   5. Fibroblast and myofibroblasts cause wound contraction during the remodeling phase.

III. **Healing in specific tissues**
   A. **Skin**
      1. In addition to production of connective tissue and wound contraction, epithelialization occurs.
      2. A single layer of cells advances from the wound edges (and adnexal structures in partial-thickness wounds), then stratifies once a single layer is complete.
      3. Partial-thickness wounds reepithelialize over the course of 1 to several weeks, depending on the depth of the wound and how many intact adnexal structures remain.
      4. If epithelialization is prolonged, as in healing by secondary intention or in a deep partial-thickness wound or burn, the inflammatory phase lasts longer, resulting in increased collagen production and contraction.

   B. **Bone**
      1. The fracture site undergoes an inflammatory phase with neutrophil and macrophage invasion.
      2. **Osteoinduction:** Precursor cells in the endosteum, periosteum, and surrounding tissue become osteoblasts.
      3. **Osteoconduction:** Osteoblasts enter the fracture site, originating from endosteum, periosteum, and surrounding tissue.
      4. A **callus** then forms, containing fibroblasts, osteoblasts, and other cells.
      5. Chondroblasts produce ground substance, fibroblasts produce collagen, and osteoblasts produce hydroxyapatite.
      6. Both apposition of bone and endochondral ossification occur.
      7. At first the callus consists of poorly organized woven bone, which is remodeled by osteoclasts and osteoblasts into lamellar bone.
      8. The more rigidly fixed and well reduced the fracture is, the less prominent callus formation and endochondral ossification are; healing occurs mainly by apposition.
      9. Once remodeling is finished, the healed bone structure is the same as normal bone, with no remaining scar.

C. Tendon

1. Tendon heals by a combination of two mechanisms: intrinsic and extrinsic healing.
2. **Intrinsic healing**
   a. The inflammatory phase is minimal.
   b. Epitenon cells move into the site of injury and begin to produce collagen, acting like fibroblasts.
   c. Intrinsic healing is increased by tendon motion.
3. **Extrinsic healing**
   a. Inflammatory, proliferative, and remodeling phases occur.
   b. After hemostasis, inflammatory cells infiltrate the wound.
   c. Fibroblasts are attracted and produce collagen, which is eventually remodeled.
   d. Adhesions form between the site of injury and surrounding tissues, and act as a pathway for cell migration and revascularization.
   e. Adhesions, and therefore extrinsic healing, are increased by immobilization.

D. Nerve

1. Axons distal to the injury are phagocytized by macrophages and Schwann cells **(Wallerian degeneration)**.
2. The proximal axons each produce one or more myelinated regenerating fibers with growth cones at the distal end of each fiber; combined, these regenerating fibers are a **regenerating unit.**
3. The regenerating unit grows distally, directed by local chemicals and factors.

E. Liver

1. The liver is the only adult organ that undergoes regeneration.
2. All hepatic cells, including hepatocytes, biliary cells, and others, are involved in recreating normal hepatic histology without scar formation.
3. Scarring (cirrhosis) occurs with chronic or severe damage.

IV. Mechanical properties

A. **Wounds have little strength during the first 2 to 3 weeks** (inflammatory and proliferative phases).

B. By the third week, the wound begins to gain strength rapidly as remodeling occurs.

C. **Wounds have 50% of their final strength at 6 weeks,** and most of their final strength a few weeks later.

D. Strength may continue to slowly increase until 6 to 12 months from the time of injury.

E. **Maximum strength is about 75% of normal tissue.**

V. Fetal wound healing

A. Skin (but not all fetal tissue) heals by regeneration without scarring. This is limited to the first two trimesters.

B. Many aspects of fetal tissue and the fetal environment may contribute to scarless healing.
   1. The fetal environment (amniotic fluid) is sterile.
   2. Amniotic fluid contains growth factors and extracellular matrix molecules.
   3. The inflammatory phase is minimal, and macrophages may or may not be the main organizing cells in the healing process in the fetus.
   4. The growth factor and cytokine milieu is different in the fetus, although the significance of any particular difference is unclear.

Factors Contributing to Impaired Wound Healing

I. Local factors

A. Arterial insufficiency

1. Local ischemia leads to inhibited collagen production and infection.

  2. Ankle-brachial index should be checked in patients who have lower extremity wounds and who are also at risk for vascular insufficiency.
  3. Correcting the underlying cause of ischemia with bypass grafting or stenting may be required before an ischemic wound will heal.
B. Venous insufficiency
  1. Increased venous pressure leads to protein extravasation and buildup, decreasing oxygen diffusion.
  2. Increased venous pressure leads to edema.
C. Edema
  1. Causes ischemia by increasing extracellular volume, decreasing oxygen diffusion and concentration.
  2. Compression and elevation are essential.
D. Infection
  1. Invasive infections are defined as having quantitative bacterial counts of 10^5 per gram of tissue or higher.
    a. Healing is impaired by many mechanisms, including increased collagen breakdown and decreased epithelialization.
    b. Hypertrophic scarring is increased.
    c. Coverage with grafts or flaps is less likely to work.
    d. An open, infected wound should be treated with appropriate antibiotics and debridement until tissue concentrations of bacteria are less than 10^5 before closure is attempted.
  2. β-Hemolytic streptococci inhibit wound healing in any concentration.
  3. Swab cultures of open wounds are meaningless; colonization does not inhibit wound healing, and may actually aid it.
E. Pressure
  1. Prolonged unrelieved tissue pressure greater than capillary arterial pressure (32 mm Hg) leads to local ischemia and plays a central role in pressure sore formation (see Chapter 47, "Pressure Sores").
  2. Pressure relief by regular position changes (with or without specialized mattresses and seat cushions) is essential to healing pressure sores.
F. Radiation
  1. Irradiated tissue often becomes relatively ischemic due to vascular fibrosis.
  2. Radiation injures fibroblasts, decreasing their ability to undergo mitosis and to produce collagen.
  3. Irradiated wounds may require skin grafting or flap closure to heal.
G. Foreign material or necrotic tissue will prevent wound healing and should be debrided.
II. Systemic factors
A. Diabetes mellitus
  1. **Microvascular and macrovascular disease** associated with diabetes leads to local ischemia.
  2. Glycosylated hemoglobin has a greater than normal oxygen affinity, and therefore **oxygen delivery is impaired.**
  3. **Neutrophil function is impaired,** and susceptibility to infection is increased.
  4. **Peripheral neuropathy** results in prolonged and increased tissue pressure because the normal signal to relieve pressure (pain) is decreased or absent.
  5. If the wound is well vascularized and glucose is well controlled (<180 mg/dL), a surgical wound in a diabetic patient should heal adequately.
B. Malnutrition
  1. **Adequate protein stores** are important to wound healing.
    a. Normal albumin level is greater then 3.5 g/dL.
    b. However, albumin half-life is 20 days and does not reflect acute changes in protein nutrition.
    c. Prealbumin level is a better measurement of acute changes in protein nutrition because of its shorter half-life (2–3 days).
    d. Prealbumin level below 17 g/dL (normal 17–45) indicates protein malnutrition.

2. Healthy, uninjured adults require **35 kcal per kilogram per day** to maintain weight, and require **0.8 to 2.0 grams of protein per kilogram per day.**
3. Caloric and protein requirements are increased with chronic wounds, large injuries, and burns.
4. In general, surgical closure of a chronic wound should not be attempted unless the patient's albumin level is above 3 g/dL.

C. Vitamin deficiency
1. Vitamin C, copper, iron, thiamine, and zinc are essential to wound healing.
2. However, supplementation of vitamins or minerals is rarely required and does not improve wound healing unless a known vitamin or mineral deficiency exists.
   a. **Vitamin C deficiency causes scurvy,** with impaired healing and wound breakdown due to decreased cross-linking of collagen.
   b. There is no evidence that vitamin C supplementation augments wound healing in patients without scurvy.
3. **Vitamin A is an exception;** supplementation may be beneficial when a deficiency does not exist. Vitamin A supplementation either orally or topically (mixed with topical antimicrobials) can reduce some of the adverse wound-healing effects of glucocorticoids.

D. Chemotherapy
1. By suppressing the bone marrow's ability to produce inflammatory cells, the inflammatory phase of healing is blunted.
2. Wound infection is also increased.

E. Smoking
1. **Smoking increases carboxyhemoglobin,** decreasing oxygen delivery to peripheral tissue.
2. **Nicotine,** including patches and gum, causes peripheral vasoconstriction.
3. Nicotine is particularly deleterious for flaps and skin grafts, where vascular supply is critical.
4. Optimally, patients should stop smoking at least 2 weeks prior to surgery and maintain cessation until wound is healed.
5. **Urine cotinine levels** can be measured preoperatively to gauge patient compliance.

F. Aging
1. **A decreased inflammatory phase** in the elderly slows the healing process.
2. Both healthy skin and wounds have decreased strength.
3. Age alone does not prevent a wound from healing, but can contribute to poor wound healing if combined with other factors.
4. Because the inflammatory phase is decreased, hypertrophic scarring is unusual.

G. Glucocorticoids
1. **Inhibit the inflammatory phase** of healing.
2. **Inhibit collagen synthesis** by fibroblasts, leading to decreased wound strength.
3. Healing can be improved with **vitamin A supplementation** (see above).

Chronic Wounds

I. **Definition:** Wounds that do not heal within 3 months are considered chronic wounds.

II. **Approach**
   A. **Adequate debridement:** Chronic wounds often have a significant amount of scar tissue, proteinaceous debris, or necrotic tissue that inhibits healing.
   B. **Treatment of infection**
   1. Infection should be suspected in a chronic wound.
   2. Tissue cultures and quantitative counts should be obtained.

C. **Appropriate wound dressings**
   1. Desiccation is a common factor contributing to poor wound healing and poor epithelialization in chronic wounds.
   2. Dressings should keep the wound moist and prevent desiccation.
   3. Dressings may also be used to debride, deliver topical antimicrobials, or absorb wound exudates as appropriate for a given wound.
D. **Treatment of the local and systemic factors** that impair wound healing, including vascular disease, edema, diabetes, malnutrition, and pressure.

Excessive Wound Healing

I. **Keloids**
   A. **Excessive scar formation:** Defined by scar tissue that extends beyond the boundaries of the incision or wound.
   B. **Etiology**
      1. Not completely understood, but growth factors certainly play a role.
      2. Keloids contain elevated levels of TGF-β.
   C. **Demographics and natural history**
      1. More common in patients of African ancestry.
      2. Tendency to form keloids is often inherited in an autosomal dominant pattern.
      3. Common in ear lobes and areas of tension.
      4. Keloids may develop months to a year after injury, and do not resolve spontaneously.
   D. **Histology**
      1. Excess collagen, and increased vascularity compared with normal scar tissue.
      2. Collagen production is many times that seen in normal scar tissue, and there is a higher proportion of type III collagen.
   E. **Treatment**
      1. Excision alone is rarely successful.
      2. Corticosteroid injection may cause some reduction in keloid size.
      3. Excision followed by corticosteroid injection locally is more successful.
      4. Excision should be followed by radiation therapy for severe cases.
      5. Recurrence is common.
II. **Hypertrophic scars**
   A. **Excessive scar formation:** Defined by scar tissue that does not extend beyond the boundaries of the incision or wound.
   B. **Etiology**
      1. Prolonged or increased inflammatory phase of healing.
      2. Increased wound tension.
   C. **Demographics and natural history**
      1. More common in patients of African ancestry.
      2. Less genetic component than keloids.
      3. Tendency decreases with age, as the inflammatory phase of healing decreases.
      4. More common in areas of tension, such as the presternal area.
      5. Develop within weeks of wounding (during the inflammatory phase), and there is usually some degree of improvement with time.
   D. **Histology**
      1. Increased collagen with collagen nodules, hypervascularity.
      2. Collagen production is increased compared with normal scar tissue, but less than in keloids.
   E. **Treatment**
      1. **Corticosteroid injection,** silicone sheeting, and pressure are often successful in reducing the degree of scar hypertrophy. Multiple treatments with corticosteroids may be required, and silicone sheeting and pressure

garments must be applied for at least 6 months before improvement is seen.

2. **Surgical excision** and reclosure may be successful if nonsurgical modalities are not working, and if the wound can be closed without tension.

Pearls

1. Vitamin E has not been shown to improve scars, whether keloid, hypertrophic, or normal.
2. Neutrophils, unlike macrophages, are not essential to wound healing; wounds will heal well without a neutrophil infiltrate.
3. Because remodeling begins at about 3 weeks, wounds do not rapidly gain strength until after this time.
4. Chronic wounds will heal if they are well debrided, infection is treated, appropriate dressings are applied, and underlying factors are corrected.
5. Nicotine, including that found in patches or gum, impairs wound healing, particularly in skin grafts and flaps.

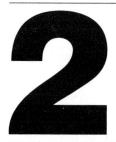

Surgical Techniques and Wound Management

Andrew P. Trussler

Management of Traumatic Wounds

I. Evaluation
  A. The management of immediately life-threatening issues always takes precedence over wound management.
  B. History of the wound should include time, mechanism, and the environmental conditions of the trauma (see below). Wounds that have remained open for over 6 to 8 hours are more likely than fresh wounds to become infected if closed. Therefore, many such wounds may be allowed to heal for delayed primary closure or by secondary closure (see below). The mechanism predicts the degree of tissue damage. The environmental conditions surrounding wounding (e.g., farm accidents) may predict a greater likelihood of contamination.
  C. Past medical history
    1. **Comorbidities:** Diabetes, vascular disease, immunosuppression, malignancy, coagulopathies, malnutrition, and valvular disease can impair wound healing.
    2. **Tetanus status:** Determine the need for prophylaxis (Table 2-1).
    3. **Past surgical history:** Document previous surgical scars, the presence of vascular bypass(es), old nonhealing wounds, and previous implants.
    4. **Medications:** Steroids and other immunosuppressants may impair wound healing.
    5. **Allergies:** Allergies to sulfa-containing drugs are a contraindication for the use of topical silver sulfadiazine (Silvadene), but not for mafenide acetate (Sulfamylon); use penicillin allergy to guide antibiotic treatment if indicated.
    6. **Tobacco use:** A significant cause of impairment of wound healing.
  D. Physical exam
    1. **Examine the wound** for active hemorrhage, foreign bodies, and surrounding tissue damage.
    2. **Evaluate for tetanus-prone wounds** (more than 6 hours old, stellate, deep punctures, crush injuries with signs of infection, devitalized tissue, or foreign body contamination).
    3. Evaluate for proximity to and damage to underlying nerves, blood vessels, bone, and muscle.
    4. **Document a complete neurovascular examination.**
    5. Probe lacrimal and parotid ducts to assess for injury, if suspected.
    6. Measure length, area, and depth of wound and describe configuration (i.e., stellate, linear, avulsion, etc.).
  E. Radiology: Evaluate underlying structures for fracture, hematoma, and gas.
II. Irrigation and debridement
  A. It is difficult to define the border between irreversibly damaged tissue and salvageable tissue in the acute setting, but a delay in debridement may cause further tissue damage and infection.
  B. Debridement involves the excision of all devitalized, contaminated tissue and foreign bodies.

Table 2-1. Tetanus prophylaxis guidelines from the Centers for Disease Control and Prevention, 1998

Tetanus Toxoid History	Clean, Minor Wounds	Contaminated or Major Wounds
<3 doses, or unknown	Tetanus toxoid	Tetanus toxoid Tetanus immunoglobulin
≥3 doses	Nothing (except tetanus toxoid if >10 yr since last booster)	Nothing (except tetanus toxoid if >10 yr since last booster; consider immunoglobulin if toxoid is not administered)

    C. In the case of a crush component, or if a large area or vital structures or both are in question, surgical débridement of grossly involved tissues, followed by aggressive dressing changes, can be initiated until further definition of the wound evolves (demarcation).

    D. Ideally, **vital structures** including nerves, blood vessels, tendons, and bones should not be debrided, if possible. However, if grossly infected or unsalvageable, they should be debrided and reconstructed.

    E. Irrigation with copious amounts of normal saline solution or lactated Ringer's via a pulsatile jet irrigator is beneficial in the reduction of bacterial counts and surface debris in acute wounds.

    F. Combinations of different debridement techniques can complement each other. **Mechanical debridement** employs both sharp and blunt excision of devitalized tissue; **gauze debridement** uses repetitive applications of moistened gauze, which desiccates and gradually removes necrotic, fibrinous debris from the wound (not used for clean wounds); and **chemical debridement** employs topical enzymes, which digest devitalized tissue.

III. Closure

    A. Closure should be attempted within 6 hours if the wound is clean, debrided, free of foreign bodies, irrigated, and hemostatic.

    B. Primary closure: Performed at the time of presentation.

    C. Secondary intention closure: Allows the wound to heal on its own.

    D. Tertiary closure (delayed primary closure): Performed after a period of secondary healing.

    E. Wounds with bacterial concentrations of greater than 10^5 organisms per gram of tissue have been shown to heal poorly without further debridement. β-Hemolytic streptococci can impair wound healing at lower concentrations.

    F. Lacerations to areas of abundant blood supply, such as the face and hands, resist bacterial proliferation, extending the window of opportunity for primary closure.

    G. Human and cat bite wounds typically have high initial virulent bacterial counts and should generally not be closed primarily.

        1. Human bite wounds are often contaminated with *Eikenella corrodens.*

        2. Cat bite wounds are prone to infection with *Pasteurella multocida.*

    H. Treatment of contaminated wounds with debridement and dressing changes decreases the bacterial concentration to facilitate safe, delayed primary closure.

IV. Classification of operative wounds

    A. Clean (Class I): Atraumatic, uninfected, with no entry into the genitourinary, gastrointestinal, or respiratory tracts; 1% to 5% infection rate.

    B. Clean-contaminated (Class II): Minor breaks in sterile technique, entry into genitourinary, gastrointestinal, or respiratory tracts without significant spillage; 8% to 11% infection rate.

    C. Contaminated (Class III): Traumatic wounds or gross spillage of enteric contents, with entry into infected tissue, bone, or fluid; 15% to 16% infection rate.

    D. Dirty (Class IV): Drainage of abscess or debridement of soft tissue infection; 28% to 40% infection rate.

V. Indications for antibiotic use
   A. Acute wounds with surrounding cellulitis or gross contamination.
   B. Human or animal bites: Directed antibiotic coverage (see organisms, discussed earlier).
   C. Contaminated wounds in immunosuppressed or diabetic patients: Consider broad-spectrum and anaerobic coverage.
   D. Significant wounds to the central face: To prevent spread to the cavernous sinus.
   E. Valvular disease: To prevent endocarditis; presence of prosthetic device: to prevent bacterial seeding.
   F. Lymphedematous extremities.
   G. Initial treatment: Broad (penicillinase-resistant or cephalosporin), with more specific therapy dictated by bacterial culture and sensitivity.
   H. Routine soft tissue infections: Usually caused by gram-positive organisms (staphylococci or streptococci), and empiric narrow coverage can be employed while observing clinical response.
   I. Crepitus or foul smell: May suggest an anaerobic infection.

VI. Dressings
   A. Partial-thickness injuries (e.g., abrasions and donor sites) heal by reepithelialization from the hair follicles.
      1. Improved healing is witnessed with adherent dressings that maintain a moist environment, such as biologic dressings (allografted or xenografted skin), synthetic biologic dressings (Integra), hydrogel dressings, and semipermeable or nonpermeable membranes (Tegaderm or OpSite).
      2. Petroleum-based antimicrobial gauze (e.g., Xeroform)
         a. May be encouraged to dry onto a partial-thickness wound to provide a matrix for scab formation. Natural scab is composed of fibrin, blood clot, and wound exudates, which protect and seal the underlying wound.
         b. Useful for split-thickness skin graft donor sites.
         c. Reliable, easy to use, and low infection rates.
         d. Reepithelialization is slower, and there is typically more pain compared with occlusive dressings.
   B. Saline-moistened gauze dressings ("normal saline wet-to-dry") theoretically debride necrotic tissue from contaminated wounds as the dressing dries. This type of dressing should not be routinely used, because the wound bed tends to become desiccated, impairing healing.
   C. Silver sulfadiazine
      1. Provides a broad topical antibiotic and helps maintain a moist environment.
      2. The mainstay of dressing care for a majority of traumatic wounds.
   D. "Wet to wet," or hydrating dressings, should be placed over exposed vessels, tendons, or nerves to prevent desiccation.
   E. Layered gauze should be maintained over sutured wounds for 48 hours to prevent bacterial contamination, protect the wound from trauma, wick moisture from the wound surface, and facilitate epithelialization.
   F. Topical antimicrobial ointments may provide an occlusive, moist environment for wound healing. These should not be used for more than a few days because prolonged use has been associated with allergic reactions and rashes, which can be difficult to distinguish from cellulitis.

Surgical Wounds

I. Incisions
   A. Skin incisions should be placed inconspicuously, and when possible, hidden from view.
   B. For example, forehead procedures may be performed via a transcoronal approach, breast procedures from an inframammary, transaxillary, or periareolar approach, and nasal procedures from a transcolumellar approach.

C. **Relaxed skin tension lines (RSTLs), or Langer's lines** (Fig. 2-1): Natural skin lines or wrinkle lines with minimal linear tension. They lie perpendicular to the lines of pull of the underlying muscles and are accentuated with muscular activity. They were demonstrated in 1861 by Langer, who punctured cadaveric skin with a rounded punch to create elliptical wounds through natural skin tension. Placement of incisions parallel to RSTLs minimizes widening and hypertrophy and helps to camouflage scars.

D. **Incisions should be made as short as possible,** while long enough to complete the procedure and minimize the amount of traction on the wound edge.

E. Placement of skin incisions should not compromise future flap design, or adequate mobilization or resection of surrounding skin.

F. **Extremity incisions should generally be made longitudinally.** Placement in the midaxial plane helps to avoid placing a scar over the flexor surface of a joint, which can lead to flexion contracture.

G. **Common hand exposures:** Facilitated by midaxial or volar zigzag (Bruner), linear dorsal intermetacarpal, and perpendicular thenar incisions.

H. **Scalp incisions** should be beveled parallel to the hair follicles to prevent incisional alopecia.

I. **Eversion of wound edges** promotes flat, nondepressed scars due to excellent approximation of the deep dermis.

J. **The triangle over the anterior chest** from the shoulders to the xiphoid has an increased tendency to form hypertrophic scars.

K. **Plantar foot incisions** commonly result in long-term postoperative pain.

II. **Handling of tissue**

A. **A sound knowledge of anatomy** and a formal preoperative plan help prevent unnecessary incision and dissection.

B. **Preoperative and intraoperative Doppler mapping** of vascular pedicles, loupe magnification, and bipolar coagulation help protect tissues.

C. **Excessive retraction and pressure** can crush tissues, resulting in ischemia, necrosis, and delayed healing. Skin should be retracted with minimal tension with hooks or fine-toothed forceps.

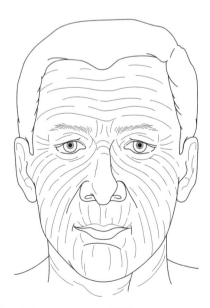

Fig. 2-1. Langer's relaxed skin tension lines (RSTLs) in the face.

   D. Moist packs and irrigation should be used liberally intraoperatively to prevent tissue desiccation.
   E. Dissection should be carried out in anatomic planes to avoid unnecessary violation of fascia, blood vessels, nerves, and muscle.
   F. Excessive traction on nerves may cause neuropraxia.
III. **Aseptic technique**
   A. Prevention of infections involves the surgeon, staff, and instrumentation, although surgical technique and host factors play major roles in preventing surgical site infection.
   B. A surgeon's hand is normally colonized by coagulase-negative staphylococci and coryneform bacteria; conversion to a moist environment beneath gloves preferentially promotes proliferation of gram-negative resident bacteria.
   C. Hand scrubbing
      1. Classically should last **2 to 5 minutes** with alcohol, iodophors, or chlorhexidine gluconate-based scrubs.
      2. **Chlorhexidine gluconate** is the most effective agent.
      3. **Chlorhexidine/alcohol "waterless" hand scrubs** have been proven effective with less scrubbing time.
   D. Operative sites can be prepared with the same agents.
   E. Avoid cleansing open wounds with scrub solutions, because they can be toxic to tissues; saline irrigation is generally sufficient.
   F. Hair should be *clipped* from the operative field prior to preparation; *shaving* is associated with increased infection rates, particularly when performed the night before surgery.
   G. Avoid hair removal in cosmetically sensitive areas, such as the scalp, eyebrows, and beard. Hair regrowth in these areas may be inhibited.
IV. **Hemostasis**
   A. Bleeding can cause ischemia and hematoma formation, which can be a nidus for infection and can compromise both wound healing and flap survival.
   B. Epinephrine, either injected or topical, can act as a potent vasoconstrictor to maintain a dry operative field. Epinephrine should not be used for digital or penile blocks for fear of terminal ischemia, and systemic signs of absorption should be monitored (tachycardia, hypertension, arrhythmias).
   C. Electrocautery can be used to thermocoagulate small blood vessels by providing a direct electrical current of high frequency and amperage and low voltage.
      1. **Unipolar electrocautery** directs current through the tissue to a grounding pad. Distribution to surrounding structures is variable.
      2. **Bipolar electrocautery** minimizes distribution to surrounding tissues and affects only the tissues between the forceps teeth.
   D. Large vessels should be clamped and tied, or suture-ligated.
   E. Topical hemostatic agents can be used on large oozing areas and vascular anastomoses. They include fibrin glue or spray, thrombin, and gelatin sponges (Gelfoam).
   F. Drains can be placed in an operative field to reduce serum and blood accumulation. These are generally removed when their output is 15 to 30 cc per day (depending on the anatomic site). Drains do not prevent hematomas!
V. **Closure materials**
   A. Closure materials include sutures, adhesives, and staples. **All provide anatomic realignment and strength during wound healing.**
   B. Suture materials are classified as natural or synthetic, absorbable or nonabsorbable, and braided or monofilament.
      1. **Natural sutures** tend to be more reactive (induce a greater inflammatory response) than **synthetics.**
      2. **Absorbable sutures** lose tensile strength as they are degraded. In children or uncooperative adults, absorbable sutures are often used for skin closure because they do not require removal.
         a. **"Gut" sutures** (ovine intestinal submucosa/bovine intestinal serosa): Moderately reactive, hydrolyzed by proteolytic enzymes within 60 days;

lose tensile strength within 7 days. If treated with chromization ("chromic gut" sutures), they will last 2 to 4 times longer. "Fast-absorbing chromic gut" is ideal for rapidly healing tissues such as oral mucosa and some pediatric lacerations and incisions.

  b. **Polyglycolic acid** (e.g., Vicryl): Synthetic, braided, minimally reactive, and absorbed within 90 days. It begins to absorb and lose tensile strength in 2 weeks. It is widely used for intradermal sutures, though it can "spit" (extrude) or become a nidus of infection.

  c. **Polydioxanone** (e.g., PDS): A synthetic monofilament, minimally reactive, and absorbed within 6 months. It loses tensile strength within 4 weeks, has a tendency to "spit," and has a low risk of infection.

  d. **Polycaprone glycolide** (e.g., Monocryl): A synthetic monofilament, minimally reactive, absorbed within 3 months, and loses tensile strength within 3 weeks.

3. **Nonabsorbable sutures**

  a. **Nylon:** A synthetic monofilament, minimally reactive, slow to resorb, maintains tensile strength for more than 2 years, has a low coefficient of friction (i.e., it is "slippery"), and is ideal for running dermal stitches.

  b. **Polypropylene** (e.g., Prolene): A synthetic monofilament, minimally reactive, maintains tensile strength longer than nylon, has a lower coefficient of friction, and is somewhat more difficult to handle than nylon. It is ideal for running suturing of vascular anastomoses and dermal closures.

  c. **Silk** (braided): Moderately reactive, undergoes significant proteolysis in 2 years with progressive tensile strength loss over 1 year; easy to use; can be a nidus for infection.

  d. **Braided polyester** (e.g., Ethibond): Moderately reactive, no absorption, maintenance of tensile strength for over 2 years, and usually becomes encapsulated in connective tissue.

  e. **Stainless steel** (braided or monofilament): Minimal reaction, excellent maintenance of tensile strength if used properly; difficult to handle.

4. **Braided sutures** have superior handling characteristics compared with **monofilament** sutures, but infection rates are slightly higher with braided sutures.

C. **Other closure materials**

  1. **Staples** create minimal reaction and are more rapid than suture closure, but less precise. They provide excellent strength and hemostasis for single-layer scalp wound closure.

  2. **Surgical tapes** (e.g., Steri-Strips) can be used alone or over sutures to help approximate, protect, and conceal the surgical wound. Excess tension can cause blistering. They can be left on the wound until they begin to peel off.

  3. **Biologic or synthetic adhesives** (e.g., cyanoacrylates) can be used with or without sutures to provide closure and protection to a low-tension wound. Cosmetically appealing and more rapid than sutures. Precision of closure is sometimes compromised.

VI. **Closure methods** (Fig. 2-2)

A. **Simple interrupted sutures:** Provide exact approximation of the wound edges with minimal manipulation or tension. This method is more time-consuming than continuous ("running") techniques.

B. **Vertical and horizontal mattress sutures:** Increase the degree of eversion of the wound edge, though they can be more ischemic (especially horizontal mattress sutures).

C. **Subcuticular continuous or interrupted sutures:** Placed in the dermis, avoiding the need for surface sutures and resulting in no external suture material and favorable scarring. An absorbable or nonabsorbable monofilament can be used. If the tails are left long and brought out through the skin, the stitch can be removed in the office once healing has begun.

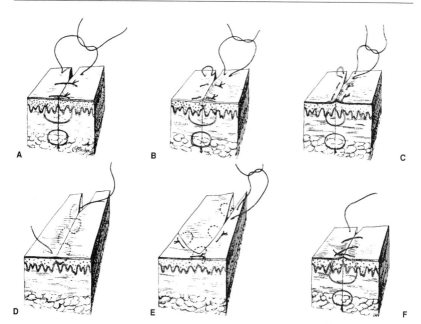

Fig. 2-2. Suture closure methods for the skin. **A:** Simple interrupted. **B:** Vertical mattress. **C:** Horizontal mattress. **D:** Continuous subcuticular. **E:** Half-buried horizontal mattress. **F:** Running. (From Place M, Herber S, and Hardesty R. Basic techniques and principles in plastic surgery. In *Grabb and Smith's Plastic Surgery*, 5th ed. Aston SJ, Beasley RW, Thorne CH, (eds) Philadelphia, Lippincott-Raven, 1997. With permission.)

   D. Continuous running sutures: Often used in place of simple interrupted sutures. Fine running sutures can replace simple interrupted sutures in low-tension wounds, and are placed much more rapidly. Locking the suture provides for improved hemostasis, although this is rarely needed.

   E. The timing of suture removal depends on the absorption rate of the suture, anatomic region, wound healing capabilities, wound tension, and desired cosmetic result. Epithelialization of the suture tract typically develops in 7 to 10 days, creating scarring.

      1. In the face, it is cosmetically optimal to remove the skin sutures in 4 to 7 days, provided that the wound has healed with sufficient tensile strength.

      2. In the extremities and trunk, skin sutures are commonly removed 1 to 2 weeks postoperatively.

3 Grafts

Edwin Y. Chang

I. **General**
   A. **Autograft:** From the same individual.
   B. **Allograft:** From another individual of the same species.
   C. **Xenograft:** From another species.
II. **Skin grafts**
   A. **Indications**
      1. **Typically the second rung** on the reconstructive ladder, after primary closure.
      2. **Lack of adjacent tissue for coverage:** Quantity, quality, location, appearance.
      3. **Uncertainty of tumor clearance** or margin control.
      4. **Morbidity, risk, and potential for complications** associated with more complicated treatment options.
      5. **Other factors:** Nutritional status, age, comorbid conditions, smoking, and compliance.
   B. **Recipient site requirements**
      1. **Viability:** Recipient surface must provide an adequate blood supply and be devoid of devitalized tissue.
      2. **Hemostasis:** Hematoma is the major cause of graft failure.
      3. **Bacterial load:** Excessive bacterial contamination will prevent graft take.
      4. **Comorbidities:** Certain systemic diseases (diabetes), effects (smoking), medications (anticoagulants, nicotine), and local conditions (irradiation, venostasis) can affect graft survival.
   C. **Delayed graft application**
      1. Harvested grafts may be stored on the donor site or at 4°C for several days.
      2. Viability of graft decreases with time.
      3. Useful for monitoring early viability of muscle flaps that would be obscured by skin graft coverage.
      4. Allows maximization of recipient site (improved hemostasis, decreased serous output).
   D. **Graft healing and survival**
      1. **Imbibition:** Plasma imbibition is responsible for skin graft survival for 2 to 3 days until angiogenesis occurs.
      2. **Revascularization**
         a. Starts in 2 to 3 days, with full circulation restored in 6 to 7 days.
         b. Theories include direct anastomoses between recipient and donor vessels (inosculation), ingrowth of vessels along channels of donor vessels, and new, random vascular ingrowths.
      3. **Regeneration of dermal appendages**
         a. Dermal appendages are more likely to regenerate in thicker grafts.
         b. Once sweat glands regenerate and reinnervation occurs, sweating assumes the characteristics of the recipient site.
         c. Sebaceous glands retain the characteristics of the donor site.
      4. **Reinnervation**
         a. Reinnervation assumes the characteristics of the recipient site.

b. Split-thickness grafts can regain sensations quicker, but full-thickness grafts regain more complete innervation.

c. Reinnervation is incomplete, and some degree of deficit will persist.

5. Pigmentation

a. Coloration is more predicable in full-thickness grafts.

b. Permanent hyperpigmentation may result from sun exposure prior to full scar maturation.

6. Primary contraction

a. Due to elastic fibers in dermis.

b. Less in split-thickness grafts (<20%).

c. Greater in full-thickness grafts (>40%).

7. Secondary contraction

a. Progresses slowly over 6 to 18 months.

b. Full-thickness grafts contract less, because dermal components suppress myofibroblast activities.

E. Split-thickness skin graft (STSG) (Table 3-1)

1. Anatomy: STSGs contain the epidermis and partial, variable thickness of dermis. (See Figure 1-1, Chapter 1.) Thicker grafts maintain more donor skin characteristics but require more optimal recipient site conditions for survival.

2. Indications: Split-thickness grafts are more robust, and larger areas can be harvested compared with full-thickness grafts.

a. Resurface large wounds, cavities, and mucosal defects.

b. Muscle flap coverage.

c. Flap donor site closure.

d. Wound coverage after tumor extirpation, when the situation requires pathologic examination for clearance prior to definitive reconstruction.

3. Donor site selection: Consider the location of the resulting scar, ease of postoperative donor site care, and adequacy of available area. Typical donor site is the anterolateral thigh, which maximizes all of these criteria. Small grafts can be taken from the upper inner arm. The scalp can be an excellent donor site, with a hidden scar and good facial skin match.

4. Technique

a. Harvest

(1) Free-hand knife (Goulian knife, Weck blade, or Blair knife) or scalpel. Grafts often have irregular edges and variable thickness. The quality of the graft is operator dependent.

(2) Drum dermatome: Useful for taking a graft from an irregular surface and for taking irregularly shaped grafts. Mentioned for historical perspective.

(3) Air- or electricity-driven dermatome: Rapid harvest of large grafts that are of consistent thickness.

Table 3-1. Comparison between split-thickness and full-thickness skin grafts

Split-Thickness Grafts	Full-Thickness Grafts
Epidermis and partial-thickness dermis	Epidermis and entire dermis
Easier take	Improved cosmesis
Less primary contraction	Greater primary contraction
Greater secondary contraction	Less secondary contraction
Donor site heals by reepithelialization	Donor site can usually be closed primarily
	Preferred for facial defects, hands, and over joints

b. Meshed grafts versus sheet grafts
 (1) Meshing increases the coverage area while minimizing the harvest area.
 (2) Meshing can improve the contour of grafts over irregular surfaces.
 (3) Meshing allows for fluid egress, reducing the chance of hematoma or seroma formation.
 (4) Meshing increases secondary wound contraction and may be desirable to decrease the size of the wound. Avoid the use of meshed grafts over joints.
 (5) Sheet grafts provide a superior aesthetic benefit and should always be used on the face and hands.

c. Donor site care
 (1) Occlusive dressings (e.g., DuoDerm), semiocclusive dressings (e.g., Tegaderm, OpSite), semiopen dressing (e.g., Xeroform), and open treatments can be used.
 (2) Semiocclusive dressings have been shown to encourage faster reepithelialization. Semiocclusive dressings are least painful and nearly maintenance free. Leakage and infection can be troublesome.
 (3) Xeroform dressings are reliable and consistent but require daily drying.

d. Recipient site care
 (1) Ideal dressings provide uniform pressure to prevent seroma formation, hematoma formation, and shear.
 (2) Bolster dressings consist of a nonadherent layer covered with mineral oil and saline-moistened cotton balls (to prevent desiccation), secured to wound with sutures or staples.
 (3) Vacuum-assisted closure (VAC) sponges can also be used.
 (4) Dressings are usually left undisturbed for 5 days unless the wound shows signs of infection.

F. Full-thickness skin graft (FTSG) (Table 3-1)
 1. Anatomy: FTSGs include the epidermis and the dermis in its entirety. (See Figure 1-1, Chapter 1.)
 2. Indications: Full-thickness grafts maintain greater semblance to normal skin and contract minimally. Their use is limited to small, uncontaminated, and well-vascularized wounds.
 3. Donor site selection
  a. Site should be inconspicuous and easily closed primarily.
  b. Arrange donor site scars to lie on the border of aesthetic units and parallel to relaxed skin tension lines (RSTLs).
  c. Recipient site characteristics are important (thickness, texture, pigmentation, and presence or absence of hair). Thicker grafts may be taken from preauricular, postauricular, supraclavicular, and groin areas.
   (1) Nose: Forehead and preauricular donor areas are usually best.
   (2) Cheek: Neck and supraclavicular areas are usually best.
   (3) Hand: The groin area is often used.
 4. Technique
  a. Wound preparation (cleansing, debridement, and hemostasis) is particularly important for full-thickness skin grafts.
  b. Harvest: Aggressive defatting is critical to improve short-term survival via imbibition.
  c. Wound care and dressing
   (1) Donor site: Typically closed primarily.
   (2) Recipient site: Bolster dressings are especially important to provide pressure ensure contact for imbibition and to prevent seroma or hematoma formation.
  d. Tissue expansion (e.g., lower abdominal/groin expansion for facial or hand coverage): May increase donor site area and allow for primary closure.

III. Bone grafts
A. Classifications
1. By composition
a. Cortical
(1) Composed of nonporous, lamellar bone.
(2) Primarily used to provide support for major bony defects.
b. Cancellous
(1) Composed of porous, highly cellular trabeculae.
(2) Used to stimulate healing, bridge smaller defects, and increase bulk.
(3) Offers little structural support.
c. Corticocancellous: Theoretically provides benefits of both
2. By vascular supply
a. Nonvascularized: Provides scaffolding and template for vascular and cellular in growth, which eventually resorbs and replaces graft (creeping substitution).
b. Pedicled vascularized bone graft
(1) Transferred on a vascular pedicle.
(2) Predominantly used in the craniofacial region.
(3) The fibula can be transferred to a tibial defect.
c. Free vascularized bone graft
(1) Allows transfer of a large segment of bone and promotes healing of the recipient site.
(2) Retains epiphyseal growth.
3. By origin
a. Autograft
(1) Maximal healing potential.
(2) Increased surgical time.
b. Allograft
(1) Decreased healing potential.
(2) Increases time for incorporation due to immunogenicity.
(3) Freeze-dried allografts have higher availability, lower immunogenicity, and lower risk for disease transfer compared with fresh frozen allografts.
B. Graft healing and function: Osteogenic, marrow, endosteal, and periosteal cells from donor bone as well as cells from the recipient site participate in bone formation.
1. Osteoconduction: Scaffold or template function that a graft provides to allow the ingrowth of capillaries, osteoprogenitor cells, and matrix components from the host tissue.
2. Osteoinduction: Recruitment and stimulation of bone- and cartilage-producing cells from the host tissue by substances present within the graft.
3. Osteogenesis: Production of new bone by cells in the graft that survive transplantation.
C. Indications
1. Promote and enhance healing: In cases of delayed union, nonunion, osteotomies, and poor healing potential.
2. Bridge bony defects: Used in comminuted defects to fill cortical defects, provide continuity, and increase healing. Grafts are also used to replace cortical segment loss from severe fracture or tumor excision.
3. Fill cavities: In cases of cysts, sequestrum, and tumor removal.
4. Arthrodesis.
D. Donor sites: Selection depends on the quantity, type, and vascularity of the graft desired. Donor site morbidity and patient characteristics also dictate donor site selection.
1. Ilium: Source of large quantity of cancellous and corticocancellous bone. The inner or both tables of the iliac crest may be harvested, with additional cancellous bone available by curettage. A vascularized graft based on the deep circumflex iliac has large vessels with a long pedicle.

       a. Advantages: Little aesthetic deficit. Use is limited in patients younger than 10 years because of incomplete ossification.

       b. Disadvantage: Donor site morbidity (pain).

    2. Cranium: Source of large quantity of cortical bone. Only the outer table is used in adults, while both the inner and outer tables can be used in children because of the osteogenic potential of the dura and the lack of a functional diploë layer in children younger than 6 or 7 years.

       a. Advantages: Low graft resorption rates. Low donor site morbidity (alopecia, contour step-off). Good aesthetic result.

       b. Disadvantages: Brittleness, which may require graft from another source to fill in the dead space. Larger bone grafts require a formal craniotomy.

    3. Ribs: Source of large quantity of cortical bone that is more porous and malleable than graft from other sources. Dominant pedicle for vascularized graft is the posterior intercostal arteries.

       a. Advantage: Malleable.

       b. Disadvantage: Difficult fixation due to its porosity.

    4. Fibula: Pedicled or free graft based on peroneal artery and venae comitantes. Suitable to bridge defect in the bong bones. Fibular head and distal quarter of fibula spared to avoid functional deficits.

       a. Advantages: Good graft length. Long pedicle.

       b. Disadvantage: Limited size.

    5. Other sites: Distal radius and proximal ulna are used as a source for cortical and cancellous bone. Free radius graft is based on the radial artery.

  E. Technique: Strict aseptic technique is employed. Minimize the time between harvest and placement. The graft should be wrapped in blood-soaked sponges. Use copious amounts of irrigation during sawing and drilling to reduce mechanical and thermal damage.

IV. Cartilage grafts

  A. Types

    1. By matrix characteristics

      a. Hyaline cartilage

        (1) Found in the trachea, larynx, nasal septum, nasal ala, and ribs.

        (2) Offers support through rigidity and resilience.

      b. Elastic cartilage

        (1) Found in the external ear, external auditory meatus, Eustachian tube, and epiglottis.

        (2) More malleable, elastic, and resistant to repeated bending than hyaline cartilage.

      c. Fibrocartilage

        (1) Found in the pubic symphysis, intervertebral discs, and ligamentous and tendonous insertions.

        (2) Resists tensile and compressive forces, but lacks flexibility.

    2. By source

      a. Autogenous cartilage: Primary and preferred source

      b. Homologous cartilage

        (1) Relatively small immune response because chondrocytes are surrounded by nonreactive extracellular matrix.

        (2) Freeze-dried, preserved cartilage further reduces inflammation and limits disease transfer.

        (3) More intense inflammation, thicker connective tissue capsule formation, and more absorption compared with autogenous cartilage.

  B. Indications

    1. Structural support and augmentation: Ear reconstruction, eyelid and tracheal support.

    2. Contour deformity: Correction of saddle nose deformity and inverted nipples, alternative to bone graft in correcting facial contour deformities.

    3. Joint repair and resurfacing: Used as spacer in temporomandibular joint (TMJ) repair or to fill defects in articular cartilage.

C. Healing and survival
1. **Both chondrocytes and extracellular matrix survive** and maintain cartilage characteristics.
2. **Avascular:** Survives by osmosis from a well-vascularized recipient site.
3. Limited inflammatory reaction with little graft resorption (<20% in autografts).
4. **Requires coverage** to prevent desiccation and infection.
5. **Scoring** and cross-cutting allows cartilage to be shaped. It will bend away from the scored side.
6. **Symmetric carving and K-wire stabilization** may prevent warping.

D. Donor sites
1. **Ear:** Source of elastic cartilage that possesses a natural curvature. Used for eyelid support and nipple reconstruction, TMJ and orbital floor repair.
   a. Advantages: Easily accessible and relatively abundant.
   b. Disadvantage: Curvature is not always desirable.
2. **Nasal septum:** Source for straight, rigid hyaline cartilage. Used for nasal reconstruction.
   a. Advantage: Easily accessible.
   b. Disadvantages: Availability is limited. Overresection can result in postoperative saddle nose deformity.
3. **Costal cartilage:** Abundant source of hyaline cartilage. Used for reconstruction requiring a large amount of cartilage (e.g., microtia and tracheal reconstruction).
   a. Advantages: Large amount of graft material; reliable. Distant donor site allows for two-team approach.
   b. Disadvantages: Tendency to warp with time, and donor site morbidity (pneumothorax, pain).

V. Fat and dermal/fat grafts
A. Graft healing and survival: Low graft viability and high graft absorption with greater than 50% of fat resorption and near 50% of dermis resorption. In dermal/fat graft, bulk is predominantly determined by the dermal layer. Overcorrection is needed to optimize the result. Survival rate decreases with infection and trauma.

B. Donor sites: Can be harvested from any fat-containing part of the body. Most common sources are the abdomen, buttock, and thigh for availability and cosmesis.

VI. Composite grafts
A. Composed of two or more tissue components, such as skin with cartilage, skin with fat, or full-thickness lip or eyelid.

B. Indications: Primarily used for reconstruction of the following.
1. **Nasal ala:** To prevent alar collapse and subsequent airway obstruction.
2. **Nasal sidewall:** To prevent nasal valve obstruction.
3. **Nasal tip:** To provide structural integrity.
4. **Ear:** To repair substantial auricular defects for cosmesis. Restoration of ear structure for glasses or hearing aid placement.
5. **Eyelid:** To prevent ectropion and lid contracture from loss of tarsal plate.

C. Donor sites: Septal cartilage, auricular cartilage, and costal cartilage.

D. Limitations and survival: Graft survival occurs via imbibition, inosculation, and then revascularization. The metabolic demand of the graft limits the size that will survive to a width of 1.0 to 1.5 cm.

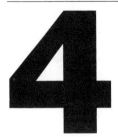

Flaps

Jenny B. Lynch

I. General
A. Definition and terms
1. A **flap** is a segment of tissue that contains a network of blood vessels that may be transferred from a donor site to reconstruct a secondary defect.
2. The base of the flap that contains the blood supply is called the **pedicle.**

B. Flaps can be categorized according to several criteria.
1. **According to the blood supply**
   a. **Random-pattern flaps:** Have no dominant blood supply.
   b. **Axial flaps:** Have a dominant feeding vessel.
   c. **Reverse-flow flaps** (also known as distal pedicle flaps or reverse axial pattern flaps): The proximal blood supply is divided, leaving the flap to survive on the intact distally based vessels (e.g., reverse radial forearm flap, reverse superficial sural artery flap).
2. **According to the proximity to the defect**
   a. **Local:** The flap shares a side with the defect (e.g., rhomboid flap).
   b. **Regional:** The flap is near, but not immediately adjacent to the defect (e.g., paramedian forehead flap).
   c. **Distant:** The flap is not near the defect (e.g., groin flap).
   d. **Free flap:** Free tissue transfer.
3. **According to the method of transfer**
   a. Advancement
   b. Transposition
   c. Rotation
   d. Interpolation
   e. Jumping
   f. Waltzing
   g. Free
4. **According to the tissue contained**
   a. Cutaneous
   b. Fasciocutaneous
   c. Musculocutaneous
   d. Osteocutaneous
   e. Osteomusculocutaneous
   f. Omentum/bowel

C. Monitoring of flaps
1. **Clinical evaluation** is the best method of flap assessment.
   a. **Temperature:** Should be body temperature.
   b. **Color:** Should be pink, neither white nor blue/purple.
   c. **Capillary refill:** Should be approximately 2 seconds.
   d. **Point bleeding:** Upon introduction of a fine-gauge needle, bleeding should be present. Blood should be red, not purple/blue.
   e. **Firmness:** Should be soft, but with some appreciable turgor.
2. **Signs of insufficient arterial supply**
   a. Cool.
   b. Pallid (white).

   c. Capillary refill slower than 2 seconds.
   d. Slow or absent point bleeding.
   e. Softer.
3. **Signs of insufficient venous return** (venous congestion)
   a. Warmer than expected.
   b. Blue to purple hue.
   c. Capillary refill faster than 2 seconds (blood pooled in venous system returns rapidly).
   d. Brisk point bleeding, with dark blood.
   e. Tense, swollen.
4. **Factors leading to flap vascular compromise**
   a. Tight dressings.
   b. Tight sutures.
   c. Pressure from positioning.
   d. Hematoma, causing increased tissue pressure, impeding inflow/outflow.
   e. Kinking of the flap or pedicle or both.
   f. Cool ambient room temperature.
   g. Nicotine, caffeine, or other vasoconstricting agents.
   h. Microvascular technical issues (see Chapter 6).
5. **Formal tests** (rarely necessary).
   a. Doppler studies.
   b. Fluorescein dye.
   c. Sensors for O_2, pH, temperature.
D. **Crane principle**
   1. A pedicled flap is used to lift, transport, and deposit subcutaneous tissue from one place to another.
   2. After 10 to 21 days, angiogenesis is sufficient from the recipient bed to support the deeper layer of the overlying flap. The top (superficial) one-half to three-fourths of the flap is then raised and returned to the original donor site.
   3. A viable subcutaneous layer is left behind, which may be covered by a split skin graft.
   4. This technique provides coverage to a local or regional area, without significant donor site morbidity.
E. **Angiosome concept**
   1. An **angiosome** is a composite unit of skin and underlying tissue supplied by a source vessel.
   2. The entire surface area of the body is composed of angiosomes.
   3. An angiosome consists of an arteriosome and a venosome.
   4. Angiosomes connect either by true anastomoses or by choke vessels (reduced-caliber vessels) that may dilate up to true anastomoses under certain circumstances, such as flap delay (see "Delay phenomenon").
   5. Explains how a flap could support more than one angiosome area under certain conditions.
F. **Delay phenomenon**
   1. **A flap is partially elevated and reset** in a separate procedure or procedures before definitive flap elevation and transfer.
   2. This allows the harvest of a larger flap because of the survival of a random cutaneous component distal to the boundaries defined by the original vasculature.
   3. **Benefits of delay** are thought to be due to the following.
      a. Changes in sympathetic ton.
      b. Increased number of vessels in the flap (angiogenesis).
      c. Dilation of previously present choke vessels.
      d. Metabolic changes in the flap, increasing tolerance.
   4. **Time recommended between delay procedures varies,** but usually 7 to 14 days between delays is sufficient.

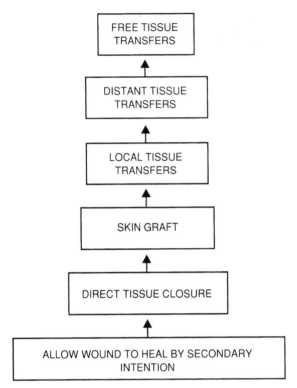

Fig. 4-1 The reconstructive ladder. (From Place M, Herber S, and Hardesty R. Basic techniques and principles in plastic surgery. In *Grabb and Smith's Plastic Surgery*, 5th ed. Aston SJ, Beasley RW, Thorne CH (eds). Philadelphia, Lippincott-Raven, 1997. With permission.)

G. Reconstructive ladder (Fig. 4-1)
  1. A systematic approach that facilitates decision making when reconstructing a defect.
  2. Progresses from simple to complex choices.
    a. Healing by secondary intention.
    b. Direct closure.
    c. Skin graft.
    d. Local tissue transfer: A flap raised immediately adjacent or near to the defect (the flap and the defect share an edge).
    e. Regional flap: A flap raised near the defect (the flap and the defect do not share an edge).
    f. Distant tissue transfer: A flap raised some distance from the primary defect.
    g. Free tissue transfer.
  3. Reconstructive "elevator": Often the best solution to a reconstructive dilemma is not the simplest, necessitating a jump up the "ladder."
H. Factors in flap decision making
  1. Location of defect
  2. Size of defect
  3. Underlying or exposed structures
  4. Potential donor sites

5. Donor site defects or disability
6. Viability of surrounding tissue
7. Shape and contour of the potential reconstruction
8. Surgeon's experience
9. Surgical goals
10. Patient's medical history
11. Patient's expectations
12. Potential complications
13. Outcome evaluation
14. Cost of care

II. Cutaneous flaps

A. Indications
1. Reconstruction of a local defect with similar, adjacent tissue.
2. Need for full-thickness tissue to cover relatively less vascular tissue such as bone or tendon without periosteum/paratenon intact (skin graft is insufficient).

B. Blood supply to the skin
1. Direct cutaneous arteries

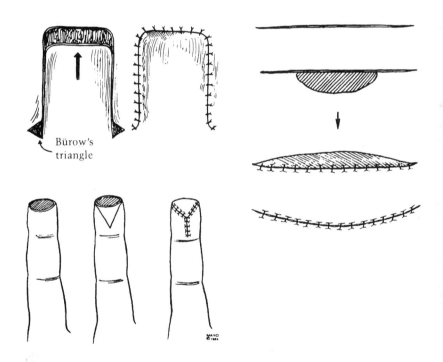

Bürow's
triangle

Fig. 4-2. Advancement flaps: **A:** Single pedicled advancement flap; **B:** Bipedicled flap; **C:** V-Y advancement flap. A from Place M, Herber S, and Hardesty R. Basic techniques and principles in plastic surgery. In *Grabb and Smith's Plastic Surgery*, 5th edition. Aston SJ, Beasley RW, Thorne CH (eds). Philadelphia, Lippincott-Raven, 1997. B and C from Fisher J and Gingrass M. Basic Principles of Skin Flaps. *Georgiade Plastic, Maxillofacial, and Reconstructive Surgery*, 3rd edition Georgiade G, Riefkohl R, Levin S (eds). Philadelphia, Williams & Wilkins, 1997. With permission.

    2. Fasciocutaneous arteries
    3. Musculocutaneous arteries
C. Types of skin flaps
  1. Random-pattern flaps
    a. Designed on a random vascular supply.
    b. Roughly dependent on a length-to-width ratio of about 2:1 in the lower extremity and 4:1 in the head and neck. Flap ischemia is expected when these guidelines are exceeded without flap delay.
  2. Axial-pattern flaps
    a. Designed along a named artery (angiosome).
    b. Can be much longer and robust than random-pattern flaps.
  3. Advancement flaps (Fig. 4-2)
    a. Single-pedicled flap: The flap is raised as a square or rectangle, and is undermined and advanced to fill the defect. Small triangles (Burow's triangles) may be made at the base of the flap to facilitate advancement.

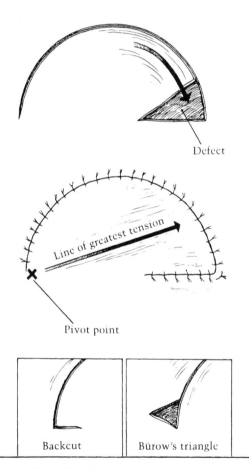

Fig. 4-3. Rotation flap. (From Place M, Herber S, and Hardesty R. Basic techniques and principles in plastic surgery. In *Grabb and Smith's Plastic Surgery*, 5th edition. Aston SJ, Beasley RW, Thorne CH. Philadelphia, Lippincott-Raven, 1997. With permission.)

b. **Bipedicled flap:** An incision parallel to the defect allows the flap to be undermined and advanced. Useful for longitudinal defects of extremities.

c. **V-Y advancement flap:** A flap is raised in a "V" shape, and advanced to fill the defect and closed as a "Y." Useful on the face and for finger tip reconstruction. A variation of this is the Y-V flap.

4. **Rotation flaps** (Fig. 4-3)

   a. **The basic rotation flap** is raised in a semicircle. It is particularly useful for scalp defects and sacral pressure sores.

   b. **Bilobed flap:** Two flaps are raised 45 to 50 degrees apart, adjacent to the defect. The first flap is rotated in to fill the primary defect. The second flap fills the donor site of the first. The donor site of the second flap is closed primarily. Useful for defects on the nose, where superior skin laxity can be stepwise transferred to the inferior (e.g., tip) region, where laxity is sparse. This flap moves the ultimate donor site to a distant position, where primary closure is possible.

5. **Transposition flaps** (Fig. 4-4)

   a. **Z-plasty:** Interpolation of two adjacent triangular flaps, which has the effect of moving lateral tissue in to increase tissue length longitudinally. It classically consists of a central component with adjacent limbs oriented at 60 degrees. All three lines are of equal length. Angles may be 30 degrees to 90 degrees. Increasing the angle increases the percent gain in length (Table 4-1). Multiple Z-plasties may be done in series. Clinical examples: Lengthen scar contractures, change scar direction, release epicanthal folds or constricting bands.

   b. **Limberg or rhomboid flap:** Used to close a rhombic-shaped (equilateral parallelogram) defect, with angles of 60 degrees and 120 degrees. To create the flap, the short diagonal of the rhombus is extended a distance equal to its length. Complete the flap by drawing a line parallel to the nearest limb of the flap. Four flaps can be drawn around the various sides of the defect.

   c. **Dufourmentel:** A variation of the Limberg flap. Used for rhomboid-like defects that have angles other than classic 60 and 120 degrees. Draw a line from the short diagonal of the rhomboid. Continue the line of one of the sides to intersect the line already drawn. Bisect these lines to get the limb of the flap, which should be equal in length to the side. Complete the flap by drawing a line parallel to the long horizontal.

   d. **Interpolation:** Also called an island flap. A skin paddle is elevated distally on a vascular pedicle proximally. The flap is then transposed into a nearby defect either over or under a skin bridge.

III. **Fasciocutaneous flaps**

   A. These are flaps that include the deep fascia, which incorporates a rich vascular network—the fascial plexus. Branches from this plexus reach the skin as direct or indirect perforators.

   1. The arc of rotation is determined by the distance from the pedicle base to the maximal safe length of the elevated flap.

   2. The pedicle of a fasciocutaneous flap may be lengthened by tracing the perforators of the flap back to the source vessel.

   3. A cutaneous nerve may be incorporated into the flap, making it sensate.

   4. Can be used as local, regional, or free tissue transfer flaps.

   B. **Classification of fasciocutaneous flaps** (Table 4-2)

   C. **Workhorse pedicled fasciocutaneous flaps** (Table 4-3)

IV. **Muscle and musculocutaneous flaps**

   A. **Indications**

   1. Need for bulk.

   2. Eradication of dead space and infection (e.g., sternal and lower extremity reconstruction).

   3. Restoration of function (e.g., gracilis transfer to the upper extremity or face).

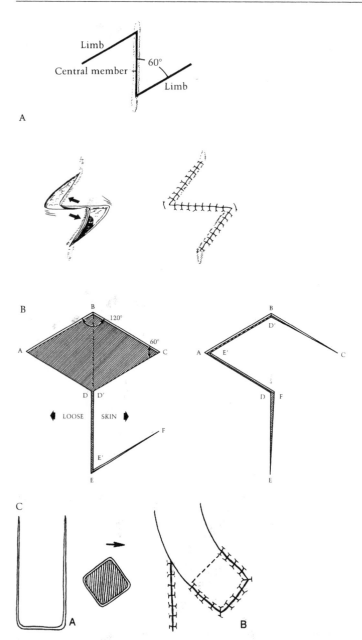

Fig. 4-4. Transposition flaps: **A:** Z plasty; **B:** Rhomboid (Limberg) flap; **C:** Interpolation flap. (A and B from Place M, Herber S, and Hardesty R. Basic techniques and principles in plastic surgery. In *Grabb and Smith's Plastic Surgery*, 5th ed. Aston SJ, Beasley RW, Thorne CH. Philadelphia, Lippincott-Raven Publishers, 1997. C from Fisher J. and Gingrass M. Basic principles of skin flaps. In the textbook, *Georgiade Plastic, Maxillofacial, and Reconstructive Surgery*, 3rd ed. Georgiade G, Riefkohl R, Levin S. (eds). Philadelphia, Williams & Wilkins, 1997. With permission.)

Table 4-1. Theoretical gain in length for Z plasty with different angles

Angle of Z Plasty (degree)	% Theoretical Gain in Length of the Central Limb
30	25
45	50
60	75
75	100
90	120

   B. Advantages
      1. Bulk to fill depth of defects.
      2. Conform to fit an irregular wound.
      3. Highly vascular.
      4. May include bone in the transfer.
      5. May be transferred with motor or sensory nerve.
   C. Disadvantage: Sacrifice of a functional muscle
   D. Classification of musculocutaneous flaps (Table 4-4 and Fig. 4-5)
   E. Workhorse muscle and musculocutaneous flaps (Table 4-5)
V. Flap modifications
   A. Free flaps (see Chapter 6, "Microsurgery")
   B. Supercharging
      1. The process of enhancing the blood supply of a pedicled flap by performing a microvascular anastomosis to a secondary pedicle in the flap.
      2. Example: A pedicled transverse rectus abdominis (TRAM) flap—addition of anastomosis or anastomoses of the deep inferior epigastric vessels to vessels in the axilla, neck, or chest.
   C. Flap prefabrication
      1. The transfer of a new vascular pedicle into an area of tissue that will later be raised as a flap.
      2. The flap, based on new vasculature, can be raised after approximately 6 weeks.
      3. Rarely used because of the availability of numerous alternative options.
   D. Prelamination
      1. The introduction of additional tissue layers into the flap prior to transfer.
      2. A two-staged procedure: Stage 1 modifies the donor flap with the introduction of additional tissue. Stage 2 raises the flap.
      3. Allows custom-made flaps for specialized areas such as the face. Clinical example: Prelaminate a forehead flap or forearm flap with cartilage and skin graft for nasal reconstruction.
   E. Vascularized bone flaps
      1. The most commonly transferred bones
         a. Radius: Based on the radial artery.
         b. Fibula: Based on the peroneal artery.
         c. Scapula: Based on either circumflex scapular or thoracodorsal artery.
         d. Iliac crest: Based on the deep circumflex iliac artery.

Table 4-2. Nahai-Mathes classification system for fasciocutaneous flaps

Type	Vessel Description	Examples
A	Direct cutaneous perforator	Temporoparietal fascial flap
B	Septocutaneous perforator	Radial artery forearm flap
C	Musculocutaneous perforator	TRAM flap

TRAM, transverse rectus abdominis muscle.

Table 4-3. Workhorse pedicled fasciocutaneous flaps

Name	Arc of Rotation (standard flap)	Pattern of Circulation	Maximum Size (cm)	Source Vessels	Sensory Nerve
Groin flap	Abdominal wall, perineum, hand, forearm	Type A	25×10	Superficial circumflex iliac	Lateral cutaneous T12
Reverse superficial sural	Foot and heel	Type A	8×12	Median superficial sural	Insensate
Radial forearm	Anterior, posterior forearm, elbow, upper arm	Type B	10×40	Radial	Medial and lateral ante brachial cutaneous
Scapular/parascapular	Shoulder, axilla, thoracic wall	Type B	20×7	Circumflex scapular (transverse and descending) branches	Cutaneous of intercostals 3, 4 and 5
Temporoparietal fascia flap	Ear, ipsilateral face, FOM	Type A	12×9	Superficial temporal	Auriculotemporal
Lateral arm	Anterior, posterior shoulder	Type B	15×8	Posterior radial collateral	Posterior brachial cutaneous
Posterior interosseus	Elbow, antecubital fossa, proximal volar forearm	Type B	18×8	Posterior interosseus	Medial, dorsal antebrachial cutaneous
Paramedian forehead flap	Nose, midface, forehead	Type C	6×8	Supratrochlear, supraorbital	Supratrochlear, supraorbital

FOM, floor of mouth.

Table 4-4. Mathes and Nahai classification of musculocutaneous flaps

Type	Description	Examples
I	One vascular pedicle	Gastrocnemius, tensor fascia lata
II	One dominant pedicle and one or more minor pedicles (flap cannot survive on the minor pedicles alone)	Biceps femoris, rectus femoris, soleus, gracilis
III	Two dominant pedicles	Gluteus maximus, rectus abdominis, serratus anterior
IV	Segmental pedicles	Extensor hallucis longus sartorius, tibialis anterior
V	One dominant pedicle and several segmental smaller pedicles (flap can survive on the minor pedicles alone)	Latissimus dorsi, pectoralis major

    2. Toe (or partial toe/joint) **transfer**
       a. Great toe: Based on the first dorsal metatarsal artery.
       b. Second toe: Also based on the first dorsal metatarsal artery.
  F. Perforator flaps: The perforating vessel or vessels are dissected down to deeper vessels, leaving the intervening tissue intact and not included in the flap. This allows thinner flaps to be harvested, and potentially reduces donor site morbidity. For example, a deep inferior epigastric perforator (DIEP) flap versus a free TRAM flap, leaving the rectus muscle intact.
  G. Innervated flaps
    1. Motor: Possible functional free tissue transfers
       a. Latissimus
       b. Serratus
       c. Pectoralis minor
       d. Gracilis

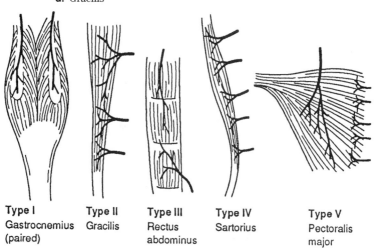

Type I Gastrocnemius (paired) **Type II** Gracilis **Type III** Rectus abdominus **Type IV** Sartorius **Type V** Pectoralis major

Fig. 4-5. Mathes and Nahai classification of muscle flaps based on vascular supply.

Table 4-5. Workhorse muscle and musculocutaneous flaps

Flap	Skin Paddle	Pattern of Circulation	Arc of Rotation	Size (cm)	Vessel	Nerve
Gastrocnemius	Possible	Type I	Suprapatellar, knee, upper one-third tibia	20×8	Sural	M: tibial; S: saphenous, sural
Soleus	No	Type II	Middle, lower one-third leg	8×28	Popliteal, posterior tibial, peroneal	M: posterior tibial, medial popliteal
Latissimus dorsi	Possible	Type V	Neck, occiput, parietal scull, face, chest, abdomen	25×35	Thoracodorsal	M: thoracodorsal; S: cutaneous intercostal
Pectoralis major	Possible	Type V	Face to orbital rim, neck, chest, upper arm	15×23	Thoracoacromial	M: pectoral; S: intercostal
Rectus abdominis	Possible	Type III	Anterior thorax, groin, perineum, inferior trunk	25×6	Superior and deep inferior epigastric	M: intercostals; S: intercostals
Gluteus maximus	Possible	Type III	Sacrum, ipsilateral ischium	24×24	Superior and inferior gluteal	M: inferior gluteal; S: L1–S3
Tensor fascia lata	Possible	Type I	Lower abdominal wall, groin, perineum	5×15	Lateral circumflex femoral (ascending branch)	M: superior gluteal; S: T12, femoral cutaneous
Gracilis	Possible	Type II	Groin, perineum, vagina, anus, ischium	6×24	Medial circumflex femoral	M: obturator; S: femoral cutaneous, obturator

M, motor; S, sensory.

2. **Sensory flaps** most commonly used
   a. Lateral arm flap with posterior brachial cutaneous nerve.
   b. Radial forearm flap with medial and lateral antebrachial cutaneous nerves.
   c. Dorsalis pedis flap with deep peroneal nerve in the first web and superficial peroneal nerve in the remainder.

H. **Delayed flaps** (see "Delay phenomenon")

I. **Tissue expansion** (see Chapter 5, "Tissue Expansion")

Pearls

1. Use a piece of suture or gauze as a template to measure the transfer distance of the flap.
2. If a flap has vascular compromise postoperatively, and it does not improve with positioning, then dressings and sutures should be removed from the flap at the bedside. If the flap does not improve, then it should be explored in the operating room.
3. There is no automated monitoring device that can substitute for a bedside evaluation by trained personnel.
4. The dressing is critical. The best reconstruction can be foiled by dressings applied in the last 20 minutes in the operating room.

5

Tissue Expansion

Jenny B. Lynch

I. Introduction

A. **Tissue expansion:** A reconstructive technique that expands tissue to attain an optimal aesthetic and functional result using local tissue when primary closure of a soft tissue defect is not possible. A tissue expander is essentially a silicone balloon that is placed subcutaneously and is slowly filled with saline. Overlying tissues are stretched, resulting in an increased area of tissue.

B. **History:** The first case, to reconstruct an ear, was described by Charles Neumann in New York in 1956. The technique was pioneered in the 1970s by Radovan (Georgetown University) and Austad (University of Michigan).

C. **Benefits of tissue expansion**
   1. Creation of additional tissue.
   2. Similar appearance and mechanical properties of donor and recipient tissues.
   3. Increased vascularity of tissue.
   4. Predictable amounts of tissue gained.
   5. Useful technique in many regions of the body.

D. **Expander shapes**
   1. Rectangular: Useful on trunk, extremities, and scalp. Gives the greatest overall tissue gain.
   2. Round: Useful in head and neck and breast reconstruction.
   3. Crescent: Expands more centrally than peripherally.
   4. Custom expanders: Specially designed for irregular defects; uncommon and expensive.

E. **Choice of expander** depends on the following.
   1. Size of defect: Maximum width and length.
   2. Availability and characteristics of donor tissue.
   3. Expected advancement of the expanded tissue: Estimated from the width of the expanded tissue.

II. Biology

A. **Epidermis:** Becomes thicker with tissue expansion.

B. **Dermis**
   1. **Papillary dermis:** Unchanged.
   2. **Reticular dermis:** Thinned.
   3. **Collagen bundles:** Thickened.
   4. **Elastic fibers:** May rupture and undergo fibrotic changes. This can manifest clinically as striae.
   5. **Dermal appendages:** Show degenerative changes.
   6. **There is a decreased appreciation of pain,** temperature, pressure, and touch in the expanded skin in 50% of cases, despite normal distribution of sensory corpuscles.
   7. **The skin is occasionally dry,** with pigment changes and thinning hair from dispersion of follicles.
   8. **Expanded skin is hypervascular.** Tissue expansion causes some of the changes typically associated with the delay phenomenon.

C. **Hypodermis:** Fat atrophy is followed by fibrosis. Clinically, this reduces the bulk of the flap.

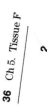
   D. Muscle injury from the expansion process can [...] (e.g., reduced brow elevation due to frontalis dama[...]

   E. Capsule
   1. Formed around the expander by foreign body [...]
   2. At time of expander removal, capsulotomy or [...] to maximize the flap area and improve the ov[...]
   3. Capsulectomy should be limited, because the [...] pattern flaps can be interrupted.

III. Indications

   A. To create donor tissue of similar color, texture, and sensation for defect closure

   B. Scalp and forehead reconstruction
   1. Expanders are placed subcutaneously or subgaleally.
   2. Expansion allows adequate recreation of the frontotemporal hairline.
   3. Ideal incisions lie within the hairline, brow line, vertical midline, and within relaxed skin tension lines.
   4. Caution should be observed regarding the frontal branch of the facial nerve.

   C. Face and neck reconstruction
   1. Expanders in the face are placed in the subcutaneous plane centrally, and over the parotidomasseteric fascia laterally.
   2. Caution should be exercised with regard to Stensen's duct and the motor or sensory nerves of the face, which may be stretched or accidentally divided.
   3. Expanders in the neck are usually placed above the platysma.

   D. Nasal reconstruction: Small defects may be reconstructed with expanded nasal skin. This is most useful for the thin, mobile skin over the root or dorsum of the nose.

   E. Auricular defects
   1. Tissue expansion is useful for auricular defects from congenital causes (e.g., microtia) or acquired causes (e.g., traumatic amputation, burns, or resection for malignancy).
   2. Tissue expansion produces skin that is thin, vascularized, and nonhair-bearing.
   3. The incision is placed in the postauricular hairline.
   4. When expansion is complete, the ear can be reconstructed with the insertion of a cartilaginous framework and covered with the expanded tissue.

   F. Upper and lower extremity
   1. The expander is placed above the level of the deep investing fascia of the muscles.
   2. Attention should be paid to sensory nerves, superficial named vessels, and lymphatics.
   3. Expansion is useful for covering defects from hypertrophic or burn scar excisions, congenital nevi, tattoo excision, and skin graft excision.
   4. There is a propensity to form keloid scars in the deltoid area.
   5. Complication (expander exposure and infection) rates increase as tissue expanders are used distally.
   6. Maintain full range of motion in joints during expansion.

   G. Abdominal and back expansion
   1. Expanders may be placed in the back or the abdominal wall.
   2. Plan the incision either in the suprapubic hair or in the groin crease for the abdomen and in the posterior axillary folds or intergluteal crease for the back.
   3. Because of the segmental innervation pattern of both the abdomen and the back, damage to cutaneous nerves is less likely to have debilitating consequences than in the extremities.

   H. Breast reconstruction (see Chapter 34, "Breast Reconstruction")
   1. Usually a two-stage procedure, in which a permanent implant is exchanged 8 to 12 weeks after expansion.

In some cases, expanders may serve as permanent implants, avoiding a second procedure.
3. Expansion is useful in both immediate and delayed reconstruction.
4. Optimal if the pectoralis major, pectoralis minor, and serratus anterior are intact.
5. Expansion is usually begun 3 weeks postoperatively.
6. Expansion may proceed during chemotherapy if blood counts are normal.

IV. **Principles of expander placement**
A. **Location and donor site characteristics**
1. **Generally the scalp, face, breast, and anterior trunk** tolerate expansion the best.
2. **Site choice for the expander**
a. Usually close to the defect.
b. Parallel to the long axis of the defect.
c. Should not impinge on joint motion during expansion.
3. **Donor tissue**
a. Free of contamination or infection.
b. Well vascularized.
c. Free of unstable scar tissue.
4. **Considerations in expander placement**
a. Patient expectations, compliance.
b. Defect size.
c. Donor tissue: Extent and characteristics.
d. Number, size, and shape of expanders.
e. Possible location of expanders.
f. Expected scar lines.
g. Expansion period.
h. Multiple expansion procedures.
5. **Caution with**
a. Irradiated tissue.
b. Insulin-dependent diabetes mellitus.
c. Vascular disease.
d. Connective tissue disease.
B. **Geometry of tissue expansion**
1. **Size of the expander:** Use the largest possible expander, limited only by the available donor tissue.
2. **Multiple expanders** are often needed, depending on available donor tissue.
3. **Incision placement**
a. Incisions are usually radial to the expander pocket.
b. Try to place incisions away from previous scars, skin grafts, thin skin, and donor tissue.
c. Design the scar to be hidden or camouflaged.
C. **Timing of inflation**
1. **Volume is infused intraoperatively** to gently fill the pocket created for the expander, thus helping to avoid hematoma or seroma formation. Avoid placing tension on the incisions at the time of the operation, which increases the risk of dehiscence and exposure.
2. **Expansion begins 1 to 3 weeks postoperatively** and usually continues on a daily or weekly basis thereafter.
3. **Fill expander according to**
a. Patient comfort or discomfort.
b. Skin blanching over the expander.
4. **Always expand more than you think you will need** (and then expand some more).
D. **Complications and treatment**
1. **Cellulitis or infection**
a. Usually results in the need for expander removal because of decreased bacterial clearance from around the expander.
b. Needs early and aggressive treatment with intravenous antibiotics.

    c. Remove the expander if the infection is periprosthetic, and irrigate site with saline solution, iodine, and/or antibacterial solution.

    d. Port infection: Exteriorize the port.

2. Exposure or extrusion of the expander

    a. May require removal of expander.

    b. Treat infection, if present.

3. Implant failure or rupture

    a. Most commonly iatrogenic.

    b. Replace the defective part.

4. Flap ischemia or skin loss: Especially common in the lower leg

    a. Avoid traumatic tissue dissection.

    b. Usually needs to be debrided and closed.

    c. Treat infection, if present.

5. Minor complications

    a. Valve turnover.

    b. Incorrect valve placement.

    c. Inadequate expansion.

    d. Valve or tubing exposure.

E. Preexpansion of flaps

  1. Axial cutaneous flaps may be preexpanded to cover a larger area.

    a. Especially useful with the deltopectoral and groin flaps.

    b. Improves chances for primary closure of the donor site.

  2. Myocutaneous flaps

    a. Latissimus dorsi and pectoralis major.

    b. Expansion of skin, subcutaneous tissue, and underlying muscle.

    c. There is experimental evidence of increased microcirculation in expanded myocutaneous flaps, which facilitates safe transfer.

F. Endoscopic tissue expander placement (see Chapter 7, "Endoscopic Plastic Surgery")

  1. Advantages

    a. Smaller incisions.

    b. Direct visualization of the pocket being dissected.

    c. Can visualize and correct problems encountered during expansion.

  2. Disadvantages

    a. Steep learning curve.

    b. Altered depth perception.

    c. Potential expander damage.

Pearls

1. **An exposed expander** can sometimes be further expanded if it is not infected.
2. **Check the expander** for leaks prior to its insertion.
3. **Coloring the contents of the expander** with methylene blue helps identify the valve correctly when filling and highlights leakage from the valve easily.
4. **Use a 23-gauge butterfly or Huber (noncutting) needle** inserted perpendicular to the expander to fill it. Bigger needles may cause the valve to leak with back pressure.
5. **Expanded tissue** can be reexpanded 3 to 6 months later.

6

Microsurgery

Gregory H. Borschel

I. Historical notes

1912	Carrel	Nobel Prize for microvascular anastomosis
1938	Cawthorne	Facial nerve coaptation
1959	Seidenberg	Free jejunum to the esophagus
1962	Malt and McKhann	Arm replantation
1969	McLean and Buncke	Free omentum to the scalp
1973	Daniel and Taylor	Free groin flap to the lower extremity
1973	O'Brien, et al.	Free groin flap to the lower extremity

II. Instrumentation

A. Magnification

1. **Microscopes**
   a. $6\times$ to $40\times$ magnification.
   b. Focal length: 200 to 275 mm.
   c. Fiberoptic lighting allows for cool illumination.
2. **Loupes**
   a. Can be used for the anastomosis of larger vessels ($>$1–2 mm), with $4\times$ or greater magnification.
   b. Dissection prior to the anastomosis is usually best accomplished with $2.5\times$ to $3.5\times$ loupes.
   c. Can be helpful in head and neck and lower extremity reconstruction because of the freedom to negotiate inherent angles, which are awkward with a scope.

B. Microsurgical instruments

1. **General requirements:** Glare free (nonreflective coatings), nonmagnetized, nonlocking, lightweight, fine tips, and well balanced.
2. **Caretaking:** Should be performed by a designated technician or the surgeon. Use of "instrument milk" (an oil-based lubricant) will prevent corrosion of tips and joints.
3. **Forceps:** Fine tips (e.g., "jeweler's," or no. 2–no. 5).
4. **Needle holder:** Some prefer to use forceps; others prefer nonlocking angled needle holders.
5. **Scissors:** Straight for adventitia and suture, curved for vessels, and serrated for nerves.
6. **Clamps:** Acland/Kleinert type (connected, adjustable double clamps); single clamps of varying sizes. Clamp pressure should be rechecked and adjusted periodically to avoid clamp trauma to vessels.
7. **Vessel dilators:** Have thin, smooth tips to avoid intimal damage.
8. **Background:** Yellow allows maximal contrast with the suture material.

C. Microsutures

1. Monofilament nylon or polypropylene.
2. **8-0:** Forearm- or wrist-sized vessels and nerves.
3. **9-0 and 10-0:** Digital vessels and nerves.
4. **11-0:** Distal digital vessels and pediatric cases.
5. **Needles:** 75 to 135 μm in diameter.

D. Solutions
  1. **Heparinized saline/lactated Ringer's solution:** 100 U/mL; should be kept warm; used for irrigation of vessel ends.
  2. **2% lidocaine:** To alleviate vasospasm.
  3. **Papaverine:** To counteract vasospasm. Papaverine will precipitate on contact with heparin, thereby clouding the operative field.

III. Preparation for microvascular procedures
  A. Setup and operator comfort
   1. Secure loose or moving limbs or parts in the field.
   2. Maintain excellent hemostasis.
   3. Use moist sponges to prevent desiccation of the operative field.
   4. Practice good ergonomics: Rest your forearms and/or hands on stacked towels adjacent to the operative field; keep your feet flat on floor and your back straight by adjusting the table, microscope, and/or stool.
   5. If the focus is first adjusted at maximum zoom, it should be maintained through the full zoom spectrum.

  B. Vessel preparation
   1. Debride all vessel segments showing evidence of trauma (this is critical to prevent thrombosis).
   2. Dissect enough vessel length to relieve anastomotic tension, but avoid excessive dissection, since that may cause vasospasm.
   3. Clean the periadventitia from the vessel ends.
   4. Check for adequate flow by releasing the clamp and visualizing the pressure head.
   5. Examine the lumen for debris, valves, or intimal injury, and flush with heparinized saline/lactated Ringer's solution.
   6. Dilate vessels *only* with smooth vessel dilators.

IV. Microvascular anastomotic techniques
  A. General
   1. The needle should enter the vessel at right angles, slightly more than one wall thickness from the cut edge of the vessel.
   2. Avoid touching the endothelial surface with pointed instruments. The only instrument that should enter the vessel lumen is a vessel dilator, which can be used as a forceps.
   3. The entire wall should be traversed by the needle, ensuring full-thickness bites.
   4. Use three throws per knot.
   5. Always visualize the lumen on each pass. This can be aided by a flush with heparinized saline/lactated Ringer's solution.
   6. Upon completing the anastomosis, release the distal clamp first, check for backflow, repair any leaks, and then release the proximal clamp.
   7. Leave the anastomosis alone after its initial completion, avoiding the urge to fuss with it. If there are no significant anastomotic leaks, place warm saline-soaked sponges over the vessel and wait at least 10 minutes without manipulation prior to assessing patency.

  B. End-to-end anastomosis
   1. **The halving technique** (Fig. 6-1)
      a. Commonly used.
      b. Two key sutures are placed approximately 160 to 180 degrees apart. One half is closed, and then the vessel is flipped over for completion of the closure.
   2. **The triangulation technique**
      a. Three key sutures are placed at 120-degree intervals.
      b. Posterior and opposite suture retraction by an assistant can prevent "backwalling."
      c. Alexis Carrel was awarded the Nobel Prize in 1912 for his work on this vascular suture technique and the transplantation of blood vessels and organs.

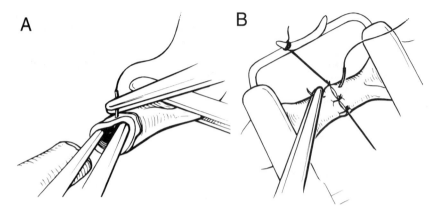

Fig. 6-1. End-to-end microvascular anastomosis, halving technique. **A:** Stay sutures are first placed at 160–180° apart (a1 and a2). **B:** Subsequent sutures are placed on the front wall at and then the a3, a4, and a5. The vessel is then turned over, and the back wall anastomosis is completed. (From Shenaq S and Sharma S. Principles of microvascular surgery. In the textbook, *Grabb and Smith's Plastic Surgery*, 5th ed. Aston SJ, Beasley RW, Thorne CH Philadelphia, Lippincott-Raven, 997. With permission.)

3. **The "back wall up" technique**
   a. Useful for tight spots or deep holes in which vessel rotation is difficult.
   b. The first suture is placed on the back wall, with subsequent sutures moving around sequentially to the top. This allows for continuous visualization of the lumen without flipping the vessel over.
C. **End-to-side anastomosis**
   1. Preserves flow in the pedicle to distal tissues.
   2. Allows anastomosis of vessels of different sizes.
   3. The side opening can be made in several ways, including the following.
      a. Slit the vessel with a no. 15 blade, and then excise an ellipse with the scissors.
      b. Lift the vessel wall with a suture and excise an ellipse with the scissors.
      c. Slit three vessels with a no. 15 blade, and then use a small vessel punch for the excision.
   4. If the vessel can be flipped from side to side, then sutures are placed at the "toe" and "heel" of the anastomosis first, and these two sutures are run continuously down each side of the anastomosis.
   5. If the vessel cannot be flipped, then the back wall is sewn first.
V. **Microvascular troubleshooting**
A. **Healthy flap characteristics**
   1. Pink
   2. Warm
   3. Dopplerable pulses
   4. Soft, but with tissue turgor present
B. **Signs of compromised arterial inflow**
   1. Pallid
   2. Cool
   3. Dopplerable arterial pulse may still be present
   4. Poor tissue turgor
C. **Signs of poor venous outflow** (more common)
   1. Tense
   2. Warm or cool
   3. Purple, bluish tinge

        4. May still have Dopplerable signals

        5. Increased tissue turgor

D. No-reflow phenomenon

    1. Follows an ischemic insult to the flap. There is a lack of perfusion in the tissues, despite reestablishment of patency in the pedicle. The process consists of a cycle of ischemia leading to edema and thrombosis, which lead to greater ischemia.

    2. Reversible damage at 4 hours.

    3. Irreversible damage at 6 to 12 hours.

E. Flap salvage

    1. Careful monitoring by trained personnel and a high index of suspicion will save failing flaps.

    2. Local factors should be considered immediately, such as constrictive dressings, inappropriate positioning, and hematoma. Dressings should be taken down at the bedside. Incisions can be released pending transport to the operating room to relieve compression from edema or hematoma or both.

    3. Immediate return to the operating room is warranted for all flaps under suspicion for failing inflow or outflow.

    4. Salvage rates are typically greater than 50%.

F. Preventive measures

    1. Meticulous technique (most important)

        a. Prevent vasospasm.

            (1) Gentle (and minimal) vascular dissection.

            (2) Warm patient, warm room.

            (3) Topical papaverine.

            (4) Avoid acidosis or alkalosis.

            (5) Communicate with anesthesia personnel to avoid vasoconstricting agents and to maintain adequate levels of hydration (best monitored via urine output).

        b. Avoid "backwalling."

        c. Avoid intraluminal intimal damage.

        d. Minimize vessel size mismatch, when possible.

    2. Anticoagulants

        a. The use of these agents is highly dependent on operator preference and the individual case presentation. There is no proof of increased patency with use of these agents. The risks and side effects of their use must be weighed against the potential benefit.

        b. 10% Dextran-40

            (1) Acts as a volume expander, and decreases the "stickiness" of platelets.

            (2) Give a 5-mL test dose first to assess for a sensitivity reaction.

            (3) Run an i.v. infusion at 25 mL/hr or give 500 mL as maintenance fluids once daily for 3 to 5 days.

            (4) No tapering is needed.

            (5) Side effects: Congestive heart failure/volume overload, allergic reactions, and renal toxicity.

        c. Aspirin: 325 mg daily for 2 weeks, with first dose given PR in the recovery room.

        d. Heparin

            (1) Indicated for some replants and anastomotic revisions.

            (2) Not used routinely.

            (3) Must be prepared to transfuse if using heparin.

VI. Microneural surgery

  A. Nerves are **coapted,** whereas vessels are **anastomosed.**

  B. Peripheral nerve anatomy (Fig. 6-2)

    1. Adventitia (paraneurium): Surrounds the nerve.

    2. Outer (epifascicular) epineurium: The connective tissue layer that invests all the fascicles in a peripheral nerve.

    3. Inner (interfascicular) epineurium: Invests individual fascicles.

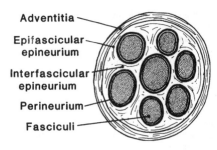

Adventitia

Epifascicular epineurium

Interfascicular epineurium

Perineurium

Fasciculi

Fig. 6-2. Peripheral neuroanatomy, cross-section. (From Millesi H. Principles of nerve grafting. In *Georgiade Plastic, Maxillofacial, and Reconstructive Surgery*, 3rd ed. Georgiade G, Riefkohl R, Levin S, (eds). Philadelphia, Williams & Wilkins, 1997. With permission.)

4. **Fascicle:** A group of axons enclosed within an epineurial sheath.
5. **Perineurium:** Deep to the inner epineurium; the strongest layer.
6. **Endoneurium:** The extracellular matrix surrounding axons; a weak layer.
C. **Types of nerve injury: Seddon classification**
  1. **Neuropraxia:** Complete spontaneous recovery is expected within days.
  2. **Axonotmesis:** Axonal disruption within intact connective tissue layers. Wallerian degeneration ensues.
  3. **Neurotmesis:** Axonal and endoneurial disruption, with possible disruption of connective tissue layers. The more layers that are disrupted, the worse the prognosis will be without repair.
D. **Types of nerve injury: Sunderland classification (as modified by MacKinnon)**
  1. **Sunderland I** (neuropraxia): As in Seddon.
  2. **Sunderland II** (axonotmesis): As in Seddon.
  3. **Sunderland III** (neurotmesis): Loss of continuity of endoneurial tubes with intact perineurium. Distal Wallerian degeneration occurs.
  4. **Sunderland IV** (neurotmesis): Loss of continuity of the perineurium. Distal Wallerian degeneration occurs.
  5. **Sunderland V** (neurotmesis): Loss of continuity of the epineurium. Distal Wallerian degeneration occurs. Without coaptation there is virtually no chance of recovery.
  6. **MacKinnon VI:** Mixed injury pattern, with various combinations of the previously listed injury types.
E. **Nerve coaptation methods**
  1. **General**
    a. Must be tension free; otherwise, a nerve graft is indicated.
    b. In most cases of transection of small peripheral nerves, no difference is seen in outcomes following the various types of repair.
  2. **Epineurial repair**
    a. Most common.
    b. Nerve edges are anatomically aligned, and then sutures are placed at regular intervals. Surface vasculature and fascicular patterns are used to guide alignment.
    c. The needle should pass through the epineurium two to three needle breadths from the cut edge, avoiding deep penetration.
    d. The first two sutures can be left long and used for manipulation.
  3. **Fascicular repair**
    a. Individual fascicles are coapted.
    b. The theoretical advantage of greater anatomic alignment has not translated into superior outcomes.

4. Group fascicular repair

    a. Indicated in the repair of larger nerves at levels that allow identification of specific branches.

    b. Individual fascicular groups are coapted at the inner epineurial level.

Pearls

1. Have a backup plan preoperatively.
2. Check equipment function before the case begins.
3. Maintain continuous, thorough communication with anesthesia colleagues.
4. Surgeon comfort is paramount:
       a. Take breaks every 2 hours or so.
       b. If you drink caffeine routinely, consume your normal amount.
       c. Relax. Listen to the music of your choice.
       d. Ergonomics: Use proper seat height and good posture.
5. Setup is key:
       a. Position the patient for maximal easy access.
       b. Arrange team members for surgeon convenience and overall efficiency.
       c. Place a stack of towels under your forearms and/or wrists to avoid fatigue.
       d. Invest the time to ensure a straightforward anastomosis.
6. Take time on splints and padding. A poorly designed dressing can ruin a well-executed operation, whereas a well-designed dressing prevents pressure on the flap and pedicle.

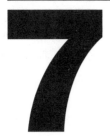

Endoscopic Plastic Surgery

Anil Mungara

I. Basic concepts
A. Endoscopic surgery is not a specialty, per se. Like microsurgery, it is merely one of many tools in the armamentarium of the plastic surgeon.

B. Definition: Operating within a cavity using minimal incisions and endoscopic visualization.

C. The endoscope is inserted via a small incision. Light is reflected to the camera, which projects the image to a video screen. Operating instruments are introduced via separate incisions.

D. Optical cavity considerations
  1. **An optical cavity** is essential for light to be reflected to the endoscope and provide visualization of the operating field.
  2. **The potential cavities of the peritoneum, joints, or thorax** can be used via gas or saline insufflation.
  3. **A subcutaneous cavity** must be created for most plastic surgery procedures, which is usually maintained by mechanical retraction.

E. Advantages of endoscopic versus open approaches
  1. Less morbidity (especially pain) through the use of smaller incisions.
  2. Improved cosmesis secondary to smaller scars.
  3. Shorter recovery time (controversial).

F. Disadvantages of endoscopic approaches
  1. Increased operating time.
  2. Technically more demanding than most open approaches.
  3. Learning curve: Results depend on surgeon experience.
  4. Additional cost of specialized equipment and extended operating room time.

G. Indications
  1. Patient preference.
  2. When minimal scarring is desired (e.g., facial aesthetic surgery).
  3. Controversial: Indications continue to evolve.

II. Instrumentation
A. Components: Endoscope, light source, camera, video monitor, endoscopic operating instruments.

B. Endoscopes
  1. **Size:** Available in 4- to 10-mm diameters. Larger endoscopes contain more fiberoptic bundles, transmitting more light and increasing image clarity; especially useful in breast and trunk procedures. Smaller endoscopes are useful for facial procedures.
  2. **Angles:** Available in 0-, 30-, and 45-degree angles. Angled endoscopes are useful for enhanced viewing around obstacles (e.g., negotiating the convexity of the frontal bone during endoscopic brow lifting).

C. Light source: Typically xenon; connected to the endoscope via a fiberoptic cable.

D. Cameras
  1. **Single-chip cameras** contain alternating pixels that sense red, green, and blue; they are smaller and less expensive than three-chip cameras.

2. **Three-chip cameras** contain separate chips dedicated to sensing each color, resulting in improved image quality.

III. **Access incisions: factors to consider**
   A. **Location:** Ideally hidden under clothing, within aesthetic unit divisions, and parallel to relaxed skin tension lines.
   B. **The optical cavity** should lie between the surgeon and the video monitor to facilitate orientation.
   C. **Anesthesiologist and operating room personnel positioning** should be considered, as well as patient positioning, in order to maximize surgeon coefficiency.

IV. **Troubleshooting**
   A. **Cloudy image**
      1. Endoscope prewarming prevents condensation from warm body tissues.
      2. Antifog solutions (surfactants) are used to disperse condensation on the lens.
   B. **Altered colors or dark image:** White balancing is performed before introduction of the endoscope by placing a gauze pad near the lens and activating the automatic white balance function.
   C. **Video interference patterns**
      1. Usually caused by electrocautery.
      2. Remedied by switching the electrocautery to a different outlet.
   D. **Insufficient smoke evacuation:** Requires enlargement of access incision or addition of another port for suctioning.

V. **Specific uses**
   A. **Transaxillary breast augmentation**
      1. Has become a relatively common procedure.
      2. Hides scars in axilla.
      3. The subpectoral space can be better visualized with endoscopy than with the relatively blind open version of the procedure.
      4. The large optical cavity of this area requires a 10-mm endoscope for adequate light transmission and visualization.
      5. Drawbacks: Lack of complete control in adjusting the inframammary fold.
   B. **Latissimus dorsi muscle harvest**
      1. Most commonly indicated for postmastectomy breast reconstruction. Also used for Poland's syndrome reconstruction and muscle harvest for free tissue transfer.
      2. Existing scars, especially those in breast or axilla, may serve as access incisions.
      3. The endoscope is most useful for elevating the most distal aspect of the latissimus dorsi muscle. The proximal portion can be elevated through a 4-cm transaxillary incision.
   C. **Tissue expander insertion**
      1. Dissection from a remote access site prevents expander extrusion and allows for early, aggressive expansion.
      2. Endoscopic visualization is superior to open procedures when dissecting from a remote access incision site.
   D. **Facial aesthetic surgery**
      1. **Brow lift**
         a. Alleviates problems associated with open brow lift, including large coronal scars, alopecia, and paresthesias.
         b. Controversy exists as to the degree of sustained lift achievable with this technique.
      2. **Midface lift:** Indicated in patients with relaxed superficial fascia and mild skin laxity. A temporal approach is used to resuspend the midface fascia.
   E. **Maxillofacial trauma**
      1. The endoscope has been used in reduction and fixation of some types of facial fractures.
      2. Nasal edema and surrounding injuries can make the diagnosis of nasal septal fractures difficult. Endoscopic examination can facilitate this diagnosis.

F. **Nerve and vein grafts:** Standard harvest of the greater saphenous vein and sural nerve involves a long leg incision or multiple "stepladder" incisions. Endoscopic harvest eliminates lengthy scars and associated wound-healing problems.

G. **Nasal airway surgery**
   1. The endoscope allows angled magnified views of the nasal airway.
   2. Visualization of the nasal airway makes endoscopic procedures superior to classic techniques in some cases. Examples include inferior turbinate surgery, and treatment of paranasal sinus disease, epistaxis, and dacryocystostenosis.

H. **Diagnostic endoscopy of the head and neck**
   1. The bony and soft tissue supports of nasopharynx, oropharynx, and larynx support an optical cavity that is amenable to endoscopic visualization.
   2. Most indications for head and neck endoscopy in plastic surgery involve head and neck cancer and structural abnormalities associated with velopharyngeal insufficiency.

I. **Harvest of jejunum, rectus abdominis, and omentum**
   1. Endoscopic techniques minimize complications associated with open harvest of these tissues, such as ileus, bowel obstruction from adhesions, and wound dehiscence.
   2. Jejunal harvest can be performed for cervical esophageal reconstruction.
   3. Rectus muscle harvest can be performed through a transperitoneal approach or through an extraperitoneal approach from within the rectus sheath.
   4. The omentum can be exteriorized using the laparoscope, and then dissected. Complete intraperitoneal dissection of the omentum is difficult.

J. **Carpal tunnel release**
   1. Endoscopic release preserves the superficial palmar fascia, the palmar fat pad, and the cross branches of the cutaneous nerves.
   2. The main disadvantage involves the small window of visualization, which increases the risk of injury to the palmar vascular arch and motor branch of the median nerve. In addition, since some of these structures are not divided, symptoms may recur.

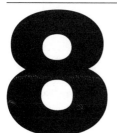

Local Anesthetics

Joon Y. Choi

Pharmacology of Local Anesthetics

I. Chemistry and mechanism of action
  A. Local anesthetic (LA) molecules consist of a lipophilic aromatic portion, an intermediate chain containing either an amide or ester group, and a hydrophilic amine group.
  B. LAs reversibly block propagation of action potentials by blocking $Na+$ channels.
    1. LAs prevent Na^+/K^+ exchange by blocking Na^+ channels, thus stabilizing the plasma membrane. Without the influx of Na^+ ions, the depolarization threshold is not reached, and action potentials are halted.
    2. Small-diameter nerve fibers are more sensitive to LAs. Larger, myelinated nerves must have several nodes of Ranvier blocked before they are affected.
    3. Local anesthetics block pain first; then the sensation of cold, heat, and light touch; and, finally, deep pressure.
II. Pharmacokinetics
  A. Potency is related to lipid solubility, since the axolemma (plasma membrane) is made up of 90% lipids. The more lipid soluble the drug, the faster it penetrates the membrane.
  B. Rate of onset
    1. The pKa of the LA molecule determines the rate of onset (the amount of lipid-soluble uncharged base determines the diffusion rate across the nerve cell membrane).
      a. The greater the concentration of nonionized LA, the faster the onset.
      b. The lower the pKa, the higher the concentration of nonionized LA at a given pH, and therefore the faster the onset.
      c. The addition of sodium bicarbonate will raise the pH, and thus speed the onset of action. This will also reduce pain upon infiltration.
        (1) Add 1 mEq to 10 mL 1% lidocaine.
        (2) Add 0.1 mEq to 10 mL 0.25% bupivacaine.
    2. Inflamed tissues have a low pH, which decreases the concentration of nonionized LA and reduces the effect.
  C. Duration
    1. Intrinsic vasodilatory effect of LAs reduces their duration of anesthesia.
      a. All LAs cause vasodilation, except cocaine, which causes vasoconstriction.
      b. Vasodilation promotes removal of LA, thus shortening the duration.
      c. Epinephrine counters the vasodilatory effects of LAs and prolongs their duration of action. Seven minutes are required for the hemostatic effect of epinephrine.
    2. Protein binding increases the duration of anesthesia.

Table 8-1. Summary of properties: Esters versus amides

Property	Esters	Amides
Metabolism	Rapid, by plasma cholinesterase	Slow, hepatic
Systemic toxicity	Less likely	More likely
Allergic reaction	Possible via PABA derivative formation; may cause malignant HTN	Very rare
Stability in solution	Breaks down in ampules (heat, sunlight)	Very stable chemically
Onset of action	Generally slow	Moderate to fast
pKa	Higher than physiologic pH (8.5–8.9)	Close to physiologic pH (7.6–8.1)

PABA, p-aminobenzoic acid; HTN, hypertensive nephropathy; pKa, measure of acid strength.

III. **Esters versus amides** (Table 8-1)
  A. **LAs containing an "i" before the "-aine" in their names are amides.**
     Examples: lidocaine, bupivacaine, etidocaine.
  B. **Metabolism**
     1. Amides and one ester (cocaine) are metabolized by the liver.
     2. Most esters are metabolized by plasma cholinesterase.
     3. Poor hepatic function or blood flow (e.g., cirrhosis, congestive heart failure, hypothermia, general anesthetics, beta blockers) alter aminoamide LA metabolism.
  C. **Allergic reaction**
     1. **Associated with esters,** not amides.
     2. **Methylparaben** is an antibacterial preservative that can cause a reaction to amides.
     3. **Amides may trigger malignant hyperthermia.**
  D. **Toxicity and treatment**
     1. **Calculation of maximum administration volume**
        a. Maximum dosage of lidocaine
           (1) Without epinephrine: 5 mg/kg patient weight.
           (2) With epinephrine: 7 mg/kg. Local epinephrine-induced vasospasm results in decreased systemic absorption of the lidocaine.
        b. Patient weight × LA concentration × maximum concentration for the specific LA used. (1% solution = 10 mg/1 cc.) For example, 1% lidocaine with epinephrine in a 70-kg man: 70 kg × 1 cc/10 mg × 7 mg/kg = 49 cc.
     2. **Central nervous system toxicity**
        a. Stimulation: Restlessness, circumoral numbness, tinnitus, visual disturbances, disorientation, shivering, tremors, and clonic convulsions.
        b. Depression of medullary center and respiratory failure, hypotension, bradycardia, ventricular arrhythmia, and coma.
        c. Treatment: Diazepam, midazolam, or thiopental i.v. For convulsions: Succinylcholine and endotracheal intubation.
     3. **Cardiovascular toxicity**
        a. Myocardial depression: Decreased contractile force, excitability, and conduction rate and increased refractory period.
        b. Arteriolar dilation (except cocaine).
        c. Treatment: Atropine for bradycardia, i.v. fluids and ephedrine to address hypotension, and epinephrine for profound cardiovascular collapse.

4. **Neuromuscular or local tissue toxicity**
   a. Caused by depression of calcium activity leading to decreased muscle excitability and contractility.
   b. Reversible myotonic effects with direct injection of LA into muscles.
5. Methemoglobinemia manifests as cyanosis; treatment is with methylene blue.

E. **Esters**
   1. **Cocaine:** Vasoconstrictor; topical use only; useful intranasally for concurrent anesthesia and hemostasis.
   2. **Chloroprocaine:** Rapidly metabolized; favored by obstetricians because of low fetal exposure.
   3. **Procaine:** Not effective topically.
   4. **Tetracaine:** Effective topically.

F. **Amides**
   1. **Bupivacaine:** Long duration—up to 24 hours; slow onset; high potency and toxicity; mixed with lidocaine for rapid onset and long-duration block. Preferentially blocks sensory rather than motor fibers.
   2. **Etidocaine:** Used for regional blocks; preference for motor over sensory fibers.
   3. **Lidocaine:** Rapid onset; moderate duration; highly stable; nonirritating; maximum dose is 5 mg/kg (plain) and 7 mg/kg with epinephrine.
   4. **Mepivacaine:** Longer duration and more rapid onset than lidocaine.
   5. **Prilocaine:** 40% less toxic acutely, but metabolites can cause methemoglobinemia.
   6. **Ropivacaine:** Similar to bupivacaine, but less potent and less cardiotoxic.

Nerve Blocks

I. **Upper extremity blocks**
   A. **Axillary block**
      1. Position the patient supine with arms abducted and forearms at right angles with the hands above the head.
      2. Feel the axillary arterial pulse and follow it proximally until it disappears under the pectoralis major.
      3. The needle is advanced with an index finger over the pulse until one of the following occurs:
         a. A distinctive "click" is heard, consistent with penetration into the plexus sheath.
         b. Paresthesia is elicited in the median, ulnar, or radial nerve distribution.
         c. Arterial blood is aspirated; inject half of the LA behind the artery by advancing the needle, and the other half in front of the artery.
         d. An attached nerve stimulator indicates needle tip placement within the sheath.
   B. **Bier block**
      1. Place a dual tourniquet on the upper arm and a peripheral i.v. line distally.
      2. Elevate the arm and exsanguinate with an Ace wrap all the way from the fingers to the tourniquet.
      3. Inflate the proximal tourniquet and then remove the Ace bandage.
      4. Slowly inject local anesthetic through the peripheral i.v. line.
      5. After 20 minutes (or sooner if patient discomfort occurs), inflate the distal tourniquet and deflate the proximal one. Anesthesia lasts as long as the tourniquet is inflated.
      6. If a procedure lasts less than 20 minutes, tourniquet deflation should be done in stages to avoid LA toxicity via i.v. bolus release of the LA.
   C. **Wrist block**
      1. **An ulnar nerve block** is performed by introducing the needle radial to the flexor carpi ulnaris (FCU) and ulnar to the ulnar artery at the proximal

wrist crease. The dorsal cutaneous nerve is blocked by subcutaneous infiltration extending from the injection site to the mid-dorsum of the wrist.

2. A median nerve block is performed by introducing the needle between the palmaris longus (PL) and the flexor carpi radialis (FCR) at the level of the ulnar styloid process or the proximal crease of the wrist. If there is no PL (in 15% of hands), inject on the ulnar side of the FCR. Avoid direct injection into the nerve substance by asking the patient to report any paresthesias.

3. The radial nerve (sensory branch) is blocked subcutaneously just proximal to the wrist, superficial to the extensor pollicis longus. Start injecting just radial to the radial artery and extend around to the midpoint of the dorsum of the wrist.

D. Digital block

1. Epinephrine is avoided due to the risk of tissue loss (controversial). Three mL is usually adequate for most digital blocks.

2. Anatomy

a. The common digital nerves branch at the distal palmar crease and lie volar to the flexor tendons. The digital arteries and nerves change orientation when entering the digits, with the nerve coming to lie volar to the artery in the digits.

b. Dorsal sensory branches should also be addressed.

3. Digital block technique

a. Dorsal approach (some think is less painful)

(1) Subcutaneous wheal over the extensor tendon to block the dorsal nerves.

(2) Two injections just proximal to the web, one on either side of the digit; advance the needle until the tip approaches the palmar skin surface, and then withdraw while injecting slowly.

b. Volar approach: A subcutaneous wheal is placed directly over the flexor tendon and then laterally near the digital neurovascular bundles.

c. Sheath approach: Insert the needle volarly, just distal to the distal palmar crease, down into the flexor tendons. With slight pressure on the syringe plunger, withdraw the needle slowly until there is a loss of resistance (indicating injection into the potential space of the flexor sheath). Inject a couple of mL of local anesthetic. Sometimes, a fluid wave can be felt distally in the finger over the sheath. This technique reliably results in digital anesthesia with one injection, but is not very effective in cases of sheath violation, such as distal amputation.

II. Facial blocks

A. Distal trigeminal blocks

1. The terminal branches of cranial nerve V lie in line with the pupil (with the eye in a midgaze position), approximately 2.5 cm off the midline.

2. Supraorbital nerve: Palpate the supraorbital notch just under the midportion of the eyebrow and inject 2 to 3 mL; avoid injection into the foramen.

3. Supratrochlear nerve: Inject just lateral to the root of the nose in the medial portion of the orbital rim.

4. Both the supraorbital and supratrochlear nerves can be blocked by horizontal infiltration 2 cm above the eyebrow.

5. Infraorbital nerve: An upper buccal sulcus or external approach may be used. Palpating the foramen may be difficult. Injection of 2 to 5 mL of 1% lidocaine with epinephrine usually lasts 60 to 90 minutes.

6. Mental nerve: May be approached transorally or transcutaneously. Enter the mucosa between the bicuspids, aiming at the apex of the second bicuspid root. The foramen location varies with a patient's age, moving more superiorly and medially with age.

B. Nose (rhinoplasty anesthesia)

1. External

a. Sensibility is supplied by the infratrochlear (V1), external nasal (V1), and infraorbital (V2) nerves.

      b. Technique
         (1) 1% lidocaine with epinephrine is injected along a line that starts from the nasolabial fold, continues lateral to the ala and along the base of the nasal sidewall, and ends at the radix.
         (2) Inject cranially and caudally for a regional block.
   2. Internal
      a. Sensibility via the inferior posterior nasal nerve, nasopalatine nerve, superior posterior nasal nerves, and branches of the ethmoidal nerves.
      b. Technique: Cotton pledgets dipped in 4% cocaine are placed directly on the nasal mucosa.
  C. Ear
   1. Nerves of the external ear
      a. Lesser occipital nerve.
      b. Great auricular nerve.
      c. Auriculotemporal nerve.
   2. Technique
      a. Field block using 1% lidocaine with epinephrine.
      b. Two injection sites cranially and caudally: Inject anteriorly and posteriorly around the ear either in a ring-like fashion or a diamond-shaped pattern.
III. Intercostal block
  A. Second through seventh intercostal nerves are anesthetized.
  B. The patient is placed supine, with the arms abducted.
  C. Injection of 3 to 5 mL inferior to each rib is performed in the midaxillary line.
  D. Additional subcutaneous infiltration is occasionally necessary.
   1. Superomedially, for superficial cervical plexus
   2. Midline, due to crossing innervation of the intercostals

---

Topical Anesthetics

I. Eutectic mixture of local anesthetics (EMLAs)
  A. No local or systemic toxicity, but methemoglobinemia is a potentially life-threatening adverse effect in neonates.
  B. Oil-in-water emulsion; consists of 2.5% prilocaine and 2.5% lidocaine.
  C. Duration and depth of pain blockade are both a direct function of the application time: EMLA is usually applied 1 hour before a procedure.
II. ELA-max
  A. Consists of 4% or 5% lidocaine, delivered in a liposomal vehicle.
  B. Faster onset and longer duration than EMLA.
III. Tetracaine and cocaine
  A. Ester based.
  B. Useful for laceration repair; absorbs through the open surface of the wound.
IV. Iontophoresis
  A. Uses a low-voltage current to drive the transdermal delivery of lidocaine.
  B. Advantages: Needle-free process, rapid onset of anesthesia (within 10 minutes), and excellent cutaneous penetration.
  C. Disadvantages: Limited to small surface area, superficial burns are possible, and the equipment is comparatively complex.

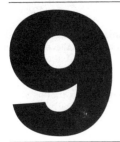

Patient Selection and Psychiatric Aspects of Plastic Surgery

Jafar S. Hasan

I. Potential impact of plastic surgery
   A. Increased self-esteem.
   B. Decreased self-consciousness.
   C. Patients may be judged as more attractive by others (potential to alter social dynamics).

II. Patient factors
   A. Patient satisfaction is determined by patients' *perceptions* of outcomes rather than true physical outcomes.
   B. Preoperative expectations influence patients' postoperative perceptions of the outcome.
   1. **Surgical:** The surgeon should attempt to guide these expectations.
   2. **Social:** Expectations of drastic social change may be a warning sign.
   3. **Psychological**
      a. Appropriate patients: Negative view specific to the feature being surgically corrected.
      b. Potentially problematic patients: Negative views are more generalized (overall body image).
   C. Patient motivations for cosmetic surgery.
   1. **Internal motivations** (positive): Desire to improve self-confidence by improving physical appearance.
   2. **External motivations** (potentially negative).
      a. Patients may attribute social problems to physical aspects alone.
      b. Failure to improve the social situation after cosmetic surgery may cause the patient to blame the surgeon.
   D. Body image
   1. Defined as a person's feelings and perceptions about his or her body.
   2. **Appropriate plastic surgery patients:** No greater body image concern than general population.
   3. **Potentially problematic patients:** Generalized body image concerns (not isolated to concern over one specific feature).

III. Examples of psychopathology
   A. Body dysmorphic disorder (BDD)
   1. **American Psychiatric Association criteria (DSM-IV)**
      a. Preoccupation with imagined defect in appearance. (If a slight physical anomaly is present, then the concern must be markedly excessive.)
      b. The preoccupation causes clinically significant distress and impairment in function (social, occupational, or other).
      c. The preoccupation is not better accounted for by another mental disorder (e.g., anorexia nervosa).
   2. **Features**
      a. Excessive grooming.
      b. Extensive efforts to "hide" the imagined defect.
      c. Frequent comparing of the "defect" with that of others.
      d. Multiple visits to plastic surgeons to correct the "defect".
   3. **Responds poorly to surgery,** and the perceived "defect" may switch to other specific body features.

B. Schizophrenia
1. May have delusions involving a perceived physical defect.
2. Perceptions of reality are skewed.
C. Anxiety disorders
1. Panic attack
a. American Psychiatric Association criteria (DSM-IV): Period of intense fear/discomfort involving four or more of the following:
(1) Palpitations
(2) Sweating
(3) Trembling/shaking
(4) Shortness of breath
(5) Feeling of choking
(6) Chest pain
(7) Nausea or abdominal distress
(8) Feeling dizzy/lightheaded
(9) Feeling of unreality
(10) Fear of going crazy
(11) Fear of dying
(12) Paresthesias
(13) Chills or hot flushes
b. Refer for psychiatric consultation.
2. Post-traumatic stress disorder (PTSD)
a. Operation may cause patient to "reexperience" a traumatic event.
b. American Psychiatric Association criteria (DSM-IV)
(1) Experienced an event that was life-threatening or associated with serious injury.
(2) Event may be "re-experienced" as
(a) Recurrent/intrusive distressing images, thoughts, or perceptions
(b) Recurrent/distressing dreams
(c) Feeling or acting as if the event were recurring
(d) Intense psychological distress
(e) Physiologic reactivity to cues that symbolize the event
(3) Persistent avoidance of stimuli associated with the event.
(4) Increased arousal (two or more of the following):
(a) Difficulty falling or staying asleep
(b) Irritability or outburst of anger
(c) Difficulty concentrating
(d) Hypervigilance
(e) Exaggerated startle response
(5) Duration of symptoms for more than 1 month.
c. The disturbance causes clinically significant distress or impairment in social, occupational, or other activities.
IV. Patient screening and selection
A. Indications for psychiatric input
1. Excessive anxiety.
2. Subjective sense of depression.
3. Potential for the operation to cause psychological harm (e.g., suspect PTSD).
4. Anticipation of postoperative psychiatric care (e.g., potential for panic attack).
5. Severe psychopathology that contraindicates surgery.
B. Screening for potential psychopathology
1. **Allow patients to fully express their reasons** for seeking cosmetic surgery.
2. **Use open-ended questions** to gain more information.
a. "Has this deformity affected your life at home or work?" is a *close-ended question* that is likely to yield little more than a yes or no response.

        b. "Tell me the various ways in which this deformity has affected your life at home and at work" is an *open-ended question*, which is more likely to reveal the patient's expectations and motivations for the operation.

C. Preoperative clues

  1. Poor prognosis

    a. History of recurrent psychiatric illness

    b. Dissatisfaction with previous procedures or surgeons

    c. History of consulting multiple plastic surgeons for either primary or secondary procedures

    d. Expectation that the operation will result in specific changes in personal life (e.g., prevention of divorce)

    e. Impulsive decision to undergo surgery

  2. Better prognosis

    a. Actual disfigurement

    b. Reasonable preoperative expectations

    c. Lack of impulsivity (long-term desire to undergo surgery)

  3. Warning signs

    a. Depression

    b. Excessive anxiety

    c. Overly demanding demeanor

    d. Poor body image and problems with self-esteem

    e. Failure to make significant long-term relationships

    f. History of sexual abuse (may have a PTSD component)

Pearls

---

1. **Get a sense of each patient's motivations.**
2. **Determine patient expectations.**
3. **Make the patient specifically state his or her concerns** about the physical feature in question. (This is very important because BDD is characterized by a level of concern that is out of proportion to the true physical "defect.").
4. **Develop a referral pattern with a psychiatrist** who has experience with cosmetic patients.
5. **Some patients may become offended by psychiatric consultation.** It is better to take that risk than to operate on patients with undiagnosed psychopathology.

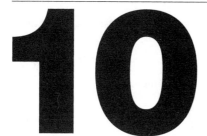

Lasers in Plastic Surgery

Christi M. Cavaliere

I. Laser physics

A. **Laser is an acronym** for **L**ight **A**mplification by **S**timulated **E**mission of **R**adiation.

B. Energy is created when atoms are excited and emit photons. A laser device consists of a cavity with mirrors that reflect and multiply photon energy.

C. Laser light is coherent (all the light waves are in phase) and monochromatic (single wavelength).

   1. Numerous elements and molecules (lasing media) can be stimulated to release photons. Each medium releases photons of a specific wavelength (measured in nanometers).

   2. Most lasers with clinical applications fall within the visible light spectrum, 400 nm to 700 nm (an exception is the carbon dioxide laser: 10,600 nm).

D. Laser light is intense, with a much higher number of photons per unit area than visible light.

E. Laser energy may be absorbed, transmitted, or refracted. The effects of clinically useful lasers depend on the specific absorption qualities.

F. Lasers are characterized by their power (watts), energy (joules), irradiance or power density (watts/cm^2), and energy density or fluence (J/cm^2).

G. **Delivery modes**

   1. Continuous wave: An uninterrupted beam.

   2. Pulsed: Beam delivered as single pulses or trains of pulses.

   3. Superpulsed or Q-switched: Extremely high-power, extremely brief pulses generating gigawatt pulses and tissue temperatures up to 300°C (single pulses measured in nanoseconds).

II. Tissue effects

A. **Selective photothermolysis**

   1. Energy of a particular wavelength is absorbed by a specific chromophore within the tissue (e.g., red chromophore reflects red light but absorbs other wavelengths).

   2. Diffusion of heat to the tissues surrounding the chromophore is limited by the exposure time (pulse width), as long as the exposure time is less than the thermal relaxation time of the tissue.

   3. Thermal relaxation time: The time needed for 50% of the heat to dissipate.

B. **Thermal effects**

   1. Most of the light energy of surgical lasers is absorbed by the target tissue. The therapeutic effect results from the heat generated.

   2. Thermal effects are controllable by adjusting the pulse duration, energy density, and heat conduction.

C. **Mechanical effects:** Thermoelastic expansion occurs when the pulse duration is shorter than the thermal relaxation time and acoustic waves are generated, potentially damaging adjacent tissues.

III. Laser safety

A. **Eye protection**

   1. All lasers can cause corneal damage.

   2. Eyewear must be wavelength specific.

   3. Laser-specific protective eye shields for patients must cover the entire orbit.

   4. Cover all doors and windows; place eyewear and signs indicating laser in use at each door.
B. Fire safety
   1. Prep with a nonflammable solution (no alcohol or chlorhexidine gluconate) and use nonflammable anesthetics.
   2. Surround treatment area with wet towels.
   3. No reflective instruments should be allowed in the treatment area.
C. Infectious disease precautions
   1. Smoke evacuator with filter: Laser vapors can contain infectious particles or tumor cells.
   2. Close-fitting, filtered laser mask: To filter out particles less than 0.1 μm in diameter.
   3. Tubing and filters must be disposed of as biohazardous waste.
IV. Laser applications (Table 10-1)
   A. Skin resurfacing: Best candidates are patients who have Fitzpatrick skin types I and II, with fine to medium wrinkles.
      1. **Histologic effects**
         a. Thermal injury to the skin with resultant wound healing.
         b. Reepithelialization: Occurs through proliferation of progenitor cells within the remaining hair follicles and sweat glands.
         c. Increased collagen synthesis: Continues for approximately 3 to 6 months. New collagen is deposited throughout the dermis, particularly in the zone of Grenz (found in sun-damaged skin—the subepidermal layer of the papillary dermis that lacks elastic fibers).
         d. Reorganization of elastic fibers that were disorganized due to aging and solar damage: Elastic fibers take on a more parallel and tightly bundled appearance.
         e. Skin contraction, due to:
            (1) Heat-induced collagen contraction.
            (2) Increased deposition of type I collagen and elastic tissue.
            (3) Reorientation of disorganized collagen and elastin fibers.
      2. **Carbon dioxide (CO_2) laser**
         a. Gas laser; 10,600-nm wavelength.
         b. Chromophore is water.
         c. Pulsed or continuous-wave modes.
         d. Improvement of fine and deeper wrinkles with a lasting result.
         e. Main side effect: Erythema for 2 to 4 months.
         f. Desired effect for skin resurfacing is tissue vaporization. The ablation threshold for skin is the energy density required to vaporize the tissue with minimal thermal damage. For the CO_2 laser, the ablation threshold is 5.5 J/cm^2.
      3. **Erbium:yttrium-aluminum-garnet (Er:YAG) laser**
         a. Solid-state laser; 2,940-nm wavelength; chromophore is water.
         b. Reduces fine, superficial wrinkles ("lunchtime peel").
         c. Can be used on areas of very thin skin, such as the dorsum of the hand.
         d. Side effects include erythema for 2 to 4 weeks.
         e. More passes are required for the same depth of penetration, compared with a CO_2 laser, with much less thermal damage. Because Er:YAG is not a coagulating laser, bleeding may occur when dermal vasculature is encountered.
         f. Ablation threshold for skin using the Er:YAG laser is 1.6 J/cm^2.
   B. Vascular lesions
      1. Selective photothermolysis targets hemoglobin and oxyhemoglobin molecules and shrinks or eliminates blood vessels.
      2. Major absorption peaks for hemoglobin and oxyhemoglobin chromophores are in the range of 500 to 1,000 nm.
      3. Laser therapy is the treatment of choice for capillary vascular malformations. Although laser therapy has been described for other vascular

Table 10-1. Indications for laser choice

Application	Laser	Wavelength (nm)	Target Chromophore	Indications	Most Common Adverse Effects
Skin resurfacing	CO_2	10,600	Water	Superficial and deep rhytides; solar pigmentation changes	Erythema for 2–4 months
	Er:YAG	2940	Water	Fine wrinkles; solar pigmentation changes	Erythema for 2–4 weeks; bleeding from dermal vessels
Vascular lesions	Pulsed-dye	585	Hemoglobin	Small, superficial vessels	Purpura for 2–3 weeks
	KTP	532	Hemoglobin	Slightly larger and deeper vessels	Purpura (rare)
Pigmented skin lesions	Q-switched ruby	694	Melanin	Pigmented areas	Results variable; poor success with melasma and café au lait macules
	Q-switched Alexandrite	755			
	Nd:YAG	1065			
	Frequency-doubled Nd:YAG	532			
	Pulsed-dye	510			
	Copper bromide or copper vapor	511 and 578	Nonspecific (epidermis and part of dermis)	Pigmented areas	
Tattoo removal					
Red and orange	Q-switched Nd:YAG	532		Red and orange pigments	Multiple treatments usually necessary; may need more than one laser to target all pigments; hypopigmentation; incomplete removal
	Pulsed dye	510		Eliminate all tattoo pigments except red and orange	
All colors except red and orange	Q-switched Alexandrite	755			
	Q-switched Ruby	694			
All colors except red, orange, and green	Q-switched Nd:YAG	1032		All tattoo pigments except red, orange, and green	
Hair removal	Long-pulse Ruby	694	Melanin	Unwanted areas of hair growth	Requires several treatments; transient erythema; hypopigmentation
	Long-pulse Alexandrite	755			
	Intense pulsed-light	590–1200	Nonspecific		

CO_2, carbon dioxide; Er:YAG, erbium:ytrrium-aluminum-garnet; KTP, potassium-titanyl-phosphate; Nd:YAG, neodymium:ytrrium-aluminum-garnet.

malformations, multimodality treatment is usually necessary and the role of the laser is not as clearly defined.

  4. **Flashlamp-pumped pulsed dye laser (FLPD)**
     a. 585 nm; earlier lasers 577 nm.
     b. Most common laser for capillary malformations; also used for telangiectasias.
     c. A flashlamp is used to excite an organic or inorganic dye to achieve a particular wavelength. The fluorescence is captured by a series of mirrors to produce a laser beam.
     d. Light absorbed by hemoglobin and oxyhemoglobin heats vessels to over 60°C for approximately 1 millisecond, causing endothelial cell contraction and vessel ablation.
     e. Minimal thermal damage occurs in surrounding tissues because the pulse duration approximates the thermal relaxation time of blood vessels.
     f. Multiple treatments are usually required. Facial telangiectasias may disappear with a single treatment. Lower extremity telangiectasias have unpredictable results, sometimes with postinflammatory hyperpigmentation. Long-pulsed tunable dye lasers are more commonly used for leg telangiectasias.
     g. May develop purpura for 2 to 3 weeks.
  5. **KTP/532** (long-pulsed frequency-doubled yttrium-aluminum-garnet laser)
     a. Solid-state laser; 532-nm wavelength.
     b. Penetration of slightly larger vessels than FLPD; better for thicker or advanced capillary and venous vascular malformations.
     c. Main advantage over FLPD laser is that purpura rarely occurs.
  6. **Argon laser:** Formerly the laser of choice for capillary malformations. It is now rarely used due to the high incidence of hypertrophic scarring and hypopigmentation.

C. **Pigmented skin lesions**
  1. Examples are solar lentigines, café au lait macules without neurofibromatosis, and nevi of Ota.
  2. The targeted chromophore is melanin. The absorption spectrum of melanin is very broad. If longer wavelengths are used (600–1,200 nm), the hemoglobin chromophore can be avoided, thereby avoiding purpura.
  3. Several lasers are available to treat pigmented lesions: Q-switched ruby (694 nm), Q-switched alexandrite (755 nm), Nd:YAG (1,064 nm), frequency-doubled Nd:YAG (532 nm), pulsed dye (510 nm), copper bromide (511 and 578 nm), and copper vapor laser (511 and 578 nm). The latter two lasers thermally destroy the epidermis and part of the dermis; melanin is not specifically targeted as a chromophore.
  4. Histologic features of a pigmented lesion previously treated with a laser may be difficult to distinguish from dysplasia or melanoma, so certainty of the dermatologic diagnosis is essential prior to laser therapy.

D. **Tattoo removal**
  1. Rapidly pulsed laser energy (Q-switched mode) penetrates to the level of the upper papillary dermis and selectively targets ink particles based on their color.
  2. Heated particles explode, producing smaller particles that can be removed by phagocytosis.
  3. Multiple treatments are usually necessary; allow approximately 3 weeks between treatments for phagocytes to clear debris.
  4. Caution: Oxidation of certain metal-containing tattoo pigments during laser treatment may lead to black discoloration instead of removal.
  5. Red and orange pigment removal: Q-switched Nd:YAG (532 nm) and pulsed dye (510 nm).
  6. Removal of all colors except red and orange: Q-switched alexandrite (755 nm) and Q-switched ruby (694 nm).
  7. All colors except red, orange, and green: Q-switched Nd:YAG (1,032 nm).

E. Hair removal
1. Melanin is the main chromophore targeted in laser hair removal; hypopigmentation is therefore a potential side effect.
2. Requires at least two or three treatments. There is often a 10% regrowth months after treatments (removes only follicles in the anagen phase of their growth cycle).
3. The laser should penetrate at least 3 mm, and must destroy both the bulge and the bulb of the hair follicle.
4. Laser types for hair removal: Long-pulse ruby (694 nm), long-pulse alexandrite (755 nm), and intense pulsed-light (EpiLight). The EpiLight system is not actually a laser (590-1,200 nm) and may be safer for darker skin colors.

F. Hair restoration
1. The high-powered CO_2 laser is used to create micrograft recipient incisions (0.6–1.2 mm).
2. Flash scanner allows rapid and uniform placement of numerous incisions.

G. Acne scarring
1. Er:YAG laser is specific for collagen and scar.
2. "Ice pick" scars show minimal improvement.
3. Isotretinoin (Accutane) treatment impairs reepithelialization after laser resurfacing. Wait at least 1 year after discontinuation of isotretinoin prior to laser treatment.

V. Adverse effects of laser therapy

A. Erythema
1. CO_2 laser resurfacing may produce erythema lasting up to 4 months.
2. More superficial laser treatment (e.g., Er:YAG) may result in erythema for up to several weeks.

B. Purpura: Most often seen with pulsed dye laser

C. Thermal burn

D. Scarring
1. Secondary to thermal burn or infection.
2. Treat keloids and hypertrophic scars with silicone sheeting, steroid injections, and/or compression.

E. Hypopigmentation and hyperpigmentation
1. Higher risk if melanin is the target chromophore.
2. Patients with Fitzpatrick skin types III, IV, V, and VI are at higher risk and are therefore poor candidates for laser resurfacing.
3. Patients with pigmentation disorders due to hormonal influence (e.g., melasma or hyperpigmentation due to birth control pills) are also at high risk.
4. Pretreatment with topical melanin-suppressing agents (lactic, azelaic, or salicylic acids) is controversial. Advocates believe hyperpigmentation is reduced by inhibiting melanin production; opponents argue that topical agents are active only in the epidermis, whereas hyperpigmentation originates in the dermis.
5. Pretreatment with sunscreen may promote sunscreen use postoperatively and help to prevent hyperpigmentation.

F. Infection: Bacterial, fungal, or viral
1. Prescribe herpes simplex prophylaxis from 48 hours preoperatively until postoperative day 14.
2. Antibiotic prophylaxis is advocated by some.

G. Focal thinning or thickening of the skin: Pretreatment with retinoids, glycolic acids, and/or hydroquinone has been debated. Advocates believe skin healing is optimized with increased fibroblast activity, whereas opponents believe retinoids may worsen telangiectasias and erythema.

H. Hypersensitivity reaction to ointments or dressings
1. In the early postoperative period, an increase in erythema signals hypersensitivity or infection.

    2. Avoid fragrances, aloe, vitamins, and other sensitizing agents. All topical agents should be hypoallergenic. Hypoallergenic cosmetics may be resumed only after complete reepithelialization.

    3. Treat with discontinuation of dressing agent in use, rule out infection, and apply topical steroid or consider a brief taper of systemic steroids.

  I. Telangiectasias: Can result from laser resurfacing; may be treated with the pulsed dye laser.

VI. Contraindications to laser resurfacing

  A. Relative: Smoking, previous resurfacing, diabetes, prior skin irradiation, active acne, hypertrophic scarring, skin hypersensitivity, and pigmentation disorders.

  B. Absolute: Keloids, scleroderma, systemic lupus erythematosus, and isotretinoin use within the previous year.

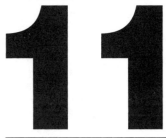

Malignant Skin and Soft Tissue Lesions

Timothy A. Janiga

Melanoma

I. Biology

A. Epidemiology
1. **Eighth most common** cancer diagnosis in the United States.
2. **Incidence is increasing** faster than any other cancer.
3. **40,000 new cases** are diagnosed per year in the United States.
4. **Lifetime risk** in general population is 0.5%.

B. Demographic risk factors
1. **Phenotypic risk factors** include fair skin (Fitzpatrick I and II) (Table 11-1), freckling, light eye color, and light hair color (stronger risk factor than eye color). Darker skin is protective against melanoma.
2. **Geographic risk factors:** High altitude and higher latitude. Extreme southern latitudes (Australia, New Zealand) experience additional ultraviolet (UV) exposure from ozone depletion.
3. **Gender:** Females have lower risk and better prognosis; the lower extremity is the most common site in females (Table 11-2). Males more commonly have lesions on the head and trunk.
4. **Prognosis is worse for African Americans** (acral lentiginous type leads to delayed diagnosis).
5. **Higher socioeconomic status** is associated with higher risk.
6. **History of ultraviolet radiation exposure** (both UVA and UVB), especially a history of blistering sunburns, sunburns in early life, and intermittent exposure to UV light.

C. Precursor lesion risk factors
1. **Melanoma is caused by multiple processes** leading to malignant transformation of melanocytes.
2. **A previous melanoma confers a 3% to 5% chance** of developing a second melanoma.
3. **Congenital nevi**
   a. Malignant potential is more dependent on histology than size.
   b. Giant hairy nevi confer a 5% to 20% lifetime risk of melanoma; most commonly occur on head or pelvic region; prophylactic excision is recommended.
4. **Acquired melanocytic nevi**
   a. Typically appear at 6 to 12 months of age; usually smaller than 5 mm.
   b. Increase in number through the fourth decade then slowly regress.
   c. The greater the number of nevi (>50), the greater the chance of melanoma.
5. **Dysplastic or atypical nevi**
   a. Appear near puberty.
   b. Larger than common nevi (5–12 mm).
   c. Commonly found in covered areas.
   d. Most likely represent both a precursor lesion and a marker for patients with increased risk for development of melanoma.

Table 11-1. Fitzpatrick classification of skin type

Class	Skin Phototype	Unexposed Areas	Tanning History
I	Never tan, always burn	Pale/milky white	Red sunburn, painful swelling, skin peels
II	Sometimes tan, usually burn	Very light brown, sometimes freckles	Usually burn; pinkish or red coloring; light brown tan gradually develops
III	Usually tan, sometimes burn	Light tan, brown, olive	Rarely burn, with moderately rapid tanning response
IV	Always tan, rarely burn	Brown, dark brown, or black	Rarely burn, with rapid tanning response

6. **Atypical junctional melanocytic hyperplasia (AJMH)** (also known as lentigo maligna, or Hutchinson freckle)
   a. Thought to represent a melanoma precursor lesion.
   b. Can be present in dysplastic nevi that tend to be more irregular and lighter in color.
   c. Needs to be fully excised; 5-mm margins are recommended, but are typically inadequate.
7. **Spitz nevus**
   a. Most commonly found in children and young adults (formerly called juvenile melanoma).
   b. Easily confused with melanoma, and almost always benign.
   c. Well circumscribed and raised, with variable pigmentation.
D. **Genetic risk factors**
   1. **Family history:** Two or more cases of melanoma in first-degree relatives. Hereditary melanoma shows autosomal dominant transference with variable penetrance.
   2. **Suppressor genes and oncogenes**
      a. p16/CDKN2A: Tumor suppressor gene that is mutated or deleted in the majority of melanoma cell lines.
      b. RB1: Tumor suppressor gene expressed in higher levels in certain melanomas. Uncommon mechanism in melanoma development.
      c. CDK4: Oncogene thought to play a role in melanoma progression in a small proportion of familial and sporadic melanomas.
   3. **Dysplastic nevus syndrome** (also known as familial atypical mole and melanoma syndrome): Patients have a first- or second-degree relative with malignant melanoma, and typically have at least 50 melanocytic nevi.
   4. **Xeroderma pigmentosum (XP):** Typically presents in childhood with early death secondary to metastatic spread of skin tumors. DNA damaged

Table 11-2. Distribution of melanomas with respect to gender

Location	Men (%)	Women (%)
Scalp	7	3
Face	12	9
Neck	5	3
Arm	13	19
Front of trunk	16	8
Back of trunk	**36**	23
Leg	9	**31**
Sole of foot	2	4

by UV light is unrepaired secondary to a defective repair mechanism. Restriction from sunlight exposure is mandatory, with aggressive treatment of skin lesions.

II. Clinical diagnosis and classification

A. A dermatologist's physical examination is only 60% to 80% sensitive for diagnosing melanoma. Full-body photography to monitor atypical nevi may increase sensitivity.

B. Common clinical features of melanoma (ABCDE mnemonic)
1. **Asymmetry**
2. **Border irregularity**
3. **Color variation (shades of blue are the most ominous)**
4. **Diameter more than 6 mm**

C. Major types of melanoma
1. **Superficial spreading melanoma**
   a. Most common type: 70% of cases.
   b. Intermediate in malignancy.
   c. Usually arises from preexisting nevus.
   d. Affects both genders equally.
   e. Median age at diagnosis: fifth decade.
   f. Most common sites: Upper back in men and lower legs in women.
   g. Irregular, asymmetric borders with color variegation.
   h. Radial growth phase early; vertical growth phase late.
2. **Nodular melanoma**
   a. Second most common: 15% to 30% of cases.
   b. Most aggressive type.
   c. Typically does not arise from preexisting nevi.
   d. Men are affected twice as frequently as women.
   e. Median age at diagnosis is 50 years.
   f. Bluish-black, with uniform, smooth borders.
   g. Vertical growth phase is a hallmark feature.
   h. Not directly associated with sunlight exposure.
   i. 5% are amelanotic—associated with a poorer prognosis because of delayed diagnosis.
3. **Lentigo maligna melanoma (LMM)**
   a. 10% to 15% of cutaneous melanomas.
   b. LMM is the least aggressive type and the only one clearly associated with sunlight exposure.
   c. Head, neck, and arms of elderly (sun-exposed areas).
   d. Women are affected more frequently than men.
   e. The median age at diagnosis is 70 years.
   f. Usually greater than 3 cm in diameter; irregular, asymmetric with color variegation; areas of regression may appear hypopigmented.
   g. Precursor lesion is lentigo maligna or Hutchinson freckle (histologically equivalent to melanoma *in situ*, or AJMH): radial growth phase only. Transition to vertical growth phase marks development of lentigo maligna melanoma.
   h. Malignant degeneration is characterized by nodular development.
4. **Acral lentiginous melanoma**
   a. 2% to 8% of melanomas in whites and 35% to 60% of melanomas in blacks, Hispanics, and Asians.
   b. Presents in palms, soles, and beneath nail plate (subungual). Note: Melanonychia is a linear pigmented streak in the nail, which is often benign and is more common in black and Asian populations. Due to the risk of melanoma, biopsy of suspect lesions should be performed.
   c. Median age at diagnosis is approximately 60 years.
   d. Irregular pigmentation is common.
   e. Large size (>3 cm).
   f. Majority involve great toe or thumb.
   g. Long radial growth phase; transition to vertical growth phase occurs with high risk of metastasis.

D. Noncutaneous melanoma

1. Mucosal melanoma

a. Mucosal melanomas represent fewer than 2% of melanomas, usually presenting within the genital tract, anorectal region, and head and neck mucosal surfaces.

b. They are usually large at diagnosis, with poor prognosis.

c. Radical excision is of questionable benefit.

2. Ocular melanoma

a. Represent 2% to 5% of melanomas (most common noncutaneous melanoma).

b. Interference with vision leads to earlier diagnosis.

c. The eye has no lymphatic drainage; therefore, no nodal metastases are seen.

d. The liver is the main site of metastatic disease.

e. Treatment is by enucleation.

E. Melanoma with an unknown primary

1. Represents 3% of melanomas.

2. Diagnosis is by exclusion.

3. Nodal metastases are the most common presentation.

4. Prognosis is similar to melanomas with a known primary.

III. Melanoma staging and prognostic factors

A. Major prognostic factors: Tumor thickness, Nodal status, and Metastases—TNM (Table 11-3).

1. **Breslow thickness** is reported in millimeters; it is more accurate than Clark's level and is a better prognostic indicator.

2. **Clark's level** is based on invasion through the histologic layers of the skin.

B. Other significant prognostic factors

1. **Anatomic location:** Trunk lesions generally carry a worse prognosis than those on the extremities.

2. **Sex:** For a given melanoma, women tend to have a better prognosis; women are also more likely to have extremity melanomas, which have a better prognosis.

3. **Ulceration** is a poor prognostic sign.

4. **Lymph node involvement** or in-transit metastases are more significant than any other prognostic factors.

C. The American Joint Committee on Cancer has developed a staging system based on TNM classification (Table 11-4).

IV. Diagnosis and treatment

A. Diagnosis of primary melanoma is made by histologic analysis of full-thickness biopsy specimens.

Table 11-3. Melanoma thickness grading

Skin	5-Year Survival (%)
Clark Level	
I–In situ	100
II–Papillary dermis	88
III–Papillar-reticular dermis	66
IV–Reticular dermis	55
V–Subcutaneous	22
Breslow Depth (mm)	
<1.00	89–95
1.01–2.00	77–89
2.01–4.00	63–79
>4.00	7–67

Table 11-4. AJCC Melanoma Staging System (2002)

TNM Definitions

Primary Tumor		*Ulceration status*
Tis	Melanoma in situ	
T1	≤1.0 mm	a: without ulceration and level II/III
		b: with ulceration or level IV/V
T2	1.01–2.0 mm	a: without ulceration
		b: with ulceration
T3	2.01–4 mm	a: without ulceration
		b: with ulceration
T4	>4.0 mm	a: without ulceration
		b: with ulceration

Regional Lymph Node Involvement		*Nodal Metastatic Mass*
N0	Negative	
N1	1 node	a: micrometastasis*
		b: macrometastasis°
N2	2–3 nodes	a: micrometastasis*
		b: macrometastasis°
		c: in-transit met(s)/satellites(s)
		without metastatic nodes
N3	4 or > metastatic nodes, or matted nodes, or in-transit met(s)/satellite(s) with metastatic node(s)	

* Micrometastases are diagnosed after sentinel or elective lymphadenectomy
° Macrometastases are defined as clinically detectable nodal metastases confirmed by therapeutic lymphadenectomy or when nodal matastasis exhibits gross extracapsular extension

Distant Metastasis		*Serum Lactate Dehydrogenase*
M0	No distinct metastasis	Normal
M1a	Distant skin, subcutaneous, or nodal mets	Normal
M1b	Lung metastases	Normal
M1c	All other visceral metastasis	Elevated
	Any distant metastasis	

Staging

Stge	0	Tis N0 M0
Stage	IA	T1a N0 M0
	IB	T1b N0 M0, T2a N0 M0
Stage	IIA	T2b N0 M0, T3a N0 M0
	IIB	T3b N0 M0, T4a N0 M0
	IIC	T4b N0 M0
Stage	IIIA	T1-4a N1a M0, T1-4a N2a M0
	IIIB	T1-4b N1 M0, T1-4b N2a M0, T1-4a N1bM0, T1-4a N2b M0, T1-4a/b N2c M0
	IIIC	T1-4b N1b M0, T1-4b N2b M0, any T N3 M0
Stage	IV	any T any N M1a, any T any N M1b, any T any N M1c

1. **Excisional biopsy** is preferred for lesions less than 1.5 cm in diameter. If possible, excise lesion with 1- to 2-mm margins.
2. **Incisional biopsy** is appropriate when suspicion is low, the lesion is large (>1.5 cm) or is located in a potentially disfiguring area (face, hands, and feet), or when it is impractical to perform complete excision. Incisional biopsy does not increase risk of metastasis or affect patient survival.
3. **Permanent sectioning** is used to determine tumor thickness.
4. **Avoid shave biopsies,** because they forfeit the ability to stage the lesion based on thickness.
5. **Do not cauterize or freeze** the specimen: Tissue destruction makes it impossible to evaluate thickness and margins.
6. **Wide local excision** for tissue diagnosis can decrease the efficacy of future lymphatic mapping because of disruption of local lymphatics. Biopsy incisions should result in scars parallel to lymphatic drainage.
7. **Orientation of biopsy** incisions should also take definitive surgical therapy into consideration.
   a. Extremity biopsies should use longitudinal incisions.
   b. Transverse incisions are sometimes preferable for preventing contractures over joints.
   c. Head and neck incisions should be placed within relaxed skin tension lines, keeping facial aesthetic units in mind.
B. **Definitive management of melanoma**
   1. **Wide local excision** is the treatment of choice.
   2. **Recommended surgical margins** depend on tumor thickness (Table 11-5).
   3. **Subungual melanoma** requires amputation proximal to the distal interphalangeal joint for fingers, and proximal to the interphalangeal joint for the thumb.
C. **Management of regional lymph nodes**
   1. **Elective lymph node dissection (ELND)** involves removal of clinically negative lymph nodes from the nodal basin. A survival benefit was demonstrated in retrospective reviews; however, no survival benefit has been seen with prospective trials except for a subgroup with 1- to 2-mm (intermediate-thickness) melanomas.
   2. **Sentinel lymph node biopsy (SLNB)**
      a. In the sentinel node theory, a sentinel node will be the first lymph node seeded by tumor cells; therefore, excision of sentinel node(s) alone is adequate to determine nodal status. The morbidity of SLNB is considerably less than ELND. Sentinel node(s) can be detected in more than 90% to 95% of patients. SLNB is now widely considered the standard of care.
      b. SLNB is performed in conjunction with wide local excision of the primary tumor. Lymphatic mapping is performed to determine the first lymph node that drains the primary tumor site (sentinel node).
      c. SLNB-positive patients undergo staged regional lymphadenectomy and may be candidates for adjuvant therapy.
      d. Preoperative nuclear imaging: Radiolabeled colloid solution (technetium 99) is injected intradermally at the primary tumor. Lymphoscintigraphic imaging localizes the sentinel node basin(s) (some tumor sites can drain to multiple basins).

Table 11-5. Recommended surgical margins for melanoma excision

Melanoma Thickness (mm)	Margin (cm)
In situ	0.5
<1	1
1–4	2
>4	2–3
	(controversial)

    e. In the operating room, blue lymphangiography dye (Lymphazurin) is injected intradermally at the periphery of the primary tumor site prior to excision of the primary tumor.

      (1) Mark edges of the lesion before injection to avoid obscuring them with the dye.

      (2) Potential sentinel nodes will appear blue when exploring the nodal basin, giving secondary confirmation to localization with Geiger counter detection of ^{99}Tc.

      (3) Dye injection may briefly interfere with pulse-oximeter readings; alert anesthesiologist at time of injection.

      (4) Caution: Risk of allergy or anaphylaxis with dye injection.

    f. Following excision of the primary tumor, drapes, instruments, gowns, and gloves are changed and the regional lymph node basin(s) identified by lymphoscintigraphy are explored. All radioactive ("hot") and/or blue nodes are excised.

    g. Histologic analysis of sentinel node(s) with immunohistochemical staining identifies micrometastases. Permanent sections are required; frozen sections cannot reliably differentiate normal from neoplastic melanocytes.

D. Surveillance and treatment of melanoma recurrence

  1. Guidelines vary depending on stage of melanoma.

  2. Asymptomatic patients should be seen every 3 to 4 months for 2 years, then every 6 months for 3 years, then annually. The most accurate way to detect metastatic disease is to take a thorough history.

  3. Chest x-ray and liver function tests (LDH and alkaline phosphatase) are usually sufficient; more extensive workups including computed tomographic (CT) scans have not altered outcomes.

  4. Local recurrence typically occurs within 5 cm of the original lesion, usually within 3 to 5 years after primary excision; most often this represents incomplete excision of the primary tumor.

  5. The most common sites of recurrence are the skin, subcutaneous tissues, distant lymph nodes, and then other sites (lung, liver, brain, bone, gastrointestinal tract).

  6. Reexcision is the primary treatment for local, small, isolated lesions.

  7. Surgery is effective for palliation in patients with isolated recurrences in skin, central nervous system, lung, or gastrointestinal tract.

  8. Chemotherapy: Complete remission is rare.

    a. Dacarbazine (DTIC), carmustine, cisplatin, and tamoxifen in combination are most frequently used.

    b. Isolated hyperthermic limb perfusion for extensive cutaneous disease (melphalan and tumor necrosis factor) is used at some centers.

  9. Immunotherapy with vaccines and cytokines is the subject of ongoing clinical trials. FDA-approved regimens include interferon-α (IFN-α) for stage III disease and interleukin 2 (IL-2) for stage IV disease.

  10. The mean survival with disseminated disease is 6 months. Respiratory failure and central nervous system complications are the most common causes of death.

Nonmelanoma Skin Cancer

Nonmelanoma skin cancers (NMSCs) are the most common malignancies, and their incidence is increasing. Twenty percent of the U.S. population will develop NMSC during their lifetime. The ratio of basal cell carcinoma (BCC) to squamous cell carcinoma (SCC) is 4:1.

I. Basal cell carcinoma

  A. Basal cell carcinoma is the most common skin cancer.

  B. Risk factors:

1. **Sun exposure** (increased with high latitude, high altitude).
2. **Advancing age.**
3. **Fair complexion.**
4. **Long-term exposure to psoralens and UVA therapy** (i.e., PUVA therapy for psoriasis).
5. **Immunosuppression.**
6. **Nevus sebaceus of Jadassohn** (a superficial skin lesion typically in the head and neck region; presents as an irregular, raised, yellow to pink, non-hairbearing mass). The lesions are usually present at birth or in early childhood, and approximately 15% undergo malignant transformation to BCC.
7. **Arsenic exposure.**

C. **Characteristics of BCC**

1. **Basal keratinocytes** are the cell of origin, residing in the basal layer of the epidermis at the dermoepidermal junction.
2. **There is no common clinical precursor lesion,** and metastasis is rare.
3. **BCC is most common** in areas with high concentrations of pilosebaceous follicles, and thus more than 90% of lesions are found on the head and neck.
4. **Morbidity** is caused by invasion of the tumor into underlying structures, including the sinuses, orbit, and brain.

D. **Types of BCC**

1. **Nodular BCC:** The most common type, usually presenting as a single lesion consisting of pearly papules with telangiectasias, pruritus, and occasional bleeding. Lesion breakdown over time leads to noduloulcerative BCC ("rodent ulcer"). Histology demonstrates palisading nuclei.
2. **Superficial spreading BCC:** Slow-growing, erythematous, with minimal induration, and located primarily on the trunk. It is easily confused with other scaly, eczematous dermatoses. The lesions are shallow with a characteristic horizontal growth pattern, and often present in multiples.
3. **Morpheaform (sclerosing, fibrosing) BCC:** Flat, often yellowish or hypopigmented, sometimes resembling scars or normal skin. The true extent of the lesion is usually greater than the clinical appearance. There is a high incidence of recurrence or incomplete excision due to fingerlike extensions. Margins of 1 cm or Mohs extirpation is warranted.
4. **Pigmented BCC:** Similar to nodular BCC; easily confused with melanoma because of its deep pigmentation and nodularity.
5. **Adnexal BCC:** Uncommon and found in older individuals. Tumors arise from sweat glands, and although they exhibit slow growth, they are locally invasive, with a high incidence of local recurrence.

E. **Syndromes associated with NMSC**

1. **Basal cell nevus syndrome (Gorlin's syndrome).**
   a. Autosomal dominant inheritance.
   b. Multiple nevi/lesions often seen early in childhood, with malignant degeneration more likely by the age of puberty.
   c. Skin pits on palms and soles, jaw cysts (odontogenic keratocysts), rib abnormalities, mental retardation.
2. **Xeroderma pigmentosum (XP):** Patients have increased incidence of BCC, SCC, and malignant melanoma (see "Melanoma").
3. **Albinism.**

II. **Squamous cell carcinoma** (also see Chapter 14, "Squamous Cell Carcinoma of the Head and Neck")

A. **Second most common skin cancer after BCC**

B. **Etiology and risk factors**

1. **Ultraviolet radiation:** Sun exposure and tanning booth use; PUVA therapy for psoriasis.
2. **Chemical exposure:** Including some pesticides, organic hydrocarbons such as coal tar, fuel oil, paraffin oil, and arsenic (in welding materials).
3. **Viral infection:** Some types of human papillomavirus (HPV); herpes simplex virus.
4. **Radiation:** Long latency between exposure and disease.

5. **Marjolin's ulcer:** SCC arising in a chronic wound (e.g., chronic burn scars and pressure sores) secondary to genetic changes caused by chronic inflammation.
6. **Impaired immunity:** Immunosuppression for transplants and from AIDS; ratio of SCC to BCC is 2:1.

C. **Characteristics and precursor lesions**
1. **Actinic keratosis** (AK, or solar keratosis)
   a. Erythematous macules and papules with coarse, adherent scale.
   b. Histologically resembles early SCC *in situ* (premalignant).
   c. AK is considered a precursor lesion; up to 4% progress to SCC.
2. **Bowen's disease** (SCC *in situ*)
   a. Exhibits full-thickness cytologic atypia of the keratinocytes.
   b. Erythroplasia of Queyrat is SCC *in situ* of the glans penis.
3. **Leukoplakia**
   a. Presents as a white patch on oral or other mucosa.
   b. Malignant transformation occurs in 15% of cases.
4. **Keratoacanthoma**
   a. Typically a benign, self-healing skin tumor that is composed of squamous cells and keratin; may clinically resemble SCC.
   b. Etiology is unknown but thought to originate from hair follicles.
   c. Typically has a rapid 6-week growth phase followed by involution over the next 6 months.
   d. Excision is the treatment of choice; may be difficult to differentiate from SCC histologically.

D. **Types of SCC**
1. **Verrucous SCC:** Slow-growing, exophytic, and less likely to metastasize.
2. **Ulcerative SCC:** Grows rapidly and is locally invasive.
   a. Ulcerative SCC has very aggressive growth characteristics, raised borders, and central ulceration.
   b. Less than 50% 5-year survival if spread to lymph nodes in head and neck.

III. **Other types of nonmelanoma skin cancer**
A. **Merkel cell carcinoma**
1. **Malignant neuroendocrine tumor** arising within the dermis from cells of neural crest origin.
2. **Aggressive, with radial spread,** high local recurrence, and regional and systemic metastasis.
3. **Presents as a purple to red papulonodule or indurated plaque;** 50% involve the head and neck, 40% involve the extremities, and 10% involve the trunk.
4. **Treatment** involves wide (up to 3 cm) margins.
5. **30–50% survival at 5 years.**

B. **Microcystic adnexal carcinoma**
1. **Follicular and eccrine differentiation.**
2. **Invasive and locally destructive.**
3. **Presents as a white to pink papule-plaque** primarily on the head and neck.

C. **Sebaceous gland carcinoma**
1. **Malignant tumor** derived from adnexal epithelium of sebaceous glands.
2. **Yellowish to pink,** slowly growing papulonodule on eyelid (resembles chalazion).

IV. **Treatment of nonmelanoma skin cancer**
A. **Standard techniques:** 90% to 95% cure rates
1. **Excision**
   a. BCC: 3- to 5-mm margins for nonaggressive types, and 7-mm margins (or Moh's) for morpheaform type.
   b. SCC: 5- to 10-mm margins are usually sufficient.
   c. Frozen sections may be used to confirm negative margins intraoperatively. False negatives are common. Surgeon must have confidence in the pathologist and laboratory to use this modality.

    2. **Mohs surgery:** Sequential horizontal excision with frozen-section testing

        a. Indications include recurrent, higher-risk NMSC (morpheaform BCC and high-risk SCC) and lesions in aesthetically sensitive areas (nose, eyelid, lip, etc.).

        b. Advantages are tissue preservation and confirmation of complete excision.

    3. **Field therapy**

        a. Curettage and electrodesiccation can be used for BCC less than 1 cm that is *not* recurrent disease or morpheaform type; however, this treatment leads to a widened scar.

        b. Cryotherapy is effective for small BCC over bone or cartilage, tip of nose, or around the eye.

        c. Radiation: Requires multiple visits. High cure rates, but recurrence is relatively common many years (10–15) later.

B. Regional lymphadenectomy

    1. **Indicated for clinically positive (palpable) nodes.**

    2. **Fine-needle aspiration (FNA):** Confirm spread of SCC to palpable lymph node.

    3. **ELND:** Indicated for a tumor extending down to parotid capsule or a large lesion contiguous with a draining nodal basin.

    4. **SLNB:** Considered for high-risk SCC without palpable nodes (controversial).

C. Indications for adjuvant radiation therapy

    1. **Cutaneous SCC** with high-risk factors.

    2. **Aggressive, deeply invasive BCC.**

Soft Tissue Sarcoma

I. Biology and epidemiology

A. Arise from mesoderm-derived tissues: Bone, fat, muscle, nerve, vasculature, synovium, fibrous tissue, and cartilage.

B. Epidemiology

    1. **6,000 to 7,000 new cases** are diagnosed annually in the United States.

    2. **1% of all malignancies** occur in adults, and 15% in children.

    3. **50% are located in the extremities.**

    4. In contrast to ectoderm-derived carcinomas, **sarcomas behave in a similar fashion regardless of the cell of origin.**

    5. **Paucity of local symptoms** often leads to advanced disease at diagnosis.

    6. **A pseudocapsule forms** as the tumor expands and compresses adjacent tissue.

    7. **Major fascial planes** typically act as barriers to local invasion.

C. Risk factors and etiology

    1. **The majority of sarcomas** have no identifiable predisposing genetic or environmental cause.

    2. **Radiation exposure**

        a. Associated with osteosarcomas and malignant fibrous histiocytomas.

        b. Typically, there is a 10- to 20-year latency period after exposure.

        c. Thorium dioxide (Thorotrast), a contrast agent used in the 1940s and 1950s for radiologic procedures, is linked with a high incidence of hepatic angiosarcoma.

    3. **Chemical exposure:** Arsenic, vinyl chloride, and dioxin (contained in the Vietnam War-era defoliant Agent Orange).

    4. **Genetic factors**

        a. Neurofibromatosis (von Recklinghausen's syndrome): 5% lifetime risk of developing neurofibroma or neurofibrosarcoma.

        b. Mutation in Rb1 tumor suppressor gene: Retinoblastoma (sarcoma of the eye).

     c. Mutation in p53 tumor suppressor gene: Li-Fraumeni syndrome (variety of sarcomas).

  5. Lymphedema

     a. Following surgical procedures, radiation therapy, or parasitic infection; may also arise idiopathically.

     b. 10- to 20-year latency for development of lymphangiosarcoma.

  6. Kaposi's sarcoma: Strongly associated with human immunodeficiency virus infection.

II. Classification

  A. Subtypes are named for the cell of origin (Table 11-6). Fibrosarcoma is the most common sarcoma in adults and the second most common in children.

  B. Histologic type has little prognostic significance; histologic grade (including frequency of mitotic figures, cellular atypia, and presence or absence of tumor necrosis) is the best guide for prognosis and therapy.

III. Diagnosis and staging

  A. Extremity sarcoma: Generally painless. Delay in diagnosis is common, and patients are often erroneously treated for a hematoma or "pulled muscle."

    1. Suspicious findings include mass larger than 5 cm, enlarging or symptomatic mass, and mass present for more than 4 weeks.

    2. Magnetic resonance imaging (MRI) is the best imaging modality.

    3. Pulmonary metastases are the most common finding with metastatic disease.

    4. The 5-year survival rate is approximately 75%.

  B. Sarcoma of the abdomen or retroperitoneum

    1. Can present with vague abdominal complaints: Fullness, early satiety, pain, weight loss, nausea, and vomiting.

    2. Metastatic disease: Most common to liver.

    3. Palpable mass in 80% of patients at the time of presentation.

    4. Median survival.

     a. Primary disease: 72 months.

     b. Recurrent disease: 28 months.

     c. Metastatic disease: 10 months.

    5. Imaging

     a. MRI with gadolinium contrast: Best technique for visualizing tumor and relationship to adjacent structures.

     b. CT scan: Valuable for evaluating chest, abdomen, and pelvis for metastatic disease, and as a staging tool.

     c. Angiography: For surgical planning.

     d. Chest x-ray: Evaluate for pulmonary metastasis.

    6. Biopsy of sarcomas: Performed for extremity lesions smaller than 5 cm.

  C. Staging criteria (Tables 11-7 and 11-8)

    1. Histologic grade is the most important prognostic indicator (see above). Low-grade tumors have less than a 15% chance of metastasis; high-grade tumors metastasize in more than 50% of cases.

Table 11-6. Tissue classification of soft-tissue sarcomas

Tissue of Origin	Benign Soft Tissue Tumor	Malignant Soft Tissue Tumor
Fat	Lipoma	Liposarcoma
Fibrous tissue	Fibroma	Fibrosarcoma
Smooth muscle	Leiomyoma	Leiomyosarcoma
Skeletal muscle	Rhabdomyoma	Rhabdomyosarcoma
Cartilage	Chondroma	Chondrosarcoma
Bone	Osteoma	Osteosarcoma
Blood vessel	Hemangioma	Angiosarcoma

Table 11-7. AJCC "GTNM" classification of soft tissue sarcomas

Classification	Description
Histologic Grade	
G1	Well differentiated
G2	Moderately well differentiated
G3	Poorly differentiated
G4	Undifferentiated
Primary Tumor Size	
T1	Tumor ≤ 5 cm in greatest diameter
T2	Tumor > 5 cm in greatest diameter
Regional Lymphatic Involvement	
N0	No known metastases to lymph nodes
N1	Verified metastases to lymph nodes
Distant Metastasis	
M0	No known distant metastases
M1	Known distant metastases

AJCC, American Joint Committee on Cancer.

2. **Tumors of larger size are more difficult to grade** and have a greater chance of recurrence and dedifferentiation.
3. **Nodal and distant metastases** are associated with a similar prognosis and are classified as stage IV disease.
4. **Five-year survival** is on the order of 80% for stage I disease, 60% for stage II, 35% for stage III, and less than 10% for stage IV.

IV. Management
  A. The extremity (especially the thigh) is the most common site for sarcoma.
    1. Surgery
      a. Complete resection with negative margins is the mainstay of treatment.
      b. The pseudocapsule should not be entered.
      c. Wide-local excision (WLE) is the standard of care, with 3- to 5-cm margins of normal tissue proximally and distally. En bloc resection of uninvolved fascial plane with tumor is performed for control of the other margins.

Table 11-8. AJCC stage groupings for soft tissue sarcomas using the "GTNM" classification

Stage	Groupings	5-Year Survival (%)
IA	G1, T1, N0, M0	80
IB	G1, T2, N0, M0	
IIA	G2, T1, N0, M0	60
IIB	G2, T2, N0, M0	
IIIA	G3-4, T1, N0, M0	35
IIIB	G3-4, T2, N0, M0	
IVA	Any G, any T, N1, M0	<10
IVB	Any G, any T, N1, M1	

      d. WLE is performed after excisional biopsy even if the margins are clear.

      e. Major neurovascular structures are generally preserved for low-grade lesions, but are sacrificed and reconstructed as needed for high-grade tumors.

      f. There is no survival benefit of amputation compared with limb-sparing procedures.

   2. Radiation therapy is not indicated for small (<5 cm) low-grade tumors because of the excellent prognosis with WLE alone. It can be used as primary therapy for patients who cannot tolerate or refuse surgery, and is also useful as combination therapy for sarcomas up to 10 cm.

   3. Chemotherapy is of undetermined benefit in soft tissue sarcoma.

B. Retroperitoneal and intraabdominal sarcomas have a uniformly poor prognosis. Excision with tumor-free margins is curative, but difficult to achieve. Radiation is rarely used because surrounding organs cannot tolerate therapeutic doses.

Pearls

---

1. **SCC commonly affects the lower lip** and upper eyelid; BCC characteristically affects the upper lip and lower eyelid.

2. **Perform a punch or excisional biopsy of pigmented lesions** rather then shaving or curettage so that the depth of the lesion can be determined if it happens to be melanoma.

3. **Lentigo maligna melanoma** is the only type of melanoma that is clearly associated with sunlight exposure.

4. **Fibrosarcoma** is generally not sensitive to chemotherapy or radiation therapy.

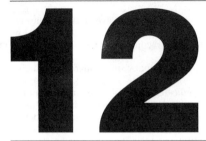

Benign Skin Lesions

Anastasia Petro

I. Definitions
   A. Macules are flat, circumscribed lesions.
   B. Papules are raised lesions, generally less than 0.5 cm in diameter.
   C. Plaques are raised lesions in which the surface area is significantly greater than the height.
   D. Nodules are raised lesions, typically larger and thicker than papules.

II. Technical considerations of cutaneous biopsy
   A. Planning: Orientation of biopsy incisions should result in the scar lying parallel to relaxed skin tension lines (RSTLs, or Langer's lines). Biopsies should be excised to the level of the subcutaneous fat.
   B. Anesthesia: Local anesthetics (e.g., lidocaine) are infiltrated after marking the planned lines of excision. Epinephrine is valuable in providing hemostasis, especially for facial biopsies (see Chapter 8, "Local Anesthetics").
   C. Biopsy techniques: Each technique can be valuable in certain circumstances.
      1. Fusiform excision: Most biopsies are amenable to fusiform excision and closure. A lesion is excised, and the resulting defect is lengthened in a 3:1 ratio to eliminate standing cutaneous deformities ("dog ears") with closure. The long axis of the excision should lie within the RSTL. Closure is performed using layered sutures (see Chapter 2, "Surgical Techniques and Wound Management").
      2. Punch biopsy: Specimens measuring 2 to 6 mm can be removed with a circular punch (similar in principle to a cookie cutter); this technique is highly effective for small lesions.
      3. Shave biopsy: Lesions with very low malignant potential can be excised in this manner. However, it leaves an open wound, which can lead to unnecessary morbidity.

III. Epidermal lesions
   A. Epidermal nevus (linear nevus)
      1. May be associated with developmental abnormalities of the ocular, central nervous, skeletal, cardiovascular, and urogenital systems.
      2. Age of onset: Birth or early childhood.
      3. Clinical appearance: Tan or brown warty papules, usually in a linear array.
      4. Location: Extremities most common.
      5. Treatment: Excision, laser therapy, dermabrasion, or cryotherapy.
   B. Inflammatory linear verrucous epidermal nevus
      1. Age of onset: Birth or early childhood.
      2. Clinical appearance: Erythematous, rough, scaly papules in a linear array.
      3. Often extremely pruritic.
      4. Location: Extremities most common.
      5. Treatment: Excision.
   C. Seborrheic keratosis
      1. Etiology is unknown.
      2. Age of onset: Middle age.

3. **Clinical appearance:** "Stuck-on" brown, warty papule or plaque.
4. **Typical location:** Trunk.
5. **Treatment:** Cryotherapy, curettage.
6. **No malignant potential.** However, many melanomas are initially misdiagnosed as seborrheic keratoses.
7. **Human papillomavirus (HPV) warts** (sexually transmitted) can mimic seborrheic keratoses in the groin and perineal areas.

D. **Actinic keratosis**
   1. **Induced by excessive sun exposure.**
   2. **Approximately 1 in 20** will develop into squamous cell carcinoma (SCC).
   3. **Actinic keratosis in transplant patients** (on chronic immunosuppression) should be aggressively treated because of high risk of transformation into SCC.
   4. **Age of onset:** Middle age.
   5. **Clinical appearance:** Erythematous, rough, or scaly macule or papule.
   6. **Location:** Sun-exposed areas, including scalp, ears, face, hands.
   7. **Treatment:** Cryotherapy, topical 5-fluorouracil (5-FU), imiquimod cream, topical tretinoin.

E. **Lentigo**
   1. **Age of onset:** Middle age.
   2. **Clinical appearance:** Tan or brown macule with slightly irregular borders.
   3. **Location:** Sun-exposed areas, including head, neck, upper trunk, and arms.
   4. **Treatment:** Cryotherapy, topical tretinoin, hydroquinone cream.

IV. **Nevocellular (melanocytic) lesions**

A. **Nevus of Ota**
   1. **Age of onset:** Appears at birth.
   2. **Typically found in patients of Asian ancestry.**
   3. **Clinical appearance:** Large, blue-gray patch.
   4. **Location:** Periocular; areas innervated by first and second trigeminal branches.
   5. **Treatment:** Laser therapy.

B. **Nevus of Ito**
   1. **Age of onset:** Appears at birth.
   2. **Typically found in patients of Asian ancestry.**
   3. **Clinical appearance:** Large, blue-gray patch.
   4. **Location:** Posterior shoulder; areas innervated by posterior supraclavicular and lateral cutaneous brachial nerves.
   5. **Treatment:** Laser therapy.

C. **Nevus spilus**
   1. **Age of onset:** Appears at birth.
   2. **Clinical appearance:** Tan patch speckled with hyperpigmented small macules and papules.
   3. **Location:** Trunk.
   4. **Treatment:** Excision if feasible, although not necessary.
   5. **No increased risk of melanoma.**

D. **Spitz nevus (benign juvenile melanoma)**
   1. **Age of onset:** Childhood to early adulthood.
   2. **Clinical appearance:** Pink or tan, dome-shaped, smooth papule.
   3. **Location:** Face (especially cheek).
   4. **Treatment:** Excision with definitive margins to decrease risk of recurrence.
   5. **May be difficult to distinguish** histopathologically from malignant melanoma.

E. **Junctional nevus**
   1. **Nevus cells are located** at the epidermal-dermal junction.
   2. **Age of onset:** Childhood to early adulthood.
   3. **Clinical appearance:** Brown, evenly pigmented macule with well-defined borders.

      4. Location: Trunk.

      5. Treatment: Excision.

      6. May be difficult to differentiate from melanoma.

F. Compound nevus

    1. Contains both junctional and intradermal components and is likely a transition between these types.

    2. Age of onset: Childhood to early adulthood.

    3. Clinical appearance: Dark brown papule with well-defined regular borders.

    4. Location: Trunk.

    5. Treatment: Excision.

G. Intradermal nevus

    1. Age of onset: Second or third decade of life.

    2. Clinical appearance: Flesh-colored or light tan papule.

    3. Location: Face or neck.

    4. Treatment: Excision.

H. Common blue nevus

    1. Age of onset: Adolescence.

    2. Clinical appearance: Blue or blue-black papule, generally less than 1 cm.

    3. Location: Head and neck and dorsum of the hands and feet.

    4. Treatment: Excision.

    5. A cutaneous metastasis of malignant melanoma can resemble a blue nevus.

I. Cellular blue nevus

    1. Age of onset: Second decade of life or older.

    2. Clinical appearance: Blue-black papule or plaque.

    3. Location: Buttocks most common.

    4. Treatment: Excision.

J. Atypical (dysplastic) nevus

    1. Age of onset: Puberty and later.

    2. Clinical appearance

      a. Classic lesion: Central brown macule surrounded by an irregular pink rim.

      b. Usually greater than 6 mm.

      c. There is a large clinical spectrum. In general, dysplastic nevi are larger than typical nevi and have more irregular pigmentation and borders compared with typical nevi.

    3. Location: Trunk most common.

    4. Treatment

      a. Excision with definitive margins to prevent recurrence.

      b. Total body skin examination (including oral, ocular, and anogenital areas) to rule out synchronous lesions.

      c. Sunscreen use and avoidance of sunburns and tanning should be strongly encouraged.

    5. Patients with dysplastic nevi and a family history of melanoma in a first-degree relative are at an especially high risk (up to 100% lifetime risk) of melanoma, and warrant regular total body skin examinations.

V. Lesions derived from epidermal appendages

A. Epidermal appendages include the sebaceous glands, hair follicles, and eccrine glands.

B. Pilomatrixoma (calcifying epithelioma of Malherbe)

    1. Derived from hair follicles, located in the lower dermis to subcutaneous fat.

    2. Age of onset: Early childhood.

    3. Clinical appearance.

      a. Extremely firm, flesh-colored nodule.

      b. Positive "tent" sign: Stretching of the overlying skin reveals multiple peaks.

    4. Location: Most commonly involves the head, neck, and upper extremities.

    5. Treatment: Excision

C. **Trichoepithelioma**
   1. **Derived from hair follicles.**
   2. **Age of onset:** Puberty or older.
   3. **Clinical appearance:**
      a. Pink or flesh-colored, shiny papule.
      b. Multiple trichoepitheliomas often coalesce to form plaques.
   4. **Location:** Most commonly involves the face.
   5. **Treatment:** Excision.
   6. **May be difficult to distinguish** clinically and microscopically from basal cell carcinoma.
   7. **Rasmussen syndrome:** Autosomal dominant disorder; triad of multiple trichoepitheliomas, cylindromas, and milia.
D. **Cylindroma ("tomato tumor," "turban tumor")**
   1. **Derived from eccrine gland structures.**
   2. **Age of onset:** Puberty or older.
   3. **Clinical appearance:** Firm, rubbery bluish-pink nodule.
   4. **Location:** Scalp.
   5. **Treatment:** Excision.
   6. **Multiple cylindromas may be present** in autosomal dominant cylindroma syndromes.
E. **Eccrine poroma**
   1. **Derived from eccrine gland structures.**
   2. **Age of onset:** Any age.
   3. **Clinical appearance:** Red, soft nodule, often pedunculated.
   4. **Location:** Sole or lateral surface of foot.
   5. **Treatment:** Excision.
F. **Syringoma**
   1. **Derived from eccrine gland structures.**
   2. **Age of onset:** Early adulthood.
   3. **Clinical appearance:** Small, clear papules.
   4. **Location:** Periocular (eyelids, upper cheek).
   5. **Treatment:** Electrodesiccation, cryotherapy, laser.
   6. Increased incidence with Down syndrome.
G. **Nevus sebaceus (of Jadassohn)**
   1. **Age of onset:** Birth.
   2. **Clinical appearance:**
      a. Before puberty: Yellow-orange, waxy smooth plaque, linear or elongated.
      b. After puberty: Rough, verrucous, orange plaque.
   3. **Location:** Scalp.
   4. **Treatment:** Excision during childhood.
   5. **May give rise to several different invasive neoplasms.**
   6. **After puberty,** approximately 10% to 15% degenerate into basal cell carcinoma.
H. **Sebaceous adenoma**
   1. **Age of onset:** Middle age.
   2. **Clinical appearance:** Yellow nodule.
   3. **Location:** Head or neck.
   4. **Treatment:** Excision.
   5. **Rare.**
   6. **Muir-Torre syndrome:** Autosomal dominant; associated with multiple keratoacanthomas and marked increase in visceral neoplasms, particularly colon carcinoma.
I. **Sebaceous hyperplasia**
   1. **Age of onset:** Middle age.
   2. **Clinical appearance:** Small, shiny, umbilicated, yellow-white papules. May be confused clinically with basal cell carcinoma.
   3. **Location:** Face.
   4. **Treatment:** Cryotherapy, electrodesiccation, or laser therapy.

VI. Cysts
A. Epidermoid cyst (epidermal inclusion cyst)
1. **Age of onset:** Adulthood.
2. **Clinical appearance**
   a. Somewhat fluctuant, flesh-colored, well-circumscribed nodule.
   b. Often with punctum.
   c. Cyst cavity filled with malodorous, keratinous debris. The term "sebaceous cyst" is a misnomer because the tumor is of epidermal and not sebaceous origin.
3. **Location:** Commonly on the face, neck, and trunk.
4. **Treatment:** Excision; if infected, incision and drainage with delayed excision after healing.

B. Dermoid cyst
1. **Age of onset:** Birth, early childhood.
2. **Clinical appearance:** Resembles epidermoid cyst, without punctum.
3. **Lined with all types of epidermal skin appendages,** usually in a vestigial form.
4. **Location:** Supraorbital ridge or lateral brow; sometimes in nasal midline.
5. **Treatment:** Excision.
6. **Differential diagnosis of a midline nasal mass** includes dermoid cyst, glioma, and meningocele. Computed tomography (CT) or magnetic resonance imaging (MRI) should be ordered prior to excision.

C. Trichilemmal cyst (pilar cyst)
1. **Age of onset:** Adulthood.
2. **Clinical appearance:** Same as epidermoid cyst.
3. **Location:** Scalp.
4. **Treatment:** Same as epidermoid cyst.

VII. Dermal lesions
A. Dermatofibroma
1. **Age of onset:** Adulthood.
2. **Clinical appearance:** Brown-red indurated papule or nodule; positive "dimple" sign.
3. **Location:** Lower extremities.
4. **Treatment:** Excision.

B. Lipoma
1. **Age of onset:** Any age.
2. **Clinical appearance:** Soft, flesh-colored nodule.
3. **Location:** Trunk, extremities.
4. **Treatment:** Excision.
5. **Generally painless,** whereas angiolipomas are more likely to be painful.

C. Dermatofibrosarcoma protuberans
1. **Age of onset:** Middle age.
2. **Clinical appearance:** Reddish-brown, firm, nodular plaque.
3. **Location:** Trunk, extremities.
4. **Treatment:** Radical excision, due to locally aggressive, infiltrative nature.
5. **Local recurrence** is common due to poorly defined clinical and histologic margins.
6. **Metastases are rare.**

D. Neurofibroma
1. **Consists of Schwann cells** and endoneurial fibroblasts.
2. **Age of onset:** Any age.
3. **Clinical appearance:** Soft, compressible, flesh-colored or pink nodule; positive "button-hole" sign.
4. **Location:** Trunk or extremities.
5. **Treatment:** Excision.

VIII. Miscellaneous
A. Granuloma annulare
1. **Age of onset:** Childhood.

  2. **Clinical appearance:** Annular plaques composed of several flesh-colored or pink firm papules.
  3. **Location:** Distal extremities.
  4. **Treatment:**
     a. Observation (lesions will often spontaneously resolve).
     b. Intralesional corticosteroids.
     c. Cryotherapy.
     d. Surgical excision.
B. **Calciphylaxis**
  1. **The cutaneous manifestation of metastatic calcification,** which leads to calcification of blood vessels and subsequent necrosis of surrounding tissue.
  2. **Usually occurs in the setting of renal failure.**
  3. **Age of onset:** Any age.
  4. **Clinical appearance:** Hemorrhagic, necrotic ulcerations with accompanying livedo reticularis, which is a red-blue mottling of the skin.
  5. **Location:** Most commonly on the trunk and extremities.
  6. **Treatment**
     a. Supportive care (patients are often systemically ill).
     b. Phosphate-binding agents.
     c. Parathyroidectomy, if appropriate.
     d. Excision is usually followed by progressive calcification in proximal tissues, creating a vicious cycle.
C. **Hidradenitis suppurativa**
  1. **Description:** Chronic inflammatory process involving cutaneous apocrine glands, often affecting the subcutaneous tissue and fascia.
  2. **Age of onset:** Puberty.
  3. **Clinical appearance:**
     a. Tender, fluctuant erythematous nodules with purulent, malodorous drainage.
     b. Extensive scarring and sinus tracts.
     c. Pain often intense.
  4. **Location:** Axillae, inframammary folds, groin, buttocks, and perineal areas.
  5. **Treatment**
     a. Meticulous cleansing with antibacterial soaps.
     b. Topical 2% clindamycin lotion twice a day.
     c. Chronic courses of oral antibiotics such as minocycline.
     d. Referral to dermatologist.
     e. Incision and drainage for localized abscess formation.
     f. Radical surgical excision of affected areas, with interim dressing changes followed by delayed skin grafting.
     g. Electron beam irradiation for severe refractory cases.

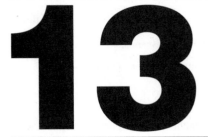

Vascular Anomalies, Lymphedema, and Tattoos

Christi M. Cavaliere

Vascular Anomalies

I. **Classification of vascular anomalies**
   A. **Historically, multiple confusing terms were used** to describe vascular anomalies.
   B. **Terms such as "cavernous" and "strawberry" have been abandoned.**
   C. **Current nomenclature** is biologically based, and includes two major classes:
      1. **Hemangioma**
      2. **Vascular malformation**
         a. Venous malformation
         b. Arterial malformation
         c. Arteriovenous malformation
         d. Capillary malformation
         e. Lymphatic malformation

II. **Hemangioma**
   A. **Pathology:** Hemangiomas are benign proliferative neoplasms of unknown etiology.
   B. **Incidence**
      1. **10% of white infants**
      2. **2% of black infants**
      3. **Higher incidence in preterm infants**
      4. **Females more commonly affected (3:1)**
   C. **Diagnosis**
      1. **Mainly clinical,** based on exam and history of vascular lesion present within the first few weeks after birth and rapidly increasing in size during the first year of life.
      2. **Ultrasound can be useful;** Doppler may distinguish high-flow from low-flow lesions when in doubt.
      3. **Magnetic resonance imaging (MRI) is the most reliable** modality for imaging involvement in adjacent structures.
   D. **Clinical characteristics**
      1. **The majority of lesions** occur on the head and neck.
      2. **Most are visible at birth** or within the first few weeks after birth.
      3. **Many begin as a pale or reddish patch;** may resemble a bruise ("herald patch").
      4. **Consider risk** of underlying abnormalities (e.g., spina bifida occulta with lumbar hemangioma).
      5. **Multiple lesions may be part of hemangiomatosis.**
         a. Mortality approximately 25%.
         b. Hepatomegaly due to liver lesions (evaluate with ultrasound or MRI).
         c. May have hemangiomas of lung or other organs.
         d. Congestive heart failure.
         e. Anemia.
      6. **Time course of hemangioma:**
         a. Rapid proliferation: 0 to 12 months.

        (1) Rapid increase in size.

        (2) May be a relatively high-flow lesion.

     b. Involution phase: 12 months to 10 years.

        (1) Often begins with central pallor, and slowly fades in color.

        (2) Decreases in size and is replaced by fibrofatty tissue.

     c. Involuted phase:

        (1) Skin ultimately becomes nearly normal in approximately 50% of cases.

        (2) Residual skin changes may include discoloration, scarring, laxity, and telangiectasia.

        (3) Fifty percent of patients show involution by age 5, 60% by age 6, and 70% by age 7.

        (4) Minimal improvement after 12 years.

E. Management

  1. Observation and reassurance ("benign neglect") is appropriate in most cases; the appearance of skin after involution is usually more favorable than the scar resulting from excision.

  2. Sequential photographs and measurements are obtained with each visit.

  3. Indications for early intervention

     a. Obstruction or malalignment of the visual axis may lead to deprivation amblyopia (1 week of obstruction during the first year of life may permanently impair development of neurologic pathways in the visual axis); may need to intermittently patch contralateral eye to promote use of the affected eye.

     b. Impending airway obstruction.

     c. Ulceration/hemorrhage.

     d. Coagulopathy/platelet sequestration: Kasabach-Merritt syndrome (KMS) was historically considered platelet sequestration and coagulopathy associated with hemangioma. More recently, KMS has been considered a feature of hemangioendothelioma or tufted angioma instead of hemangioma. If KMS is suspected with hemangioma, biopsy will likely indicate hemangioendothelioma or tufted angioma. Mortality with KMS is approximately 40%.

     e. Congestive heart failure, especially with large hepatic lesions.

     f. Progressive deformation of adjacent structures.

  4. Treatment

     a. Mild ulceration without bleeding: Standard wound care.

     b. Systemic corticosteroids (per previously noted indications)

        (1) Prednisone or prednisolone taper.

        (2) Response usually occurs in less than 2 weeks.

        (3) Approximately one-third of lesions show significant improvement, one-third stabilize, and one-third continue to worsen.

     c. Interferon alpha 2a may be considered if the hemangioma does not respond to steroids.

     d. Pulsed dye laser may improve superficial lesions (effect is limited to 1 mm depth).

     e. Embolization may be used in some instances.

     f. Excision

        (1) Generally achieves best cosmetic outcome if lesion is allowed to involute first.

        (2) If excision will clearly be necessary even after involution, consider excising earlier.

        (3) Visible lesion in school-aged child may be a source of social stress; weigh benefits and drawbacks of early excision.

     g. Use aspirin or other antiplatelet therapy for platelet sequestration.

III. Vascular malformations

  A. Common characteristics

    1. Vessels in vascular malformations are structurally abnormal due to an embryologic error, whereas hemangiomas are true neoplasms.

2. **Present at birth,** but often first noticed months to years later.
3. **Grow proportionately** with the child and do not regress or involute.
4. **Equal sex ratio.**
5. **Diagnostic imaging**
   a. Doppler ultrasound: Can differentiate high-flow from low-flow lesions.
   b. MRI and/or magnetic resonance angiography (MRA): The most useful study for assessing the extent of the lesion and the degree of involvement with surrounding structures.
   c. Angiography: Useful in some cases.

B. Capillary malformation ("port wine stain")
   1. **Differentiate from nevus flammeus neonatorum** ("stork bite," "salmon patch," or "angel's kiss"), which typically fades.
   2. **Incidence:** 0.3% of live births.
   3. **Clinical characteristics**
      a. Two-thirds develop hyperplastic skin changes (cobblestoning) by adulthood.
      b. Lesions may be present on any body part. In the face, distribution typically follows the trigeminal nerve distribution (cranial nerve V).
      c. May be a marker of underlying soft tissue or skeletal abnormality (usually hypertrophic).
   4. **Syndromes involving capillary malformation**
      a. **Sturge-Weber syndrome:**
         (1) Characteristic features include a capillary malformation in the V1 distribution of the trigeminal nerve along with vascular malformation of the underlying meninges.
         (2) Diagnosis should be considered with any capillary malformation involving the V1 distribution.
         (3) Baseline ophthalmologic examination, with follow-up every 6 months until puberty to evaluate for abnormalities of the choroid.
         (4) Seizures are possible due to vascular anomalies of the meninges.
         (5) All patients with V1 involvement require computed tomography (CT) or MRI to evaluate for Sturge-Weber syndrome.
      b. **Klippel-Trenaunay-Weber syndrome:**
         (1) Capillary malformation and/or lymphatic-venous malformation of an extremity.
         (2) Skeletal hypertrophy of involved limb is possible.
         (3) Edema, thrombosis, and pain are frequent.
         (4) May be difficult to treat; lymphatic-venous malformations are often too extensive for complete resection. Compression garments or pumps are helpful.
         (5) Resection or amputation may be indicated in rare cases.
      c. **Cobb syndrome:**
         (1) Capillary malformation in trunk area.
         (2) Associated with spinal arteriovenous malformation.
   5. **Treatment**
      a. Pulsed dye laser treatment during childhood. Requires a general anesthetic and multiple treatments. Significant improvement can usually be achieved.
      b. Argon laser treatment during adulthood; results are typically not as favorable as in children.

C. Venous malformation
   1. **Typically sporadic,** but autosomal dominant inheritance has been reported.
   2. **Incidence:** Approximately 4%.
   3. **Diagnosis is made clinically.**
   4. **MRI** is necessary for surgical planning.
   5. **Characteristic features**
      a. Bluish discoloration of skin; compressible/spongy with slow refill.
      b. Engorgement/swelling: Caused by dependent position.

  c. Changes in hormonal status may cause enlargement.

  d. May affect growth and development of adjacent structures, including overgrowth and undergrowth.

  e. May develop coagulopathy.

  f. Thrombosis causes pain and acute swelling; managed with warm compresses and elevation.

  g. Calcified thrombus (phlebolith) may be seen on x-ray.

 6. Treatment

  a. Compression therapy: may relieve pain and edema.

  b. Percutaneous sclerosis

   (1) May be performed with hypertonic saline, 100% alcohol, or sodium tetradecyl sulfate.

   (2) High recurrence rate; multiple treatments are necessary.

   (3) Most common complication is skin necrosis.

  c. Surgical excision: Preoperative embolization or sclerosis facilitates intraoperative hemostasis.

D. Lymphatic malformation

 1. The term "cystic hygroma" is no longer accepted nomenclature.

 2. Lymphatic malformations (LMs) are classified as microcystic or macrocystic.

 3. LMs may anastomose with the venous system or have a component of venous malformation.

 4. Clinical characteristics

  a. The head and neck region or the axillae are affected in the majority of cases.

  b. Neck masses may extend into the mediastinum or prepectoral area.

  c. LMs are the most common cause of congenital macroglossia, macrocheilia (lip enlargement), and macrotia.

  d. Skeletal involvement may cause distortion.

 5. Treatment

  a. Tracheostomy may be warranted for some head and neck lesions.

  b. Antibiotics are indicated for secondary infections.

  c. Percutaneous aspiration followed by sclerosis may provide short-term improvement; usually requires additional treatment.

  d. Surgical excision

   (1) Difficult dissection, especially for head and neck lesions.

   (2) Often requires multiple, staged procedures.

   (3) Technically easier as child grows; consider waiting until at least 3 years of age.

E. Arterial malformation

 1. Arterial malformations (AMs) represent abnormal development of arterial structures, including stenosis or hypoplasia, duplication, and/or tortuosity.

 2. AMs are often asymptomatic, presenting as incidental findings.

 3. Treat only if symptomatic.

F. Arteriovenous malformation

 1. Arteriovenous malformations (AVMs) are high-flow lesions characterized by abnormal connections between arteries and veins without an intervening capillary bed.

 2. Clinical characteristics

  a. Present at birth but may not become evident until late childhood.

  b. Examine for thrill, increased surface temperature, pulsation, and a bruit.

  c. AVMs may present with a rapid increase in size, especially during puberty.

  d. High cardiac output is possible with significant shunting.

  e. Vascular steal may occur in limbs, causing ischemia.

  f. May develop growth disturbance or skeletal distortion.

  g. Risk of consumptive coagulopathy.

3. Treatment
   a. Sclerosis: Rarely effective.
   b. Embolization: Ligation or embolization of feeding vessels often results in rapid enlargement of collateral vessels, increasing the size of the lesion.
   c. Resection:
   - **(1)** Preoperative embolization the day before surgery can improve hemostasis.
   - **(2)** Angiograms are valuable for mapping prior to resection.
   - **(3)** Often requires extensive skin and soft tissue resection with free-flap coverage.
   - **(4)** Complete cure is rare.

4. AVM syndromes
   a. Parkes Weber syndrome:
   - **(1)** Shares features with Klippel-Trenaunay-Weber syndrome, with multiple AVMs, usually involving a single extremity.
   - **(2)** May require amputation in rare cases.
   b. Hereditary hemorrhagic telangiectasia (HHT), also known as Osler-Weber-Rendu syndrome.
   - **(1)** Associated with multiple cutaneous, visceral, and mucosal AVMs.
   - **(2)** Autosomal dominant inheritance.

Lymphedema

I. Normal lymphatic system
A. Structure
   1. Superficial lymphatic vessels
   a. Primary lymphatics: A fine dermal network of small vessels made up of only endothelium without valves.
   b. Secondary lymphatics: A subdermal network parallel to superficial skin vessels; contain a smooth muscle layer and valves. Eventually, these join deeper lymphatic vessels at the level of the deep fascia.
   2. Deep lymphatic vessels
   a. Course through the deep fascia, paralleling larger blood vessels, eventually draining into regional nodal basin.
   b. Contain smooth muscle and valves.
B. Function
   1. Return of interstitial fluid and proteins to the venous system.
   2. Carries foreign particulate matter or proteins to lymph nodes as part of the humoral immune system.
   3. Part of the pathway for transport of fats from the gastrointestinal tract to the vascular system.
C. Mechanism of lymphatic flow
   1. Pressure differential: Lymphatic pressure varies from 0 to 16 mm Hg less than tissue pressure, favoring fluid and protein flow into lymphatic vessels.
   2. Smooth muscle within the lymphatic vessel wall may exert a pumping action.
   3. Skeletal muscle contraction and the pulsation of adjacent vessels aid in lymphatic flow.
II. Classification of lymphedema
A. Primary lymphedema
   1. Usually idiopathic, but onset may be noted after minor trauma or infection.
   2. Lymphangiogram may demonstrate lymphatic hyperplasia, hypoplasia, incompetent valves, and/or lymphatic varicosities.

3. **Categorized based on age of onset**
    a. Congenital lymphedema:
        (1) 15% of cases of primary lymphedema.
        (2) May affect isolated limb.
        (3) Milroy's disease: Familial form, with females more commonly affected. Usually affects lower extremity.
    b. Lymphedema praecox:
        (1) Onset generally before the mid 30s.
        (2) Most common form of primary lymphedema (75% of cases).
        (3) Females more commonly affected.
        (4) Usually affects lower extremity.
    c. Lymphedema tarda or Meige disease: Onset after age 35 years.
B. **Secondary lymphedema**
    1. **Represents a mechanical obstruction** of an otherwise normal lymphatic system.
    2. **Causes**
        a. Filariasis (parasitic infection with *Wuchereria bancrofti*): The most common cause of lymphedema worldwide.
        b. Iatrogenic resection of or damage to lymphatic vessels, especially axillary node dissection and pelvic surgery.
        c. Metastatic tumor, trauma, or radiation.
    3. **Usually not immediately apparent;** may develop more than 1 year after insult.
III. **Pathophysiology**
    A. **Abnormal lymphatic flow or obstruction of lymphatic vessels** leads to lymphatic stasis and prevents the return of interstitial fluid to the systemic circulation.
    B. **Protein and interstitial fluid accumulate in the tissues.**
    C. **Protein buildup triggers** an inflammatory response, resulting in collagen deposition and fibrosis of interstitium and lymphatic vessels.
    D. **Due to edema,** cells are separated from capillaries and become hypoxic, leading to further inflammation (a vicious cycle).
IV. **Diagnosis**
    A. **Differential diagnosis of extremity edema**
        1. **Venous thrombosis** or extrinsic venous compression
        2. **Venous stasis disease**
        3. **Congestive heart failure or total body fluid overload**
        4. **Low-protein state**
        5. **Factitious use of tourniquets**
        6. **Lymphedema**
    B. **Clinical evaluation**
        1. **History**
            a. Inciting factors, time course, and symptoms.
            b. Prior treatments and efficacy.
        2. **Physical examination**
            a. Extremities: Measure circumference at a fixed point (e.g., 10 cm inferior to the patella), or perform water displacement test.
            b. Neurovascular status and skin integrity and character are noted.
    C. **Imaging studies**
        1. **Doppler ultrasound:** Can visualize venous flow; may detect obstruction.
        2. **CT scan:** Signs of lymphedema include honeycomb appearance of soft tissue and thickened skin.
        3. **MRI:** Honeycombing muscle edema.
        4. **Lymphangiography and lymphatic dye injection studies:** Should be avoided due to stasis and local vessel irritation, as they may actually worsen lymphedema.
V. **Treatment**
    A. **Nonoperative management is appropriate for most patients.**
        1. **Extremity elevation.**

2. **Compression garment:** By prescription, with custom fit; must be replaced frequently to assure good compression.
3. **Pneumatic compression devices:** Can be highly effective.
4. **Exercise:** Increases lymphatic return by a mechanical pump effect.
5. **Avoid limb injury;** substantial susceptibility to cellulitis even to minor trauma.
   a. Appropriate antibiotics; avoid compression during infection.
   b. Consider suppressive antibiotics in cases of recurrent infection.
6. **For obese patients,** lymphedema may improve with weight loss.

B. **Surgical management** is of limited benefit.
1. **Practical considerations**
   a. Reduce edema as much as possible preoperatively.
   b. Consider Z- or W-plasty over joints.
   c. Foot often remains problematic; verrucous changes and edema of skin grafts may develop.
   d. Strict limb elevation postoperatively.
   e. Will likely continue to require compression garments postoperatively.
2. **Limb reduction procedures**
   a. Staged excision of skin and subcutaneous tissue with primary closure.
   b. Radical excision of skin, subcutaneous tissue, and fascia with split- or full-thickness skin graft coverage (Charles technique).
   c. Excision of subcutaneous tissue with a deepithelialized dermal flap buried in muscle in an attempt to establish a communication between the superficial and deep lymphatic systems.
3. **Lymphatic procedures (not reliably effective)**
   a. Microlymphaticovenous anastomosis.
      (1) Microanastomosis between lymphatic vessel and a small vein.
      (2) Improvement within 24 hours.
   b. Lymph node-venous anastomosis: Associated with transient improvement and a poor success rate.
   c. Microlymphatic grafting: To bypass a discrete blockage.

VI. **Complications**
A. **Recurrent cellulitis occurs in 30% of cases** of primary lymphedema and contributes to disease progression (usually *Staphylococcus* or *Streptococcus*).
B. **Ulceration.**
C. **Verrucous skin changes.**
D. **Increased risk of squamous cell carcinoma;** biopsy any suspicious lesions.
E. **Lymphangiosarcoma:** Rare (less than 1%), but carries a poor prognosis.
F. **Kaposi's sarcoma:** Rare, but reported.

Tattoos

I. **Tattoo biology**
A. **Tattoo ink** consists of particles of approximately 3 to 5 micrometers, which are engulfed by, and reside mainly within, dermal fibroblasts.
B. **Decorative tattoos**
1. **Black color** is usually created with carbon; other pigment colors are derived from a variety of metals.
2. **Professional decorative tattoos** tend to have uniform pigment depth (upper papillary dermis) and a uniform particle size. This makes them easier, more reliable targets for laser removal.
3. **Amateur decorative tattoos** tend to have variable depth (may extend to the subcutaneous tissue) and variable particle size, making them more difficult to eradicate with a laser.
C. **Cosmetic tattoos** (e.g., permanent eyeliner and lip liner). Results are variable; oxidation may darken pigment over time.

D. **Tattoos in reconstructive surgery**
  1. **Nipple reconstruction**
      a. Intradermal tattooing is useful to obtain color and size match.
      b. Wait approximately 1 month after breast reconstruction, or until healing is complete.
      c. Consider tattooing contralateral areola as well if color match is difficult.
  2. May be an alternative in brow and lip reconstruction.
E. **Traumatic tattoos**
  1. **Particulate matter** embedded in the skin may remain permanently visible.
  2. **Meticulous wound débridement** is mandatory to prevent tattooing, especially with "road rash" and powder burns. Consider surgical scrubbrush or meticulous operative debridement.
II. **Tattoo removal**
  A. **Laser removal:** Based on tattoo pigments (see Chapter 10, "Lasers in Plastic Surgery").
  B. **Dermabrasion:** Performed with a wire brush or diamond fraise; may result in scarring and pigment changes.
  C. **Excision**
    1. **Small tattoos** are easily excised.
    2. **Large tattoos** may require tissue expansion or serial excision.
    3. Patients must be willing to accept **resultant scarring** in exchange for tattoo removal.

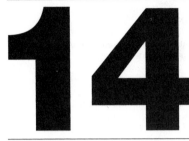

Squamous Cell Carcinoma of the Head and Neck

Cecelia E. Schmalbach

Introduction

I. Epidemiology
  A. **Squamous cell carcinoma (SCC)** is the most common cancer involving head and neck **mucosal** sites (accounts for 90% of malignancies).
  B. **Most often occurs** in the sixth and seventh decades of life.
  C. **Incidence increases** with age.
  D. **Male-to-female ratio** is approximately 2:1.
  E. **Risk factors**
      1. **Tobacco** (including smokeless or chewing tobacco).
      2. **Alcohol:** Synergizes with tobacco; increases risk by 10- to 15-fold.
      3. **Human papillomavirus (HPV).**
      4. **Epstein-Barr virus (EBV):** Associated with nasopharyngeal SCC.
      5. **Poor dental hygiene.**
      6. **Chronic irritation** (e.g., ill-fitting dentures).
      7. **Plummer-Vinson syndrome** (achlorhydria, iron deficiency anemia, dysphagia, mucosal atrophy).
      8. **Syphilis.**
      9. **Lichen planus.**
      10. **Chronic immunosuppression.**
      11. **Betel nuts:** Common in Indian population.

II. Pathology
  A. **Premalignant lesions**
      1. **Require close follow-up;** biopsy required to rule out invasive component.
      2. **Leukoplakia:** Non-pathologic, nonhistologic description of white patchy mucosa.
          a. Clinical description only.
          b. Represents epithelial hyperplasia, usually secondary to trauma.
          c. May harbor dysplasia, carcinoma *in situ*, or invasive SCC.
      3. **Erythroplakia:** Clinical description of red, "velvet-like" mucosal patches.
          a. Higher incidence of associated SCC compared with leukoplakia.
          b. Biopsy required to rule out SCC.
      4. **Lichen planus**
          a. White, flat inflammatory papule involving oral mucosa.
          b. Rarely undergoes malignant transformation.
  B. **Gross Variants of SCC**
      1. **Ulcerative type:** Most common type of oral cavity SCC.
      2. **Infiltrative type**
          a. Often found in tongue SCC.
          b. Diagnosis requires careful palpation.
      3. **Exophytic type**
          a. Least common variant.
          b. Spreads superficially.
          c. Less aggressive; least likely to metastasize.

C. SCC histology

1. **Three histologic variants:** Well, moderately, and poorly differentiated.
2. **Well-differentiated lesions** have increased amounts of keratin and predict a better prognosis.
3. **Nasopharyngeal carcinoma** has a separate World Health Organization (WHO) classification.
    a. WHO type I: SCC; represents 25% of nasopharyngeal carcinomas.
    b. WHO type II: Nonkeratinizing, transitional cell carcinoma; 12% of tumors.
    c. WHO type III: Undifferentiated carcinoma; more than 60% of tumors.
4. **Verrucous carcinoma** (Ackerman's tumor).
    a. Rare variant of SCC.
    b. Most often involves buccal mucosa followed by gingival mucosa.
    c. Exophytic; papillary morphology.
    d. Deep infiltration and metastasis uncommon.
    e. Treatment:
       (1) Surgical excision with only a few millimeters of margin.
       (2) Serial sectioning of pathology specimen necessary to rule out harboring invasive SCC.
       (3) Role of radiation controversial due to potential for transformation into an anaplastic/aggressive lesion.

D. Metastatic disease

1. **Regional spread** to cervical lymph nodes.
    a. Follows a fairly predictable pattern depending on location of primary tumor.
    b. Midline tumors can drain to bilateral nodal basins.
    c. Poor prognostic factors include multiple lymph node involvement, involvement of low neck levels, matted nodes, and presence of extracapsular spread.
2. **Distant metastasis** is most often to lung, and sometimes to bone.

III. Anatomy

A. Oral cavity

1. **Extends from the skin–vermilion lip junction** posteriorly to the junction of the hard and soft palate and circumvallate papillae.
2. **The oral cavity is divided into a number of subsites.**
    a. Lips
    b. Buccal mucosa
    c. Upper and lower alveolar ridge
    d. Retromolar trigone (RMT)
    e. Floor of mouth (FOM)
    f. Hard palate
    g. Anterior two-thirds of tongue

B. Pharynx: Three subsites

1. **Nasopharynx:** Extends from the skull base superiorly to the soft and hard palate inferiorly; from the nasal choanae/septum to the posterior pharyngeal wall. Subsites of the nasopharynx include the following.
    a. Fossa of Rosenmüller.
    b. Torus and orifice of the eustachian tube.
    c. Lateral and posterior walls.
2. **Oropharynx:** Subsites include the following.
    a. Anterior border: Circumvallate papillae.
    b. Lateral borders: Tonsil, tonsillar fossa, and tonsillar pillars.
    c. Posterior border: Posterior pharyngeal wall.
    d. Inferior border: Floor of vallecula (space between base of tongue and epiglottis).
    e. Superior border: Soft palate.
    f. The tonsil and tonsillar fossa are the most common locations of SCC within the oropharynx.
3. **Hypopharynx:** Extends from floor of vallecula and aryepiglottic folds to inferior border of cricoid cartilage; contains three subsites.

      a. Postcricoid region/pharyngoesophageal junction.

      b. Pyriform sinuses.

      c. Posterior pharyngeal wall.

C. Larynx: Three subsites

  1. Supraglottis (30% of laryngeal SCC)

    a. Separated from glottis by horizontal plane through ventricle (space between true and false vocal cords).

    b. Includes epiglottis, aryepiglottic folds, arytenoids, false vocal cords, and ventricles.

  2. Glottis (50%–70% of laryngeal SCC)

    a. Extends from ventricle to 1 cm below the free edge of the true vocal cord.

    b. Includes true vocal cords, anterior and posterior commissure.

    c. "Transglottic" tumors cross glottis in continuity with another site.

  3. Subglottis: Extends from glottis to inferior border of cricoid ring.

D. Other spaces

  1. Preepiglottic space

    a. Bound superiorly by the hyoepiglottic ligament and vallecula, anteriorly by the thyrohyoid ligament, and posteriorly by the epiglottis and thyroepiglottic ligament.

    b. The infrahyoid epiglottis has numerous holes in the cartilage, allowing cancer to easily spread from the larynx to this space.

  2. Paraglottic space

    a. Potential space between the thyroid cartilage and medial mucosa wall of the pyriform sinus.

    b. Continuous with preepiglottic space anterior and superiorly.

  3. Reinke's space: Between true vocal cord epithelium and thyroarytenoid muscle.

E. Lymphatic drainage levels of the neck (Fig. 14-1)

  1. Level I (submental/submandibular triangle): Bound by anterior and posterior bellies of the digastric, inferior hyoid bone, and body of the mandible.

  2. Level II (upper jugular): Bound by skull base, inferior border of hyoid, stylohyoid muscle, and lateral border of sternocleidomastoid muscle (SCM).

  3. Level III (mid-jugular): Bound by inferior border of hyoid, inferior border of cricoid cartilage, lateral border of sternohyoid, and lateral SCM.

  4. Level IV (lower jugular): Bound by inferior border of cricoid cartilage, clavicle, lateral border of sternohyoid muscle, and lateral border of SCM.

  5. Level V (posterior triangle): Bound by apex of SCM and trapezius muscle, clavicle, posterior border of SCM, and anterior border of trapezius muscle.

  6. Level VI (upper mediastinum): Bound by the hyoid bone, suprasternal notch, and common carotid arteries.

IV. Tumor, node, metastasis (TNM) staging system

A. Clinical staging system

  1. Stage is denoted by Roman numeral (Table 14-1).

  2. Takes into account T, N, and M levels to give a clinical stage.

  3. Treatment and prognosis are determined by stage.

B. Primary tumor (T)

  1. Oral cavity

    a. TX: Cannot assess

    b. T0: No evidence of tumor

    c. Tis: Carcinoma *in situ*

    d. T1: ≤2 cm

    e. T2: >2 cm but ≤4 cm

    f. T3: >4 cm

    g. T4a: Invades adjacent structures (cortical bone, extrinsic tongue musculature, maxillary sinus, facial skin)

    h. T4b: Invades masticator space, pterygoid plates, or skull base, or encases internal carotid artery

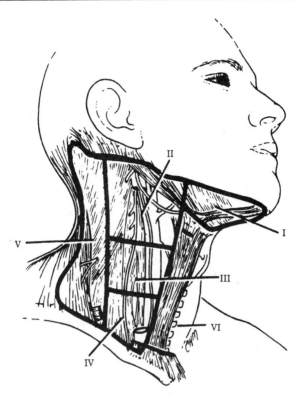

Fig. 14-1. Lymphatic drainage levels of the neck. Level I, submental and submandibular lymph node groups; level II, upper jugular group; level III, middle jugular groups; level IV, lower jugular group; level V, posterior triangle group; level VI, anterior compartment group. (From Milas K. Carcinoma of the head and neck. In *The M.D. Anderson Surgical Oncology Handbook*, 3rd ed. Feig BW, Berger DH, Fuhrman GM. Philadelphia, Lippincott Williams & Wilkins, 2003. With permission.)

2. Oropharynx
   a. T1: ≤2 cm
   b. T2: >2 cm but ≤4 cm
   c. T3: >4 cm
   d. T4a: Invades larynx, extrinsic tongue musculature, medial pterygoid muscle, hard palate, or mandible
   e. T4b: Invades lateral pterygoid muscle, pterygoid plate, lateral nasopharynx, or skull base, or encases carotid artery

Table 14-1. TNM staging system for squamous cell carcinoma of the hypopharynx and nasopharynx

	N0	N1	N2–3 or any N with M1
T1	I		
T2	II		
T3		III	
T4			IV

3. Hypopharynx
a. T1: Tumor limited to one subsite *and* is ≤2 cm.
b. T2: Tumor involves more than one subsite *or* is >2 cm but ≤4 cm without hypopharynx fixation.
c. T3: >4 cm or hypopharynx fixation.
d. T4a: Invades thyroid/cricoid cartilage, hyoid bone, thyroid gland, esophagus, strap muscles/subcutaneous tissue.
e. T4b: Invades prevertebral fascia or mediastinum, or encases carotid artery.

4. Nasopharynx
a. T1: Confined to nasopharynx.
b. T2a: Extends to soft tissues of oropharynx/nasal cavity without parapharyngeal extension.
c. T2b: Any tumor with parapharyngeal extension.
d. T3: Involves bony structures or paranasal sinuses.
e. T4: Intracranial extension, cranial nerve involvement, infratemporal fossa, hypopharynx, orbit or masticator space.

5. Supraglottis
a. T1: Limited to one subsite with normal vocal cord movement.
b. T2: Invades mucosa of more than one adjacent supraglottic or glottic subsite or region outside supraglottis (base of tongue, vallecula, medial wall of pyriform sinus) without larynx fixation.
c. T3: Tumor limited to larynx *with* vocal cord fixation or invasion of postcricoid area, preepiglottic space, paraglottic space, or inner cortex thyroid cartilage.
d. T4a: Invasion through thyroid cartilage or invasion beyond larynx (i.e., trachea, deep extrinsic tongue musculature, strap muscles, thyroid gland, or esophagus).
e. T4b: Invades prevertebral space or mediastinum, or encases carotid artery.

6. Glottis
a. T1a: Limited to one vocal cord with normal mobility.
b. T1b: Involves both vocal cords with normal mobility.
c. T2: Extension to supraglottis or subglottis or impaired vocal cord mobility
d. T3: Tumor limited to larynx with vocal cord fixation; invasion of paraglottic space or inner cortex thyroid cartilage.
e. T4a: Invasion through thyroid cartilage or invasion beyond larynx (i.e., trachea, deep extrinsic tongue musculature, strap muscles, thyroid gland, or esophagus).
f. T4b: Invades prevertebral space or mediastinum, or encases carotid artery.

7. Subglottis
a. T1: Limited to subglottis.
b. T2: Extends to vocal cord(s) with normal or impaired mobility.
c. T3: Limited to larynx with vocal cord fixation.
d. T4a: Invasion through thyroid cartilage or invasion beyond larynx (i.e., trachea, deep extrinsic tongue musculature, strap muscles, thyroid gland, or esophagus).
e. T4b: Invades prevertebral space, mediastinum, or encases carotid artery.

C. Regional lymph nodes (N)
1. **NX:** Cannot assess
2. **N0:** No regional involvement
3. **N1:** Ipsilateral lymph node ≤3 cm
4. **N2a:** Single ipsilateral lymph node >3 cm but ≤6 cm
5. **N2b:** Multiple ipsilateral lymph nodes all ≤6 cm
6. **N2c:** Bilateral or contralateral lymph node ≤6 cm
7. **N3:** Lymph node >6 cm

D. Distant metastasis (M)
1. **MX:** Cannot assess
2. **M0:** No distant metastasis
3. **M1:** Distant metastasis

Evaluation

I. History

    A. Duration of lesion or mass, and rapidity of enlargement, should be determined.

    B. Associated symptoms may include the following.

        1. **Localized pain**

        2. **Referred otalgia (ear pain)**

        3. **Dysphagia (difficulty swallowing)**

        4. **Odynophagia (painful swallowing)**

        5. **Weight loss**

        6. **Hoarseness** (indicating glottic involvement)

        7. **Shortness of breath**

    C. Social history

        1. **Tobacco use** (type; number of years).

        2. **Alcohol** (type; daily amount consumed): Patient may require prophylaxis with benzodiazepines or alcohol drip to prevent delirium tremens if hospitalization is planned.

    D. Past medical history

        1. **Past history of head and neck SCC**

        2. **Previous exposure to radiation**

II. Physical examination

    A. Tympanic membranes: Middle ear effusion may indicate nasopharyngeal mass.

    B. Oral cavity

        1. **State of dentition** is important for radiation and reconstructive considerations. Teeth may need to be extracted if they have excessive caries prior to radiation therapy.

        2. **Note size and location** of suspicious lesions.

        3. **Comment on fixation** of lesion to surrounding bone.

        4. **Describe extension** of tumor by noting all structures involved.

        5. **Deviation of tongue on protrusion** indicates involvement of hypoglossal nerve (cranial nerve XII) ipsilateral to the deviation.

        6. **Trismus** (inability to fully open mouth) indicates possible involvement of pterygoid muscle, masseter muscle, and/or infratemporal fossa.

    C. Oropharynx

        1. **Note size and location of suspicious lesions.**

        2. **Comment on fixation to surrounding bone.**

        3. **Describe extension of tumor.**

        4. **Palpate base of tongue** and RMT because lesions can infiltrate or be difficult to visualize, or both.

    D. Larynx

        1. **Perform indirect examination with mirror visualization.**

        2. **Direct visualization** with flexible nasopharyngoscope should be performed.

        3. **Assess airway, nasal portion of the soft palate, vocal cord mobility, orifice to pyriform sinuses, epiglottis, and vallecula.**

    E. Neck

        1. **Carefully palpate** for cervical lymphadenopathy.

            a. Comment on node size, location, and fixation.

            b. "Lymph nodes" greater than 3 cm are likely matted nodes.

        2. **A neck mass** can also represent direct tumor extension.

        3. **Fixation of the larynx** (loss of laryngeal crepitus and ability to move larynx side-to-side) is indicative of extralaryngeal tumor extension.

III. Laboratory studies

    A. Complete blood count.

    B. Coagulation studies (prothrombin time, partial thromboplastin time).

    C. Electrolyte panel.

    D. Liver enzymes, including alkaline phosphatase.

IV. Radiographic studies

A. Computed tomographic (CT) scan of the neck with contrast (axial and coronal).
   1. **Evaluate tumor extension.**
   2. **Assess bony and cartilaginous invasion.**
   3. **Evaluate cervical lymph node involvement.**

B. Magnetic resonance imaging (MRI) is helpful in evaluating skull base involvement and neural invasion.

C. Panorex is useful for evaluating mandibular bone involvement if the CT scan is equivocal.

D. Chest x-ray is used to screen for pulmonary metastases.
   1. **Any nodule** requires further evaluation with chest CT.
   2. **Many surgeons advocate chest CT** for any patient with recurrent SCC or with advanced stage III/IV disease because it is more sensitive than chest x-ray.

E. Positron emission tomography (PET)
   1. **Tissues** with high metabolic rates (such as tumors) demonstrate increased uptake of radioactive 18-fluorodeoxyglucose.
   2. **May be helpful in differentiating postradiation changes** from tumor, and in working up occult nodal disease, pulmonary metastasis, and secondary primaries.

F. Bone scan evaluates for metastatic lesions in patients with elevated alkaline phosphatase levels, recent fracture, or bone pain.

G. Barium swallow is used to evaluate cervical esophageal involvement if rigid esophagoscopy cannot be performed.

V. Histologic diagnosis

A. Biopsy of the primary tumor can be done in a clinic setting with local anesthesia or in an operating room under general anesthesia, depending on anatomic location.

B. Fine-needle aspiration (FNA) of neck masses is used to assess cervical metastasis.

VI. Direct laryngoscopy

A. Formal evaluation of tumor extension under general anesthesia.

B. Often provides better visualization than clinic exam because head and neck musculature is relaxed.

C. Rigid esophagoscopy and rigid/flexible bronchoscopy can be performed at the same time to evaluate synchronous primary lesions.

VII. Additional considerations

A. Cardiac clearance by cardiology team

B. Nutritional exam
   1. **Adequate nutrition** is imperative for postoperative healing.
   2. **Patient may require supplemental nutrition.**
   3. **If dysphagia or odynophagia** is problematic, consider nasogastric feeding tube placement.
   4. **If long-term nutrition** will likely be a problem, consider percutaneous endoscopic gastrostomy tube.

C. Dental exam: Patients undergoing radiation therapy will need poor dentition extracted in order to avoid caries, abscess formation, and osteoradionecrosis.

D. Pulmonary function tests are required if patient is being considered for con-servation laryngectomy.

Treatment

I. Multidisciplinary team members

A. Surgical extirpative team

B. Surgical reconstructive team

C. Medical oncologist

    D. Radiation oncologist

    E. Radiologist

    F. Dentist/Prosthodontist

    G. Speech therapist

    H. Nutritionist

    I. Physical therapist

    J. Social worker

II. Oral cavity and pharynx (excluding nasopharynx)

    A. Single-modality treatment (radiation therapy *or* surgery) for T1/T2 lesions; equal efficacy.

        1. Surgery is favored for small oral cavity tumors.

            a. Spares patient radiation side effects (see "Complications").

            b. Reserves the use of radiation for recurrence.

        2. Radiation is favored for oropharynx lesions (especially soft palate and tonsil).

            a. Speech and swallowing function are better preserved.

            b. Patient compliance is imperative when selecting candidates.

            c. Early lesions with a high rate of occult nodal metastasis (e.g., oropharynx) should include radiation to neck fields.

            d. Disadvantages: The patient will miss approximately 2 months of work and activity, and tumor recurrence may be difficult to detect in the setting of postradiation changes.

    B. Multimodality treatment for T3/T4 lesions.

        1. Surgery with radiation therapy (usually postoperative).

        2. Organ preservation protocols involving chemotherapy (usually cisplatin and 5-flurouracil) and radiation.

        3. Patients should be educated on available clinical trials.

III. Larynx

    A. Glottic SCC *in situ*

        1. Initially can be treated with vocal cord stripping and close follow-up.

        2. Recurrence requires repeat stripping, microlaryngeal excision, radiation, or partial laryngectomy depending on patient history and tumor size.

    B. Glottic T1/T2 SCC

        1. Primary radiation with 50 to 70 Gy over 5 to 8 weeks preserves voice quality better than surgery.

        2. Surgery with laser microexcision or partial laryngectomy has an overall cure rate of 80% to 85%.

        3. Neck metastases are rare (8%) because of the limited lymphatics in the glottic region.

    C. T3/T4 laryngeal tumors

        1. Vertical partial laryngectomy versus total laryngectomy (depending on tumor location and pulmonary status) with postoperative radiation.

        2. Organ preservation protocols involving chemotherapy (usually cisplatin and 5-flurouracil) and radiation have equal survival rates versus primary surgery with postoperative radiation.

    D. Subglottic SCC

        1. Nodal and cartilage involvement is common because presentation is late (presentation often involves airway obstruction).

        2. Total laryngectomy with bilateral neck dissections is usually required.

        3. Postoperative radiation is often necessary given a late presentation and advanced disease.

        4. Stomal recurrence is common.

    E. Speech rehabilitation

        1. Esophageal speech: Air released from esophagus vibrates against posterior pharyngeal wall to produce speech.

        2. Tracheoesophageal puncture

            a. A one-way valve is placed through posterior tracheal wall (at superior border of stoma) into the esophagus.

        b. Pulmonary air is diverted through the valve to vibrate against esophageal-pharyngeal wall and produce speech.

        c. Superior voice quality compared with esophageal speech.

        d. Contraindication: Poor patient vision or dexterity; poor patient motivation.

        e. Potential complications include leakage, granulation tissue formation, and *Candida* infections.

    3. Artificial larynx (electrolarynx) electronically modulates and amplifies remaining vocal sounds to simulate speech.

IV. Nasopharynx

    A. Radiation to primary lesion and bilateral necks.

    B. Concomitant chemotherapy decreases development of distant metastasis and improves both disease-free and overall survival for advanced disease.

    C. Salvage neck dissection required for persistent nodal disease following chemotherapy and radiation.

V. Management of the neck

    A. Selective neck dissection

        1. Neck dissection with preservation of one or more lymph node groups.

        2. Indication: Used as a staging procedure in a patient without clinical evidence of nodal metastasis (N0 neck) in order to determine the need for postoperative neck radiation.

    B. Modified radical neck dissection

        1. Removal of all ipsilateral cervical lymph node groups (levels I–V).

        2. Preserves at least one of the following vital structures: the internal jugular vein, sternocleidomastoid muscle, or spinal accessory nerve (cranial nerve XI).

        3. Indication: Treatment of known cervical lymph node metastasis in which the internal jugular vein, SCM, and spinal accessory nerve are not directly involved.

    C. Radical neck dissection

        1. Removal of all ipsilateral cervical lymph node groups (levels I–V).

        2. Removal of all three vital structures: internal jugular vein, sternocleidomastoid muscle, and spinal accessory nerve (cranial nerve XI).

        3. Indication: Treatment of advanced cervical disease including multiple, fixed lymph node metastases invading neck structures.

    D. Extended neck dissection: Involves additional lymph node groups beyond levels I to V or nonlymphatic structures such as the hypoglossal nerve.

VI. Reconstruction (See Chapter 16, "Principles of Head and Neck Reconstruction")

VII. Complications

    A. Surgical

        1. Bleeding.

        2. Infection, wound breakdown, potential for carotid artery exposure.

        3. Scarring.

        4. Nerve paresis or paralysis (especially marginal mandibular branch of cranial nerve VII, spinal accessory nerve, and submental nerve).

        5. Fistula formation.

        6. Chronic aspiration.

        7. Trismus (limited mouth opening).

    B. Radiation

        1. Xerostomia (dry mouth secondary to salivary gland dysfunction; may be palliated with prosalivatory topical medications).

        2. Mucositis: Patient may require percutaneous endoscopic gastrostomy or Dobbhoff tube for nutrition.

        3. Pharyngitis.

        4. Laryngeal and esophageal scarring or stenosis.

        5. Osteoradionecrosis: Treatment requires hyperbaric oxygen therapy or surgery, or both.

        6. Dental caries.

        7. Chronic aspiration.

VIII. Follow-up
- **A. Routine appointments** are imperative because head and neck SCC has a high rate of locoregional recurrence and of second primary tumor development.
  1. **First year:** Every 1 to 2 months
  2. **Second year:** Every 2 to 3 months
  3. **Third year:** Every 3 to 4 months
  4. **Fourth and fifth year:** Every 4 to 6 months
  5. **Yearly thereafter**
- **B. Yearly chest x-ray** to evaluate pulmonary metastasis.
- **C. Radiated patients** require yearly evaluation of thyroid-stimulating hormone level because of risk for hypothyroidism.

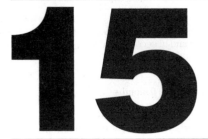

Neck Masses and Salivary Gland Neoplasms

Brent B. Ward

Evaluation of a Neck Mass

I. **History**
   A. **Age of patient**
      1. **Young patients** are more frequently associated with congenital and inflammatory processes.
      2. **Older patients** more frequently have neoplastic and malignant processes.
   B. **Duration and pattern**
      1. **Date first noted.**
      2. **Growth pattern:** Intermittent presence and fluctuations in size suggest a nonneoplastic process; slow growth followed by rapid growth suggests a neoplastic process.
   C. **Significant symptoms** that may accompany a neck mass include the following.
      1. **Otalgia, dysphonia, odynophagia, dysphagia, and generalized pain**
      2. **Constitutional symptoms:** Fever, chills, night sweats, or weight loss
      3. **Hyper- or hypothyroid symptoms:** Changes in energy level, mood, or temperature sensitivity.
   D. **Potential associations or causal agents**
      1. **Exposure history:** Tuberculosis, animals, radiation, or nickel.
      2. **Recent infections:** Upper respiratory tract infection, sinusitis, dental problems, or recent dental procedures.
   E. **Family history**
      1. **Inherited syndromes.**
         a. Multiple endocrine neoplasia type I (MEN-I): Thyroid medullary carcinoma, parathyroid hyperplasia, and pituitary tumors.
         b. Li-Fraumeni syndrome: Sarcoma and other malignancies.
         c. Basal cell nevus (Gorlin's) syndrome: Multiple basal cell carcinomas and odontogenic keratocysts.
         d. Neurofibromatosis.
      2. **Nonsyndromic family history** of benign or malignant disease.
   F. **Social history**
      1. **Tobacco:** Head and neck squamous cell carcinoma is six times more likely in smokers.
      2. **Alcohol:** A potentiator, especially in patients with a positive tobacco history.
II. **Physical examination** (requires a complete examination of head and neck; see also Chapter 14, "Squamous Cell Carcinoma of the Head and Neck")
   A. **Skin:** Examine the scalp, ears, face, and neck for lesions or masses.
   B. **Eye:** Proptosis, visual acuity disturbances, or extraocular movement changes may be a sign of an orbital mass.
   C. **Ear:** Masses or effusions may indicate eustachian tube obstruction.
   D. **Nose:** Inspect for nasal mucosa lesions and sinus discharge.
   E. **Oral cavity**
      1. **Inspect tonsillar pillars** and posterior pharyngeal wall, and perform mirror laryngoscopy or flexible laryngoscopy.

2. **Palpate and inspect palate, tongue (dorsal, ventral, and base), floor of mouth, gingiva, buccal mucosa, and lips.**
3. **Evaluate salivary flow** (Stensen's and Wharton's ducts).

F. **Neck**
   1. **Inspection**
      a. Evaluation for symmetry and visible masses or lesions.
      b. Activation of musculature and symmetry on repose and while swallowing.
      c. Jugular venous distension may be seen with upper neck masses.
   2. **Palpation**
      a. Anterior and posterior triangles (anterior and posterior to the sternoclei-domastoid muscle), including lymph node areas 1 to 5 (see Fig. 14-1).
      b. All lymph node chains are examined for the following:
         (1) Mobile versus fixed nodes.
         (2) Soft or doughy versus hard nodes.
         (3) Tenderness on palpation.
   3. **Salivary gland palpation** (see "Salivary Gland Neoplasms")
   4. **Thyroid palpation**
      a. Performed from both anterior and posterior positioning.
      b. Palpate in repose and on swallowing.
      c. Evaluate size, symmetry, and consistency.

G. **Neurologic evaluation of cranial nerve function**
   1. **May assist in detection** of an unknown primary.
   2. **Nerve involvement** may be an indicator of an aggressive neoplastic process.

III. **Differential diagnosis of neck masses**
   A. **80% rule**
      1. **80% of nonthyroid neck masses** in adults are neoplastic, and 80% of these are malignant, and 80% of these are metastases, and 80% of these are from primaries above the clavicles.
      2. **80% of neck masses** in children are inflammatory or benign.
   B. **The type of neck mass** is predicted by location.
      1. **Midline:** Teratoma, dermoid or thyroglossal duct cyst.
      2. **Anterior triangle:** Branchial cleft anomaly or lymph node (site for nodal drainage of intra- and extraoral sites).
      3. **Posterior triangle:** Lymph node (site for nodal drainage of intra- and extraoral sites).
      4. **Regional sites suggestive of local disease process**
         a. Thyroid.
         b. Salivary gland (parotid, submandibular, and sublingual).
   C. **Adenitis**
      1. **Nodes greater than 1.5 cm** in diameter are considered abnormal.
      2. **Bacterial etiologies** include *Streptococcus*, *Staphylococcus*, *Mycobacterium*, cat-scratch fever (*Bartonella*), tularemia, and *Actinomyces*.
      3. **Viral causes** include Epstein-Barr virus (EBV), cytomegalovirus (CMV), herpes simplex virus (HSV), human immunodeficiency virus (HIV), rhinovirus, and adenovirus.
      4. **Fungal infections** are likely caused by coccidioidomycosis.
      5. **Parasitic adenitis** is often caused by toxoplasmosis.
      6. **Empiric therapy** with antibiotics for 10 days to 2 weeks is indicated if the mass is inflammatory.
         a. Treat the most common causes in the differential diagnosis based on history, physical exam, and appropriate diagnostic studies.
         b. Close follow-up of empiric treatment is required.
         c. Persistence of adenitis for greater than 2 weeks requires additional workup and treatment.
   D. **Congenital neck masses**
      1. **Branchial cleft anomalies**
         a. Arise from primitive branchial arches, clefts, and pouches.
         b. May include cysts, fistulae, or sinuses.

      c. Includes first, second (most common), third, and fourth branchial cleft anomalies.

      d. Treated by excision of the cyst or sinus; may be complex in some cases of second branchial arch cysts, and may course around the carotid artery.

  2. Thyroglossal duct cyst

      a. Remnant of thyroglossal duct epithelium.

      b. Occurs anywhere from the foramen cecum of the tongue to the suprasternal notch.

      c. Most commonly diagnosed in the first two decades of life.

      d. Treated by complete excision of the cyst tract.

  3. Dermoid cyst

      a. Teratoma-like cysts contain two rather then three (teratoma) germ layers.

      b. Often presents as a midline doughy mass; most common in young adults.

      c. Usually amenable to local excision.

E. Thyroid masses

  1. Solitary nodule: Cyst, benign, or malignant neoplasm.

  2. Multinodular goiter: Toxic or nontoxic.

  3. Inflammatory/autoimmune: Reidel's, Hashimoto's, and De Quervain's thyroiditis.

  4. Malignancy: Papillary adenocarcinoma, follicular carcinoma, Hürthle cell tumors, medullary carcinoma, anaplastic carcinoma. The majority of thyroid cancers are low grade (papillary and follicular) and amenable to surgical excision. Anaplastic tumors are associated with high mortality and are usually not treated surgically.

F. Neoplastic neck masses

  1. Benign

      a. Mesenchymal: Fibroma, lipoma, leiomyoma, rhabdomyoma, and neural tumors are usually amenable to resection.

      b. Salivary gland masses: See "Salivary Gland Neoplasms."

      c. Vascular masses: Vascular malformation (not a neoplasm; actually a congenital anomaly), hemangioma, lymphangioma. (See Chapter 13, "Vascular Anomalies, Lymphedema, and Tattoos.").

  2. Malignant

      a. Sarcoma: Fibrosarcoma, liposarcoma, neurofibrosarcoma, and angiosarcoma. Usually amenable to surgical management with or without radiotherapy. (See Chapter 11, "Malignant Skin and Soft Tissue Lesions.").

      b. Salivary tumors: See "Salivary Gland Neoplasms."

      c. Lymphoma.

  3. Metastases

      a. Primary regional site for head and neck malignancy spread is to cervical lymph nodes.

      b. Esophageal and lung tumors.

IV. Diagnostic studies

A. Ultrasound with Doppler: Useful for determination of cystic versus complex versus solid; shows association with adjacent structures (thyroid, lymph nodes); provides guidance for fine-needle aspiration (FNA). Ultrasound is excellent for diagnostic imaging of thyroid disorders.

B. Magnetic resonance imaging (MRI): Best for evaluation of primary lesions of tonsillar fossae, floor of mouth, tongue, and retro- and parapharyngeal spaces.

C. Computed tomography (CT) with contrast: Evaluation of nodes larger than 1 to 1.5 cm, especially with a necrotic center of greater than 3 mm; evaluation of extracapsular extension of nodal disease.

D. FNA: Especially useful for thyroid masses and solid masses of the neck. Accuracy is highly dependent on operator and cytopathologist experience.

E. **Nuclear medicine studies:** Thyroid uptake scans can by useful for determining if a mass is actively sequestering iodine (and therefore likely benign). Salivary gland scans (see "Salivary Gland Neoplasms").

F. **Indications for open biopsy** of a neck mass
   1. **Persistent for more than 2 to 4 weeks**
   2. **Likely metastatic without evidence of primary tumor**
   3. **Negative endoscopy with multiple random biopsies**
   4. **Negative FNA**
   5. **Probable lymphoma**

Salivary Gland Neoplasms

I. **Salivary gland anatomy**
   A. **Glands develop during the sixth to eighth week of gestation** as oral ectoderm and nasopharyngeal endoderm.
   B. **Parotid gland**
      1. **The parotid is located in the preauricular upper neck** (tail) with deep and superficial lobes. The facial nerve separates the lobes.
      2. **The surrounding fascia of the gland** is an extension of the superficial layer of the deep cervical fascia.
      3. **The gland consists predominantly of serous acini.**
      4. **Stensen's duct** arises from the anterior border of the parotid and enters the oral cavity at the level of the maxillary second molar.
   C. **Submandibular (submaxillary) gland**
      1. **Located in the submandibular triangle.**
      2. **Surrounded by the splitting of the superficial layer** of deep cervical fascia.
      3. **Mucous and serous acini.**
      4. **Wharton's duct** arises from the medial gland and enters the oral cavity in the anterior floor of mouth.
      5. **Closely associated with the lingual nerve,** which sends autonomic fibers to the gland.
   D. **Sublingual gland**
      1. **Located in anterior floor of mouth** just below the mucosa.
      2. **No fascial covering.**
      3. **Mucous acini.**
      4. **Drained by multiple ducts of Rivinus** along its superior aspect entering the oral cavity. Occasionally a coalescence of these ducts form the Bartholin's duct, which empties into Wharton's duct.
   E. **Minor salivary glands**
      1. **600 to 1,000 glands** are located just below the submucosal layer of the oral cavity.
      2. **No fascial covering.**
      3. **Mainly mucus-secreting glands.**
      4. **Simple ductal system** that empties directly into the oral cavity.
II. **Diagnosis of salivary gland pathology**
   A. **History**
      1. **Findings favoring a diagnosis of neoplasm**
         a. Presence over an extended period of weeks to months.
         b. Pain is usually a sign of advanced disease.
         c. Slow but persistent growth or slow growth with a sudden rapid phase indicates possible malignant transformation or secondary infection with malignancy.
      2. **Findings favoring an infectious process:** Rapid onset with signs of inflammation (warmth, erythema, and edema), repeated episodes of inflammation, alcohol abuse, autoimmune diseases (e.g., Sjögren's syndrome), HIV, xerostomia, dehydration.

B. Physical examination findings
  1. Findings favoring neoplasm
    a. Discretely palpable firm mass, especially when fixed to adjacent tissue.
    b. Facial nerve involvement is a sign of advanced disease.
  2. Findings favoring an infectious process: Tenderness on palpation, evidence of duct obstruction, presence of a stone, purulent discharge.
III. Diagnostic studies
  A. Fine-needle aspiration
    1. Accuracy is dependent on operator and cytopathologist experience.
    2. Accuracy in distinguishing benign versus malignant tumors approaches 90% specificity.
    3. Indicated only if results may change decision to operate or extent of operation.
  B. Magnetic resonance imaging
    1. Helpful for larger tumors (>3 cm), especially where there is question of deep lobe parotid involvement.
    2. Visualizes delineation of poorly defined versus sharp margins (useful for distinguishing benign versus malignant processes).
    3. In general, benign lesions demonstrate low T_1-weighted signal intensity but high T_2 signal due to seromucinous content. Malignant lesions show low T_1 and T_2 signal intensities.
    4. Perineural invasion, nodal metastases, and dural involvement may be demonstrated.
  C. Computed tomography
    1. CT is of limited usefulness for neoplastic salivary disease; it may demonstrate bony invasion.
    2. Helpful for stone identification in duct obstruction (usually visible on plain x-ray also).
  D. Nuclear medicine studies
    1. Of historical interest; of minimal use currently for salivary gland disease.
    2. Warthin's tumor and oncocytoma usually have positive uptake of technetium 99.
IV. Benign salivary neoplasms
  A. Pleomorphic adenoma
    1. Pleomorphic adenoma is the most common salivary gland tumor (the most common *malignant* salivary tumor is mucoepidermoid carcinoma).
    2. Represents 65% of parotid and submandibular tumors and 40% of minor gland tumors.
    3. Usually occurs in patients 30 to 50 years old, presenting as a painless, slowly growing mass.
    4. Treated with excision—usually a superficial parotidectomy or extracapsular (5-mm margin) excision, submandibular gland removal, or local excision of minor gland tumors. A cure rate of 95% can be expected when excised with clear surgical margins.
  B. Canalicular and basal cell adenoma (previously known as monomorphic adenoma)
    1. Rule of 75%: Canalicular adenomas present in the upper lip in 75% of cases. Basal cell adenomas present in the parotid gland in 75% of cases.
    2. Female predilection 2:1.
    3. May resemble a mucocele, which is rare in the upper lip.
    4. Surgical excision is usually curative. Recurrence is rare and may actually represent multifocal disease.
  C. Warthin's tumor (papillary cystadenoma lymphomatosum)
    1. Most common site is the parotid gland.
    2. Rule of 10s (a gross simplification)
      a. 10% of all parotid neoplasms are Warthin's tumors.
      b. 10% are bilateral.
      c. 10 times risk in smokers.

d. 10:1 male-to-female ratio.

e. 10% are malignant.

3. **Usually Warthin's tumors are treated with local excision** with minimal margins, or with superficial parotidectomy.

D. Oncocytoma

1. **Rare neoplasm** (<1% of all salivary tumors), predominantly found in older adults.

2. **Usually presents in the major salivary glands,** with 80% arising in the parotid.

3. **Surgical excision is usually curative,** with minimal surrounding tissue taken to establish clear margins.

V. Malignant salivary neoplasms

A. Mucoepidermoid carcinoma

1. **Most common salivary malignancy** (however, the most common salivary *neoplasm* is pleomorphic adenoma).

2. **Mucoepidermoid tumors represent 10% of parotid and submandibular neoplasms,** and 20% of minor gland neoplasms.

3. **Most (70%) are found in the parotid gland,** but they may also arise in the submandibular and minor salivary glands and intraosseous locations.

4. **Classified as low, intermediate, and high grade** based on histopathology.

5. **Treatment is based on grade.**

    a. Low: Surgical excision with narrow margin; 90% cure rate.

    b. High: Treat like squamous cell carcinoma; 30% cure rate with neck dissection and postoperative radiation therapy.

B. Adenoid cystic carcinoma

1. **Represents approximately 10%** of all salivary malignancies and 40% of minor gland malignancies.

2. **Rare in the parotid;** most common malignancy in the submandibular gland.

3. **Composed of** cribriform, tubular, and solid histopathologic types.

4. **Perineural and sometimes intraneural** invasion is present.

5. **Perineural spread** is common, which may include skip lesions (breaks in continuum) that are best seen preoperatively with MRI.

6. **Treat with surgical excision** and radiotherapy; 5-year survival is 70%, but 15-year survival is approximately 10%.

C. Polymorphous low-grade adenocarcinoma

1. **Almost exclusively found in minor salivary glands.**

2. **Presents in hard/soft palate in 60%;** also presents commonly in upper lip and buccal mucosa.

3. **70% occur in women;** commonly presents in sixth to eighth decade of life.

4. **Perineural invasion is common.**

5. **Wide surgical excision** is indicated, including bone when involved.

D. Acinic cell carcinoma

1. **Rare (1%),** low-grade malignancy; metastasis is unlikely.

2. **95% arise** within the parotid gland.

3. **Broad age range** of presentation, from third to eighth decade of life.

4. **Excision** with superficial versus total parotidectomy; submandibular gland removal or wide local excision of minor glands is usually curative.

5. **Radiation therapy** may increase local control.

E. Malignant mixed tumor (carcinoma ex pleomorphic adenoma)

1. **Results from malignant degeneration** of pleomorphic adenoma.

2. **Often presents with rapid growth** in previous slow-growing lesion.

3. **Pain and facial nerve** involvement often present.

4. **Treated with excision,** neck dissection, and radiation therapy. Five-year survival is 50%.

VI. Management of malignant neoplasms

A. Surgical treatment of local disease is usually accomplished with primary tumor control:

1. **Total parotidectomy**

2. **Partial parotidectomy**

       3. **Submandibular gland removal**
       4. **Sublingual/minor gland removal**
  B. Indications for neck dissection
       1. **Dependent on clinical presentation.**
       2. **FNA is indicated for nodes** greater than 10 mm in diameter.
       3. **Primary lesion size** greater than 4 cm increases the likelihood of nodal disease and the need for neck dissection.
  C. Postoperative radiation therapy
       1. **Increases locoregional control** in larger malignancies or close margins.
       2. **60 to 65 Gy** usually administered postoperatively.
  D. Postoperative complications of salivary tumor excision
       1. **Sialocele**
         a. Presents as postoperative swelling with fluid collection.
         b. Aspiration with placement of pressure dressing is usually successful for treatment.
         c. Botulinum toxin injection may be useful for resistant sialoceles.
       2. **Facial nerve damage** (see Chapter 22, "Facial Paralysis")
         a. Damaged nerves should be immediately repaired if transection is noted intraoperatively, or grafted if a branch is intentionally resected for malignant disease.
         b. Loss of the marginal mandibular or temporal branches results in the most significant longstanding deformity due to lack of arborization; the zygomatic and buccal branches have extensive arborization, and distal branches will often recover function.
         c. The zygomatic branch is most important for eye closure and needs consideration for reconstruction if there is evidence of inadequate arborization from the buccal branch.
       3. **Frey's syndrome** (auriculotemporal syndrome)
         a. Caused by reinnervation of sympathetic sudomotor (sweat) fibers by severed parasympathetic (salivomotor) fibers normally directed to parotid gland.
         b. Results in preauricular gustatory sweating (sweating in response to salivary stimulation).
         c. Demonstrated by Minor's starch-iodine test (topical starch/iodine powder mixture turns blue with sweating).
         d. May be relatively common (up to 30%) in patients with parotidectomy.
         e. Initial treatment is topical antiperspirant prior to meals.
         f. Long-term treatment may require botulinum toxin (Botox) injections for control.

Pearls

---

1. **Eighty percent of nonthyroid neck masses** in adults are neoplastic, and of those, 80% are malignant. However, 80% of neck masses in children are benign.
2. **Indications for open biopsy** of a neck mass are as follows:
    a. Persistent for more than 2 to 4 weeks.
    b. Likely metastatic without evidence of primary tumor.
    c. Negative endoscopy with multiple random biopsies.
    d. Negative FNA.
    e. Probable lymphoma.
3. **Slow-growing salivary gland lesions** that suddenly begin rapid enlargement are often carcinoma.
4. **Lower lip masses:** Think mucocele. **Upper lip masses:** Think tumor.
5. **Rule of 10s** for Warthin's tumors:
    a. Comprise 10% of all parotid neoplasms.
    b. 10% are bilateral.
    c. 10 times risk in smokers.
    d. 10:1 male-to-female ratio.

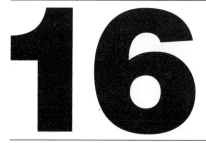

Principles of Head and Neck Reconstruction

Keith G. Wolter

I. Reconstructive goals

A. Patients requiring head and neck reconstructive procedures are often debilitated, and long-term survival is often poor. Many cancer patients must undergo additional radiotherapy or chemotherapy. Therefore, the goal is **rapid reconstruction with optimization of function and low morbidity.** When possible, this is accomplished as a one-stage procedure.

B. For head and neck cancer patients, a **multidisciplinary approach** is best. The reconstructive surgeon is part of a team that includes medical, radiation, and surgical oncologists; pathologists; nutritionists and psychiatrists; and, when needed, dentists, otologists, ophthalmologists, and speech therapists.

C. Specific principles guide head and neck reconstruction planning:

1. **Attempt to restore symmetry.**
2. **Maintain structural integrity of the nose and ears,** for both aesthetic and functional reasons (e.g., support for glasses, nasal airflow).
3. **Maintain competence of the oral and ocular openings,** with particular attention paid to the risk of late scar contractures.
4. **Replace entire anatomic subunits** when reconstructing larger defects for the best aesthetic outcome.
5. **Maintain or restore independent speech,** breathing, and swallowing functions whenever possible.

II. Reconstruction by anatomic region

A. Cutaneous defects of the head and neck (see section IV, "Facial Reconstruction")

B. Midface

1. **Goals**
   a. **Restore the contour** and projection of the region.
   b. **Recreate the maxilla and occlusive surfaces.**
   c. **Separate the oral and nasal cavities.**
   d. Provide support for the eye **or a prosthetic replacement.**
   e. **Maintain flow through the lacrimal system.**
2. **Prosthetics** traditionally have been used extensively in the midface. They may be used alone or in combination with tissue transfers. Maxillectomy defects that do not involve the buttresses or the orbit can be managed effectively with a palatal obturator.
3. **Regional flaps:** The deltopectoral flap, the temporalis muscle flap, and the forehead flap can be used to address small defects.
4. **Nonvascularized bone grafts:** Can be used to fill bony gaps. However, the graft must be covered with adequate, vascularized tissue, and must be rigidly fixed in position.
5. **Free tissue transfer**
   a. The **radial forearm osteocutaneous** flap: A vascularized piece of radius up to 10 cm in length can be harvested with the flap and used for bony support.
   b. **Scapular osteocutaneous** flaps, with or without a skin paddle, may include a portion of the latissimus muscle. They are based either on

the descending or transverse branches of the circumflex scapular artery and the angular branch thereof.

c. **The fibula,** rectus abdominis muscle, and omentum may also be useful in the midface.

C. Mandible

1. **Goals**
   a. **Restore facial contour.**
   b. **Maintain tongue mobility.**
   c. **Restore mastication and speech.**

2. **Reconstruction of large defects** can either be immediate or delayed. The trend is toward immediate reconstruction using a separate surgical team. However, if there is a question regarding surgical margin, or if the patient's health demands it, a delay before reconstruction may be advisable.

3. **Choice of reconstructive technique** depends on the defect size and location. Small bone defects, especially lateral ones, may be subject to either no repair or autologous bone grafts. However, nonvascularized bone grafts tolerate radiation poorly. Metallic implants (such as mandibular reconstruction bars) can serve as spacers to maintain position, but in the long term they are likely to fail or cause complications.

4. **A vascularized bone flap** is the method of choice for fixing most bony defects, particularly anterior ones. These flaps promote bone healing, resist radiation, and permit dental restoration with osseointegrated implants.
   a. **Free fibula flap:** The workhorse vascularized bone flap. A segment of sturdy bone up to 26 cm long can be provided, along with the overlying skin. Based on perforators from the peroneal artery, this flap causes minimal functional deformity. The skin paddle is somewhat unreliable, however. Angiography should be used preoperatively to assess the arterial anatomy and rule out congenital variations that would preclude fibular harvest (although this is somewhat controversial). The left leg is usually chosen as the donor side, because it is used less for certain activities (e.g., driving).
   b. **Iliac crest bone flaps**, based on the deep circumflex iliac artery, have a natural curve resembling the mandible. Both iliac crests can be used to perform a total mandibular reconstruction. **Radius, rib, scapula, and metatarsal** are other donor options for vascularized bone transfers to the mandible.

D. Neck

1. **Goal:** Protect vital neck structure, i.e., vessels, nerves, and airway.

2. **Pedicled pectoralis major flap:** Useful for neck coverage. Maximal mobilization is achieved by dividing the insertion and clavicular attachments. The primary pedicle is the thoracoacromial artery. Overlying skin may be transferred with the flap. The flap is hardy, but bulky.

3. **Pedicled latissimus dorsi flap:** Another useful regional flap. It is a thinner flap than the pectoralis, and the skin paddle is more likely hairless. The donor defect is favorable, and a paddle up to 10 cm can be harvested with primary closure of the skin. A disadvantage is the need for positioning changes when used for anterior neck wounds. Based on the thoracodorsal branch of the subscapular artery, the flap may be tunneled either below the pectoralis major or subcutaneously along the anterior chest. A common problem with this flap is seroma formation at the donor site; drains are mandatory.

4. **Trapezius flap:** Three different flaps can be raised.
   a. **Superior trapezius flap:** Based on the occipital artery and paravertebral perforators. It is the most reliable. Its skin paddle extends laterally across the top of the scapula.
   b. **Inferior trapezius flap:** Relies on the descending branch of the transverse cervical artery. It can be used as either a muscle or a myocutaneous flap. Its point of rotation is posterior, at the base of the neck.

      c. Lateral trapezius flap: Based on the transverse cervical artery over the acromion. It can be useful for small lateral defects.

    5. Deltopectoral flap: Based on perforators arising from the internal mammary artery. A delay procedure will permit more lateral skin to be used safely. This flap is thin and can reach the mouth, but leaves an unattractive donor site.

E. Oral cavity

    1. Goals

      a. Maintain oral competence.

      b. Provide support for the floor of the mouth.

      c. Prevent aspiration by maintaining or restoring sensation and mobility.

    2. Tongue flaps: Can be used for closure of small intraoral defects, as long as care is taken not to tether the tongue.

    3. Palatal or palatopharyngeal flaps: Can be used to fix small defects in the palate.

    4. Free radial forearm flap: The first choice for larger intraoral defects. Based on the radial artery and venae comitantes and/or cephalic/basilic veins, it is ideal for intraoral lining because of flap thinness. It can be made sensate by attaching the lingual nerve to the lateral antebrachial cutaneous nerve.

    5. Pedicled latissimus dorsi flap: Can be used for extensive oral cavity defects. This flap has the advantage of large size, but the arc of rotation can limit its use in the oral cavity. Alternatively, it can be used as a free flap.

    6. Gastroomental free flap: Provides a secreting mucosal surface useful in preventing postradiation xerostomia.

F. Tongue

    1. Goal: Recapture mobility to preserve speech and swallowing functions.

    2. The tongue heals exceptionally well. Infection, scarring, and tissue loss are rare.

    3. Partial tongue loss: Can be repaired with "setback" procedures, using the contralateral anterior tongue to provide bulk and support to the tongue base. Outcomes from these procedures are typically excellent, provided that at least one hypoglossal nerve is maintained.

    4. Total tongue reconstruction following glossectomy usually yields less than perfect results. Goals for the neotongue are airway protection, swallowing, and articulation. Bulk placement in the oral cavity can aid in food propulsion and form a seal against the palate. Choices for reconstruction are as follows.

      a. Rectus abdominis free flap: The large volume of the flap permits the creation of two or three separate cutaneous islands for complex reconstructions.

      b. Latissimus dorsi: Can be used as either a free or pedicled flap.

G. Hypopharynx

    1. Hypopharyngeal and esophagopharyngeal defects are characterized as either partial or circumferential (total).

    2. For partial defects, the hypopharynx can be restored in a number of ways.

      a. Primary closure: Care must be taken not to narrow the lumen excessively (the pharynx must permit passage of at least a 34 French catheter in order to permit swallowing).

      b. Skin or dermal grafts may be used for partial defects of the lining of esophagus or pharynx. They are initially secured with a stent to allow adherence and prevent stricture formation.

      c. The pectoralis, latissimus, and trapezius can be used to "patch" holes.

    3. Circumferential reconstruction

      a. Free jejunum: The flap of choice. A proximal segment is isolated on its mesentery and transferred to the neck, where it is placed in an isoperistaltic orientation. Endoscopic jejunum harvest is possible. Complications include a "wet" voice, halitosis, and dysphagia.

    b. Tubed radial forearm flap: Particularly useful when jejunal harvest is not advisable. This reconstruction is associated with a high incidence of stricture formation.

    c. Gastric transposition: For patients with tumors that extend below the cervical esophagus.

Pearls

1. **Feeding via gastrostomy or jejunostomy tubes** may be necessary for long-term management, particularly for patients who will require radiation therapy.
2. **Feeding tubes** should be placed at the time of reconstruction.
3. **A reliable speech therapist** is invaluable for postoperative care of head and neck reconstruction patients.

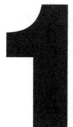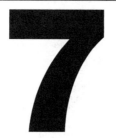

Eyelid Reconstruction

Adam S. Hassan

I. Eyelid anatomy (Figs. 17-1 and 17-2)

  A. Eyelid skin is the thinnest in the body.

  B. Lid protractor (constrictor) muscles

  1. **The orbicularis oculi** is the main protractor of the eyelids. Innervated by cranial nerve (CN) VII (underside of muscle).

   a. The pretarsal orbicularis lies over the tarsus and is involved in involuntary eyelid closure (blinking). It encircles the canaliculi, facilitating tear drainage.

   b. The preseptal orbicularis lies over the septum. It is involved in involuntary eyelid closure (blinking).

   c. The orbital orbicularis lies over the orbital rims and is involved in forced closure of the eyelids.

  2. **The corrugator supercilii muscle** originates from the supranasal orbital rim and inserts in the medial portion of the eyebrow. It is responsible for vertical furrows of the glabella.

  3. **The procerus muscle** originates from the frontal bone of the glabella and inserts into the skin of the glabella, producing horizontal furrows over the bridge of the nose.

  C. The orbital septum consists of multilayered fibrous tissue and arises from the periosteum of the superior and inferior orbital rims. It fuses with the levator aponeurosis in the upper lid and the capsulopalpebral fascia in the lower lid, forming the anatomic boundary between the eyelid and the orbit.

  D. Orbital fat is present posterior to the septum and anterior to the eyelid retractors.

  E. Lid retractor muscles

  1. **Upper eyelid retractors**

   a. The levator muscle is the main retractor of the upper eyelid. It is innervated by the superior division of CN III. It originates at the orbital apex; the muscular portion travels 40 mm, then transitions to aponeurotic portion at Whitnall's ligament (fulcrum for levator muscle), and then travels 14 to 20 mm before inserting on the anterior surface of the lower one-half of the tarsal plate. Anterior fibers travel through the orbicularis to the skin, creating the upper eyelid crease. The lateral horn of the aponeurosis divides the lacrimal gland into orbital and palpebral lobes.

   b. Müller's muscle provides 2 mm of upper eyelid elevation and is sympathetically innervated. It originates from the undersurface of the levator aponeurosis at the level of Whitnall's ligament and inserts on the superior tarsal margin. The peripheral arterial arcade is between the levator aponeurosis and Müller's muscle just above the superior tarsal border.

  2. **Lower eyelid retractors**

   a. The capsulopalpebral fascia is analogous to the levator aponeurosis in the upper eyelid. Originates from inferior rectus muscle, travels anteriorly, and splits to surround the inferior oblique muscle. The split portions of the fascia reunite as Lockwood's suspensory ligament (equivalent to Whitnall's ligament).

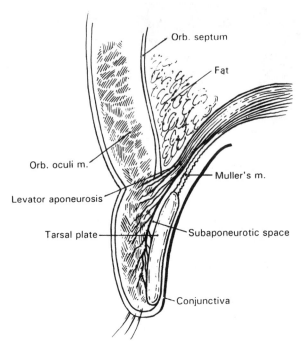

Fig. 17-1. Upper eyelid anatomy. Cross-section of the upper lid. The levator aponeurosis insertion is on top of the tarsus and into the orbicularis muscle. The conjunctiva is inseparable from the tarsal plate at that point. (From Carraway J. Reconstruction of the eyelids and correction of ptosis of the eyelid. In *Grabb and Smith's Plastic Surgery*, 5th ed. Aston SJ, Beasley RW, Thorne CH. Philadelphia, Lippincott-Raven Publishers, 1997. With permission.)

   b. The inferior tarsal muscle is comparable to Müller's muscle. It is located posterior to capsulopalpebral fascia and inserts on the inferior tarsus.
F. The tarsal plate is made of dense connective tissue that provides structural support to the eyelids.
   1. The upper lid tarsus measures 10 to 12 mm.
   2. The lower lid tarsus measures 4 mm.
   3. In the upper eyelid the marginal arcade runs 2 mm superior to the lid margin and anterior to the tarsus.
   4. Oil-secreting meibomian glands are present within the tarsi.
G. Conjunctiva: Nonkeratinized squamous epithelium provides the posterior layer of the eyelid.
H. Canthal tendons
   1. Medial canthal tendon: Two limbs originate from the anterior and posterior lacrimal crest, fusing lateral to the lacrimal sac and again splitting to attach to the upper and lower tarsal plates.
   2. Lateral canthal tendon: Begins at the lateral orbital tubercle on the inner aspect of the lateral orbital rim. It splits into superior and inferior limbs, attaching to the upper and lower tarsal plates.
I. Vascular supply: Supplied by two main sources that anastomose, forming the marginal and peripheral arcades.
   1. Internal carotid, by way of the ophthalmic artery and its branches (the supraorbital and lacrimal arteries)
   2. External carotid, by way of the angular and temporal arteries

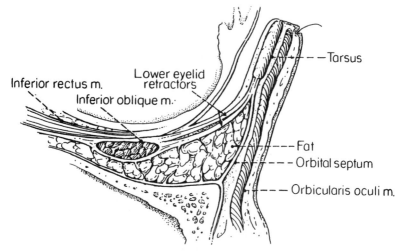

Fig. 17-2. Lower eyelid anatomy. (From Shamoun J and Ellenbogen R Blepharoplasty, forehead, and eyebrow lift. In the textbook, *Plastic, Maxillofacial, and Reconstructive Surgery*, 3rd ed. Georgiade G, Riefkohl R, Levin S (eds). Philadelphia, Williams & Wilkins, 1997. With permission.)

    J. Innervation
        1. Sensory: CN V
            a. Upper eyelid: V1
            b. Lower eyelid: V2
        2. Motor
            a. CN III
            b. CN VII
            c. Sympathetic innervation
  II. Clinical eyelid measurements
    A. Palpebral fissure: Distance between upper and lower lid margins (normal 10 mm).
    B. Marginal reflex distance: Distance from pupillary light reflex to upper eyelid margin (normal 4 mm).
    C. Levator muscle excursion: Excursion of upper lid from downgaze to upgaze (normal 12–15 mm).
    D. Lid crease: Distance from lash line to upper eyelid crease (variable).
  III. Entropion: Inversion of the lid margin
    A. Congenital
        1. Rare condition that is primarily the result of developmental aberrations such as lower eyelid retractor dysgenesis and structural abnormalities of the tarsus.
        2. Treatment: Typically surgical.
    B. Acute spastic
        1. Occurs after ocular irritation or inflammation. Sustained orbicularis muscle contraction causes inversion of the margin.
        2. Treatment: Temporizing by taping the eyelid. Botulinum toxin to the overriding orbicularis muscle. Surgical repair may be necessary.
    C. Involutional
        1. Factors
            a. Horizontal laxity
            b. Disinsertion of eyelid retractors
            c. Overriding of preseptal orbicularis

      2. Occurs more commonly in the lower eyelid
      3. Treatment
        a. Temporizing measures: Quickert sutures to evert the margin.
        b. Horizontal tightening of the lateral canthal tendon.
        c. Reinsertion of the lower eyelid retractors to the tarsus.
        d. Eyelid margin rotation with procedure such as full-thickness Wies repair.

  D. Cicatricial
    1. Scarring and contracture of tarsus and conjunctiva
      a. Autoimmune: Ocular cicatricial pemphigoid.
      b. Inflammatory: Stevens-Johnson syndrome.
      c. Infectious: Herpes zoster, trachoma.
      d. Postsurgical scarring.
      e. Trauma.
      f. Burn (chemical or thermal).
      g. Glaucoma medications.
    2. Treatment
      a. Control inflammation with immunosuppression.
      b. Marginal rotation if inflammation is controlled.
      c. Do not violate conjunctiva if there is active inflammation.
      d. Tarsus may need to be replaced with a tarsoconjunctival graft, oral mucous membrane, hard palate, or ear cartilage.

IV. Ectropion: Outward turning of the eyelid
  A. Congenital
    1. Primarily associated with blepharophimosis syndrome.
    2. Rarely isolated.
    3. If severe may require surgical repair.
  B. Involutional
    1. Occurs secondary to horizontal eyelid laxity.
    2. Commonly lateral and medial canthal tendon laxity.
    3. Usually affects lower eyelid.
    4. Treatment
      a. Mild punctal ectropion: Treated with conjunctival cautery or an excision of conjunctiva and lower eyelid retractors closed with inverting sutures (medial spindle procedure).
      b. Moderate to severe ectropion: Treated with horizontal shortening, lateral or medial canthal tightening, and lateral canthoplasty or reinsertion of lower eyelid retractors.
      c. Frequently a combination of procedures is performed.
  C. Paralytic
    1. Secondary to CN VII palsy.
    2. Corneal sensation should be assessed to rule out associated neurotrophic keratitis.
    3. Treatment
      a. Aggressive lubrication.
      b. Horizontal eyelid tightening, medial or lateral.
      c. Temporary tarsorrhaphy (medial or lateral) with permanent suture (1–3 weeks) depending on potential of return of VII nerve function.
      d. Permanent tarsorhaphy with removal of epithelium and use of absorbable sutures to secure upper and lower eyelid tarsal plates together.
      e. Elevation of lower eyelid (with hard palate graft if necessary).
      f. Gold weights to pretarsal upper lid to eliminate upper lid lagophthalmos.
  D. Cicatricial
    1. Etiologies
      a. Chronic inflammation of the skin (e.g., rosacea, atopic dermatitis, herpes zoster, eczema).
      b. Actinic skin changes.
      c. Chemical or thermal burns.
      d. Surgical or mechanical trauma.

2. Treatment
  a. Treat underlying etiology.
  b. Surgical incision of cicatricial scarring with vertical lengthening of eyelid with full-thickness skin graft.
  c. Lower eyelid may need concomitant horizontal shortening.

E. Mechanical
  1. Secondary to gravity acting upon large tumors or excess lower eyelid skin and prolapsing orbital fat.
  2. Treatment involves removing mechanical component.

V. Ptosis of the eyelid (blepharoptosis)
A. Myogenic
  1. Congenital: Dysgenesis of levator muscle.
  a. Fatty infiltration of muscle belly.
  b. When associated with a poor Bell's phenomenon or decreased supraduction and a vertical strabismus, it is termed double elevator palsy.
  2. Acquired (diffuse muscle disease): Etiologies include muscular dystrophy, chronic progressive external ophthalmoplegia, myasthenia gravis, or oculopharyngeal dystrophy.
  3. Treatment.
  a. Surgical treatment is based on levator function.
  b. Levator excursion greater than 5 mm may be amenable to levator resection.
  c. Levator excursion less than 5 mm typically requires frontalis suspension.

B. Aponeurotic
  1. Congenital: Failure of aponeurosis to insert to tarsal plate; may be associated with birth trauma.
  2. Acquired: Dehiscence of levator aponeurosis from normal insertion.
  a. Most common form of ptosis.
  b. Caused by involutional changes.
  c. May be exacerbated by ocular surgery.
  d. Associated with high, indistinct lid crease.
  e. Good levator muscle function is usually present.
  3. Treatment: Levator advancement surgery
  a. External incision through the lid crease. Identify levator aponeurosis and secure it to the tarsal plate.
  b. Transconjunctival approach may be used, resecting Müller's muscle, levator, or tarsus.
  c. Fasanella-Servat procedure: Resection of conjunctiva, superior tarsal border, and Müller's muscle.

C. Neurogenic
  1. Congenital: Innervation deficiencies during embryologic development
  a. CN III palsy: Typically associated with inability to elevate, depress, or adduct the globe. Rarely an isolated finding. Primarily requires frontalis suspension.
  b. Horner's syndrome: Secondary to decreased sympathetic innervation to Müller's muscle. Has associated miosis. Pharmacologic testing can be used to identify which order neuron is responsible for the deficit.
  c. Synkinetic neurogenic ptosis (most commonly "Marcus Gunn jaw-winking"): Unilateral ptotic eyelid elevates when the jaw is opened. Results from an aberrant connection between the motor division of CN V and the levator muscle.
  2. Acquired
  a. CN III palsy: Vasculopathic or compressive. If pupil dilation is associated, a compressive lesion must be ruled out. The most common cause is vasculopathic and is usually associated with systemic disease such as diabetes, hypertension, and atherosclerosis.
  b. Horner's syndrome: Identify order neuron with deficit.
  c. Myasthenia gravis: Reserve surgical repair to those failing medical management.

   D. Mechanical: Secondary to gravity exerting downward force on tumor associated with the upper eyelid.

   E. Traumatic: If upper eyelid laceration has associated prolapsing orbital fat, then injury to the levator muscle or aponeurosis should be suspected. Exploration may be undertaken at the time of repair. If ptosis is present after a repair, then wait 6 months for possible return of full levator function.

VI. Eyelid and canthal reconstruction

  A. Lid margin laceration repair

    1. Align the lid margin.

    2. Suture the tarsal plate together with partial-thickness passes with no exposure on the conjunctival surface.

    3. Suture the lid margin with a vertical mattress closure.

    4. Close the skin.

  B. Upper eyelid reconstruction

    1. Defect of 33% or less: Primary eyelid closure with appropriate margin repair.

    2. Defect of 33% to 50%: Lateral canthotomy and cantholysis to release lateral aspect of the lid with advancement of lateral myocutaneous flap.

    3. Defect of 50% to 75%: Tenzel semicircular flap—involves performing a lateral canthotomy and cantholysis, and then advancing a myocutaneous flap designed in the shape of an arch.

    4. Defect of greater than 75%

      a. Cutler-Beard procedure: A full-thickness lower eyelid flap advanced beneath the lower eyelid margin and secured in the upper eyelid defect (requires two stages, with division of the flap from the lower lid in 2 to 3 weeks).

      b. Free tarsoconjunctival graft taken from contralateral upper eyelid and then covered with any remaining upper eyelid skin.

  C. Lower eyelid defects

    1. Defect of 33% or less: Primary eyelid closure with appropriate margin repair.

    2. Defect of 33% to 50%: Lateral canthotomy and cantholysis with advancement of lateral myocutaneous flap.

    3. Defect of 50% to 75%

      a. Tenzel semicircular flap: Involves performing a lateral canthotomy and cantholysis and then advancing a myocutaneous flap designed in the shape of an arch.

      b. Mustarde cheek rotation flap: A large myocutaneous advancement flap that needs to be placed over a tarsoconjunctival graft, giving posterior eyelid support.

    4. Defect of greater than 75%: Hughes procedure is a tarsoconjunctival flap from the upper eyelid that contains its own blood supply. The flap must be covered with a full-thickness skin graft or a myocutaneous advancement flap. A second stage is required to open the flap, creating the new lower eyelid margin.

  D. Medial canthal defects

    1. Explore lacrimal drainage system and perform specialized repair with silicone tube intubation if violated.

    2. Secure the medial canthal tendon if it has been disrupted.

      a. Anterior limb to frontal process of maxilla.

      b. Posterior limb to posterior lacrimal crest.

    3. Address skin deficit.

      a. Small defects heal well secondarily.

      b. Full-thickness skin grafts may be used for larger defects.

      c. Median forehead flap may be used for even larger defects.

  E. Lateral canthal defects

    1. A lateral tarsal strip can be used to secure lower eyelid tarsus to the periosteum of the lateral orbital rim.

2. **A periosteal flap** can be extended from the lateral orbital rim to the remaining lateral eyelids.
3. **Myocutaneous advancement flaps** or full-thickness skin grafts are used for skin and muscle deficit.

Pearls

1. **In Graves' eye disease** rehabilitation, first perform orbital decompression, followed by strabismus surgery and finally eyelid surgery.
2. **When operating on the eyelid,** do not attempt to close the orbital septum.
3. **When reconstructing the lower eyelid,** do not allow vertical tension on your closure in order to avoid ectropion.
4. **Take preoperative photographs** before all cases, including trauma cases.
5. **Mark incision lines** with a marking pen prior to injecting local anesthetic.

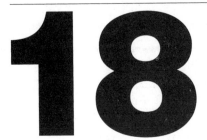

Nasal Reconstruction

J. Jason Wendel

I. History
  A. "Indian method"
    1. 600 BCE: Sushruta Samhita (forehead and cheek flaps).
    2. 1440 CE: Kanghiara family (forehead flap).
    3. 1816: Carpue reported the "Indian method" in the English literature.
  B. "French method": Cheek flaps
  C. "Italian method"
    1. 15th century: The Brancas of Sicily used cheek and arm flaps.
    2. 1597: Gaspare Tagliacozzi used the arm flap.
II. Nasal anatomy
  A. The nose is divided into thirds, according to the underlying support.
    1. Proximal third: Nasal bones and bony septum.
    2. Middle third: Upper lateral cartilages and septum.
    3. Distal third: Cartilaginous septum and alar cartilages.
      a. Medial crura.
      b. Alar domes.
      c. Lower lateral cartilages.
  B. The soft tissue envelope conforms to the underlying structures.
    1. The zone of thin skin (dorsum and columella) is loose and mobile, with few sebaceous glands.
    2. The zone of thick skin (nasal tip and ala) is fixed to the underlying cartilage and is oily, with many sebaceous glands.
  C. Vascular anatomy
    1. Arterial anatomy
      a. The angular arteries supply each side of the nose, as continuations of the facial arteries.
      b. The superior labial artery sends branches to the lower borders of the alae and the nasal septum.
      c. The dorsal nasal branch of the ophthalmic artery supplies the dorsum and the sides of the nose.
      d. The infraorbital branch of the internal maxillary artery also sends vessels to the dorsum and sides.
    2. Venous anatomy: The venous drainage of the nose parallels its arterial supply. Of note, the angular vein becomes the anterior facial vein, which has communication with the ophthalmic veins, which ultimately communicate with the cavernous sinus.
  D. Sensory innervation: Derived from the trigeminal nerve (cranial nerve V)
    1. Ophthalmic division (V1).
      a. Nasociliary nerve: Directly to the nose.
      b. Infratrochlear nerve: Provides indirect sensation to the nose.
      c. External branch of anterior ethmoidal nerve.
    2. Maxillary division (V2): Sends branches via the infraorbital nerve to the nasal sides and caudal septum.
  E. Motor innervation: The muscles of the nose are innervated by the facial nerve (cranial nerve VII). These muscles include the procerus, depressor septi nasi, and the nasalis.

III. Basics of nasal reconstruction

A. Goals: Maintain a patent airway and achieve an optimal aesthetic appearance.

B. Adequate reconstruction demands the replacement of all missing layers with similar tissue, including the following:
1. **Nasal lining**
2. **Architectural support (bone and cartilage)**
3. **Skin/soft tissue coverage**

C. Timing: Immediate reconstruction is undertaken unless
1. Tumor margins are questionable.
2. Aggressive tumor histology warrants observation or intermediate reconstructive efforts.
3. Deep bony and/or perineural invasion is present.
4. Radiation therapy is planned.

IV. Principles of aesthetic units (Fig. 18-1)

A. Burget and Menick characterized nine topographic subunits of the nose.
1. Dorsum
2. Tip
3. Columella
4. Sidewall (two)
5. Ala (two)
6. Soft triangle (two)

B. The tip, ala, sill, and columella compose the nasal lobule.

C. If possible, incisions should be designed along the borders of adjacent subunits for camouflage.

D. As a general rule, if the defect occupies more than 50% of a subunit, enlarge the defect to incorporate the entire subunit. Reconstruction of an entire subunit is generally aesthetically more pleasing.

E. If available, use an undamaged contralateral subunit as a model on which to pattern the missing subunit.

F. Divide large defects into multiple subunits and address each with a separate graft or flap; avoid the temptation to reconstruct multiple subunits with one large flap.

V. Reconstructing nasal skin cover

A. Goals
1. **Replace skin with a similar color, thickness, and texture** to that surrounding the defect.

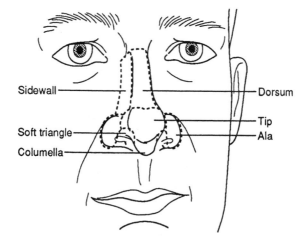

Fig. 18-1. Aesthetic subunits of the nose.

2. Design the reconstruction to fit the various unique locations of the nose by respecting the aesthetic units (e.g., dorsum and lateral sidewalls, nasal tip and alae, and the columella).

3. Follow the reconstructive ladder.

B. **Healing by secondary intention**

1. Defects of the glabella and medial canthus will usually heal favorably by secondary intention.

2. Defects of the nasal tip and alae that are allowed to heal by secondary intention usually cause distortion and notching.

C. **Split-thickness skin graft**

1. Prone to contraction and distortion.

2. A possible option when surveillance is necessary for recurrence of a high-grade lesion.

D. **Full-thickness skin graft**

1. Postauricular grafts: Good match; donor site is hidden.

2. Preauricular grafts: Also a good match and relatively well hidden.

3. Nasolabial fold: Good match for color and texture; donor scar is more noticeable.

4. Supraclavicular area: Good match for texture, and color is acceptable, but the donor scar is prominent.

E. **Chondrocutaneous grafts (composite):** Suited for small defects of all three layers at the alar rim or columella. Composite grafts are harvested from the helical root, helical margins, and concha. Their survival depends on a well-vascularized wound edge; they do not do well in an irradiated field. The maximum recommended composite graft width is 1.5 cm.

F. **Local flaps** exploit the laxity of the upper two-thirds of the nose to cover the lower one-third. In general, they are good for defects of up to 2 cm in diameter.

1. **Banner flap** (Fig. 18-2A): Essentially a transposition flap. Its use is usually limited to defects less than 1.2 cm in diameter.

2. **Bilobed (Zitelli) flap** (Fig. 18-2B): Designed at 90 to 100 degrees to exploit the laxity of skin in the upper third of the nose for reconstruction of more caudal defects.

3. **Glabellar flap:** Transfers skin from the loose area of the glabella to the nasal radix to repair defects in this area. Incisions can be well hidden in glabellar furrows.

4. **Dorsonasal flap (Rieger flap)** (Fig. 18-2C): This sickle-shaped flap is based laterally and is elevated to include the angular vessel on one side. The entire skin from the nasal dorsum is rotated and advanced caudally. It is limited to defects less than 2 cm, and will not reach the columella.

5. **Nasalis V-Y flap:** A sliding flap from the upper alar crease may be advanced to cover small defects of the lateral nasal tip.

6. **Nasolabial flap:** A versatile flap primarily used to reconstruct portions of the lobule and the nasal sidewall (Fig. 18-3A, B). It can be pedicled (superiorly or inferiorly), tunneled, made into an island, or turned over to create nasal lining. The donor site is closed primarily and heals very well. Two stages are generally required for division and inset, and a third may be needed for debulking.

7. **Cheek flap:** Best suited for replacement of the nasal sidewalls.

G. **Regional flaps:** Good for defects larger than 2 cm in diameter and for total nasal reconstruction.

1. **Forehead flap:** Paramedian or midline forehead flaps (Fig. 18-3C, D) can be elevated on either the supraorbital or supratrochlear vessels from one or both sides. The typical forehead flap is based on a single supratrochlear pedicle. It is the workhorse flap for large tip defects and for subtotal and total nasal reconstruction. The residual donor site defect is allowed to heal by secondary intention, with excellent aesthetic results. Tissue expansion should be avoided.

2. **Scalping flap:** This flap reliably delivers a large amount of skin from the forehead to the nose to repair large defects. It is raised through a coronal

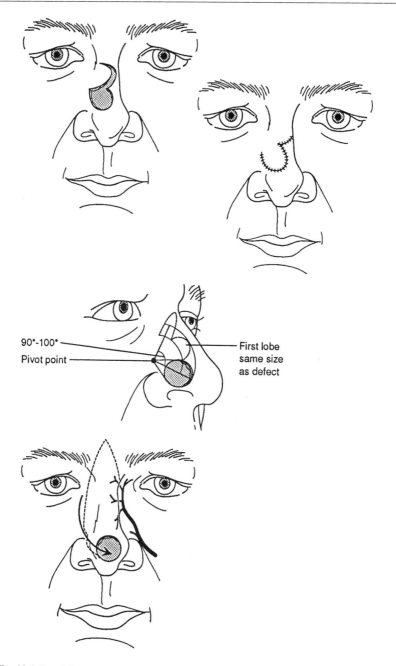

Fig. 18-2. Local flaps for nasal skin cover exploit the laxity of the upper two-thirds of the nose to cover the lower one-third, as in these examples. **A:** The Banner flap is a transpositional flap suitable for small defects of the dorsum or sidewall. **B:** The bilobed flap is a double transposition flap. The second flap is designed at 90 to 100 degrees from the first. **C:** The Rieger (sickle-shaped dorsonasal) flap is based laterally on the angular artery.

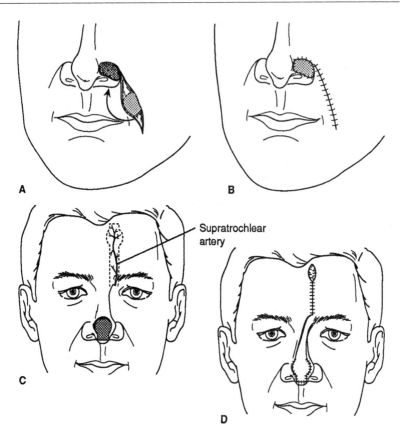

Fig. 18-3. A, B: Nasolabial flap. Two stages are required for division and inset, and a third may be needed for debulking. **C, D:** Paramedian forehead flap before and following inset. The forehead flap is a versatile workhorse flap for nasal reconstruction.

incision posterior to the superficial temporal artery, and the skin paddle extends to the contralateral forehead. The forehead donor site is closed with a skin graft, and the temporary scalp defect is kept moist with a temporary dressing. The flap is divided and inset in a second stage, with the scalp pedicle being returned to its original position. This flap provides a good color and texture match, but the donor site deformity is significant.

    3. Temporomastoid (Washio) flap: The posterior auricular skin is carried to the nose, based on the superficial temporal artery. This brings in thin, pliable postauricular skin and/or thicker mastoid skin. The skin is hairless and ample for complete nasal coverage. Some auricular cartilage may be included with the flap.

  H. Distant flaps (free tissue transfer): The flap may be prelaminated prior to transfer. In general, free flaps are bulky, with poor color match. The facial or labial vessels are often used as recipient vessels.

VI. Reconstructing nasal support
  A. Goals: Provide the foundation for nasal projection, airway patency, and appearance.
  B. Two distinct components
    1. Midline support.
      a. Nasal bones, leading edge of septal cartilage, and the medial crura.

   b. Should be fairly rigid.

   c. Provides tip projection and elevation, as well as tip definition.

  2. Lateral support.

   a. Nasal bones, upper lateral cartilages, and alar cartilages

   b. Should be flexible.

   c. Plays a role in internal nasal valve competency; keeps nostrils open, and prevents cephalad contraction.

C. Reconstruction of midline support

 1. L-strut: A longitudinal piece of bone or cartilage is seated on the radix and extends along the dorsum to the nasal tip. It then bends sharply to rest on the anterior nasal spine. This "hockey stick" configuration is usually carved from rib and results in a thickened columella. It has poor lateral stability.

 2. Hinged septal flap: Described by Millard in 1967, an L-shaped flap of septum is hinged superiorly on the caudal end of the nasal bones and swung anteriorly to support the dorsum and the tip.

 3. Septal pivot flap: Described by Gillies in 1920 as a composite flap, the entire septum is rotated forward based on a narrow pedicle caudally centered over the septal branch of the superior labial artery.

 4. Cantilever graft: A strip of bone is rigidly fixed to the nasal or the frontal bones, and is placed along the dorsum. If possible, the cartilaginous portion of the rib is used to restore the pliability of the nasal tip.

 5. Alloplastic materials: Materials such as vitallium and titanium mesh and porous polyethylene have been used as substitutes in the absence of adequate bone and cartilage; however, there is a high risk of implant exposure and infection.

D. Reconstruction of lateral support

 1. Alar cartilages: A 4- to 6-mm wide strip of cartilage can be carved from septal or conchal donor sites to replace one or both alae. Further tip definition can be achieved by adding grafts to the tip (i.e., Peck-style tip grafts).

 2. Upper lateral cartilages and nasal bones: Trapezoidal cartilage and rib grafts can be positioned on the nasal sidewall to support the middle vault against collapse and also serve as a platform for eyewear.

 3. Alar batten grafts: Additional strips of cartilage 4 to 6 mm in width can be tunneled or fastened to the leading edge of the alar rim from the alar base to the tip. This helps to resist alar notching and collapse.

E. Cartilage and bone grafts

 1. Require a well-vascularized bed to remain viable.

 2. Should be introduced at the time of reconstruction of the lining and skin.

 3. Sources of cartilage: Nasal septum, auricle, or rib.

 4. Sources of bone: Rib, calvarium, iliac crest, metatarsal, tibia, or ulna.

VII. Reconstructing nasal lining

A. Goals: Replace lining to protect structural support and prevent deformity by contraction.

B. Turn-in flaps: Hinged on the edge of the defect and flipped over to provide lining. These flaps are particularly useful when skeletal support needs to be introduced at a later time because they allow for two independently vascularized surfaces.

C. Folded regional flaps: A forehead flap can be turned over to provide lining. External coverage is accomplished with a full-thickness skin graft, another forehead flap, or a cheek flap.

D. Skin graft to forehead flap: A full-thickness skin graft is placed on the undersurface of a forehead flap to serve as nasal lining.

 1. Gillies described using a composite graft of skin and cartilage from the ear.

 2. Converse grafted a chondromucosal segment from the nasal septum onto the tip of a forehead flap.

E. Septal door flap: This technique involves folding down of septal mucosa ipsilateral to the defect and dissection of an appropriately sized flap of septal cartilage with contralateral mucosa attached. A "septal door" is then swung with the dorsal hinge toward the reconstructive side. A sufficient amount of septum has to be left in place along the dorsum to support the midline, prevent collapse, and help with nasal projection.

F. Septal mucoperichondrial flap: A large, caudally based rectangle of mucosa or a composite of mucosa and perichondrium is elevated, based on the septal branch of the superior labial artery. The flap pivots on an anterior, inferior point near the nasal spine and folds outward to furnish lining for the nasal domes.

G. Mucosal advancement flap: A bipedicled mucosal advancement flap is based medially on the remaining septum and laterally on the piriform aperture. The vascularized mucosa can immediately support a cartilage graft to give support to the alar rim. The donor site can be covered with a contralateral chondromucosal flap or with a flap from the ipsilateral nasal septum.

H. Timing

   1. Immediate: It is preferable to provide nasal lining, structural support, and soft tissue coverage in the same operation. This promotes even healing and offers maximum flexibility of the tissues before scar contraction takes place. In the event of partial tissue necrosis of the lining or support, secondary contracture will cause distortion.

   2. Staged: When large defects in nasal lining exist, some surgeons stage the reconstruction and attach the lining to a regional flap as a preliminary procedure. Once the lining has vascularized, the entire flap is then transferred. This is a safe, conservative maneuver; however, cicatricial stiffening limits flexibility and inhibits later sculpting of the tissues.

VIII. Reconstruction by prosthesis

   A. Indicated in the nonsurgical candidate.

   B. Osseointegrated implants placed in conjunction with a prosthesis can be quite successful.

   C. Prostheses can also be suspended from eyeglasses, providing a relatively natural appearance.

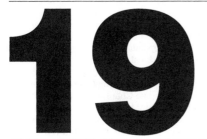

Lip and Cheek Reconstruction

Timothy A. Janiga

Lip Reconstruction

I. **Lip anatomy and physiology**
  A. **Topography**
    1. **The Cupid's bow** is the upper central vermilion border at the base of the philtral columns.
    2. **The vermilion border** (mucocutaneous line, or white roll) is the transition between the mucosa of the lip and skin.
    3. **The normal intercommissural distance** in an adult at rest is 6 cm.
  B. **Aesthetic units:** The lip is divided into four units.
    1. **Lateral wings:** Between the philtral columns and nasolabial folds.
    2. **Philtrum:** Between the philtral columns.
    3. **Lower lip:** Between the vermilion and labiomental fold.
    4. **Vermilion:** Between the vermilion border and dry-wet line.
  C. **Muscular anatomy** and motor innervation.
    1. **The facial nerve:** Exits the skull via the stylomastoid foramen, traverses the parotid gland (dividing it into the superficial and deep lobes), and innervates the muscles of facial expression on the deep surface (except for the mentalis, levator angularis superioris, and buccinator muscles). It divides into five main branches: temporal, zygomatic, buccal, mandibular, and cervical.
    2. **The marginal mandibular branch:** Runs below the angle of the mandible deep to the platysma. Proximally it lies superficial to the upper part of the digastric triangle and then turns superior and medial across the body of the mandible deep to the depressor anguli oris, where it innervates the muscles of the lower lip and chin, particularly the depressor anguli oris. Injury to this branch results in an abnormally elevated side of the lower lip while smiling.
    3. **The temporal branch:** Travels along a line 0.5 cm below the tragus to 1.5 cm above the lateral end of the eyebrow. Inferior to the zygomatic arch the nerve runs between the superficial and deep layers of the deep temporal fascia in the buccal fat pad. Above this level the nerve becomes more superficial and runs superficial to the superficial temporal fascia.
  D. **Sensory innervation**
    1. **Upper lip:** Superior labial nerve from the infraorbital nerve from the trigeminal nerve (cranial nerve V2).
    2. **Lower lip:** Mental nerve from the inferior alveolar nerve from the trigeminal nerve (cranial nerve V3). The mental nerve exits in the middle of the height of the mandible, inferior to the second premolar.
  E. **Blood supply:** Superior and inferior labial arteries arise from the facial artery. They are located 1 mm posterior to the white roll and 1 mm deep to the mucosa of the lip. The labial arteries lie deep to the orbicularis oris muscle.
  F. **Lymphatic drainage:** Upper and lower lateral lip drain into the submandibular nodes. The central lower lip drains into the submental nodes.

II. Functional considerations

    A. Oral competence: Compromise results in drooling; seen with a loss of sensation, innervation, and depth of lower lip sulcus.

    B. Microstomia can lead to difficulty with eating, denture use, and cleaning and repairing teeth. This can be treated with stretching appliances.

    C. Communication: Lip surgery usually has few long-term effects on speech.

III. Etiology and pathology of lip defects (see Chapter 14, "Squamous Cell Carcinoma of the Head and Neck," and Chapter 11, "Malignant Skin and Soft Tissue Lesions"): Neoplasm is responsible for most cases (>95%), but other etiologies include trauma, congenital nevi, hemangiomas, infections, and vasculitis.

IV. Superficial lip defects

    A. Reconstructive ladder

        1. Split-thickness skin grafts (STSGs): Should only be used as a temporary closure because of problems with contracture and scarring.

        2. Full-thickness skin grafts (FTSGs): Superior to STSGs.

        3. Local flaps are the best option.

            a. Nasolabial and cheek advancement flaps for skin replacement

            b. Labial mucosa flaps for vermilion replacement

    B. Vermilion

        1. Mark above and below the white roll with methylene blue on the tip of a needle. This provides a landmark after local infiltration with anesthetic.

        2. A vertical elliptical excision is preferred. Incisions should cross the vermilion at a 90-degree angle in order to run parallel to relaxed skin tension lines (RSTLs).

        3. Place first sutures immediately above and below the white roll to line it up.

    C. Mucosal reconstruction

        1. Musculomucosal V-Y advancement: Can be used for small defects, tubercle deficiency, and notch and whistle deformities.

        2. Axial musculovermilion advancement: Based on the axial labial artery and can be used for full-thickness lower lip defects less than one-third of the length of the lip.

Defect Size

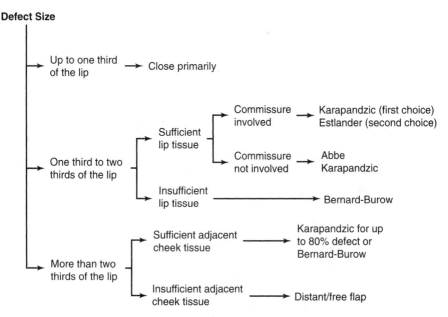

Fig. 19-1. Reconstruction algorithm for the lower lip.

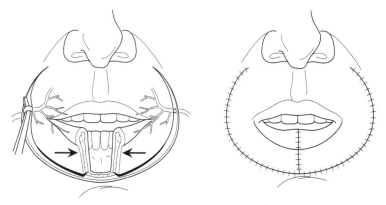

Fig. 19-2. Karapandzic flap.

    3. Labial buccal advancement: Can be used after resection of the anterior vermilion for premalignant and superficial malignant disease. Dissection should be deep to the minor salivary glands and just above the orbicularis oris to preserve the labial artery.

    4. Cross-lip mucosal flap: Can be used for large vermilion volume deficiency (hemifacial atrophy). This is a two-stage procedure.

    5. Tongue flap: Primarily for larger mucosal defects. This is rarely used due to the unpleasant cosmetic outcome.

    6. Total vermilionectomy ("lip shave operation"): Inner mucosa is advanced out in a bipedicled fashion to cover the vermilion defect. Can be used for diffuse actinic damage. This procedure is becoming less common due to the advent of CO_2 lasers.

V. Lower lip reconstruction (see algorithm, Fig. 19-1)

  A. Defects of up to one-third of the lip can be closed primarily.

    1. W-shaped excision.

    2. V-shaped excision: Both upper and lower lip.

    3. Shield excision: Provides larger margins with shorter closure lines.

    4. Single- and double-barrel excision: Burow's triangles should not be full thickness.

  B. Defects of one-third to two-thirds of lower lip

    1. Karapandzic flap (Fig. 19-2): Generally the first choice when there is sufficient lip tissue with commissure involvement.

      a. The circumoral incision width should be equal to the defect height.

      b. Dissection beneath the skin and subcutaneous tissue is a spreading motion, to preserve innervation and vascularity to the orbicularis.

      c. Reattachment of the modiolus to the orbicularis will improve oral function.

      d. Provides a sensate flap in a single stage; intact sphincter provides improved oral competence. However, use of the Karapandzic flap may lead to microstomia and prominent scars.

    2. Estlander flap (Fig. 19-3): Generally the second choice when there is sufficient lip tissue with commissure involvement.

      a. Flap width should be one-third to one-half the size of the defect (provides for proportional width reduction of both lips). Design the flap so that it lies with the melolabial sulcus; this provides easier rotation and better scar camouflage.

      b. Flap height should be equal to the defect height.

      c. Results in a rounded commissure (may have to perform commissuroplasty at a later date) and an increased incidence of insensate lip (can lead to drooling).

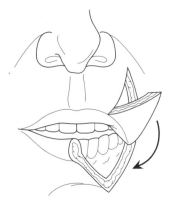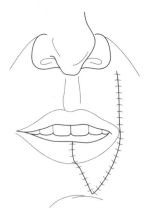

Fig. 19-3. Estlander flap.

3. **Abbe flap** (Fig.19-4): Generally the first choice when there is sufficient lip tissue with no commissure involvement.
   a. Used with both upper and lower lip defects. Philtrum makes upper lip reconstruction more difficult.
   b. Design the upper donor site with an edge at the junction of the middle and lateral thirds of the lip (width should be no greater than 2–3 cm). The height of the flap should be equal to the height of the defect. The width of the flap traditionally was designed to be half the size of the defect, but better results may come from a flap design that is equal to the defect size.
   c. The pedicle can be medial or lateral. Use a paper template for the flap design to plan the arc of rotation so that it includes tissue movement with donor site closure.
   d. Allows partial muscle recovery and acceptable cosmesis.
   e. Requires two stages (release at 2–3 weeks).
4. **Bernard procedure** (as originally described): Can be used when there is insufficient lip tissue.
   a. Full-thickness excision of the upper triangles is necessary.
   b. Lip tissue is recruited from the cheek, and consequently there is a lower incidence of microstomia.
   c. However, there is disruption of the nasolabial and labiomental folds, and an insensate lower lip can lead to drooling.
5. **Modified Bernard-Burow procedure** (Fig. 19-5): Can be used when there is insufficient lip tissue with defects greater than two-thirds of the lip length.
   a. Triangular nasolabial excisions are partial thickness and within the nasolabial fold.
   b. Buccal mucosa is used to reconstruct the vermilion.
   c. Many modifications of this flap exist.
   d. Produces less microstomia, avoids labiomental fold, and yields better sensation.
   e. Results in incomplete sensation and mobility, possible drooling.
C. **Defects involving two-thirds of the lower lip and greater**
   1. **Sufficient adjacent cheek tissue**
      a. Karapandzic flap can be used for defects of up to 80% of the lower lip. The patient's age, tissue elasticity, and resulting microstomia must be taken into consideration.
      b. Bernard-Burow procedure.

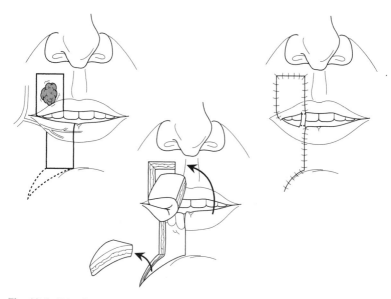

Fig. 19-4. Abbe flap.

    2. Insufficient adjacent cheek tissue: Distant flaps
       a. The pectoralis major musculocutaneous flap can be performed in a single stage and provides enough tissue to reconstruct the anterior aspect of the mouth or inner aspect of the lips.
       b. Free tissue transfer (e.g., radial forearm free flap).
VI. Upper lip reconstruction (see algorithm, Fig. 19-6)
  A. Defects of up to one-third of upper lip
    1. Lateral defects should be closed primarily.
    2. Central defects are closed by perialar crescentic excision with cheek advancement. Crescents are full-thickness skin excisions and can be either bilateral or unilateral.
    3. If the vermilion is intact, a nasolabial flap works well for small defects and can be done in one or two stages depending on size. It can produce an unsightly standing cutaneous deformity and distort the nasolabial fold, however.
  B. Defects from one-third to two-thirds of the upper lip
    1. Central defects
       a. Combined perialar crescentic advancements and an Abbe flap result in less distortion than a Karapandzic flap and produce better scars, but require two stages, with risk of flap failure.
       b. Upper lip Karapandzic flaps can be used. The circumoral incisions can typically end at the commissures.
    2. Lateral defects
       a. If no commissure involvement: Abbe flap.
       b. Commissure involvement: Estlander flap.
       c. Commissure and philtrum involvement: Estlander flap with contralateral perialar crescentic excision.
  C. Defects greater than two-thirds of the upper lip
    1. Sufficient cheek tissue
       a. Central defect.
         (1) Bernard-Burow.

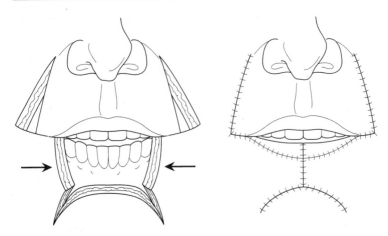

Fig. 19-5. Modified Bernard-Burow procedure.

> **(2)** Gillies: A single-stage full-thickness flap. Rotate the melolabial tissue into the defect with the lateral portion of the flap recreating the melolabial crease. This flap can provide a large amount of tissue but usually results in incomplete sensory and motor function, leading to decreased oral competence.
>
> **b.** Lateral defect: Ipsilateral Bernard-Burow with contralateral perialar crescentic excisions.

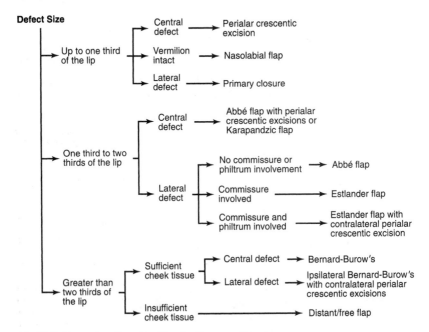

Fig.19-6. Reconstruction algorithm for the upper lip.

2. **Insufficient cheek tissue:** Temporal forehead flap, regional flap, or free flap.

Cheek Reconstruction

I. **Anatomy and physiology**
  A. **The cheek** is defined medially by the nasofacial groove, melolabial crease, and labiomental sulcus; laterally by the preauricular crease; superiorly by the infraorbital rim and superior border of the zygomatic arch; and inferiorly by the mandibular border. It is considered a single aesthetic unit that is divided into three overlapping zones.
    1. **Zone I:** Suborbital (between nasolabial fold and anterior sideburn, lower eyelid and gingival sulcus). Can further be divided into three subunits.
    2. **Zone II:** Preauricular (between ear and malar eminence, including masseteric and parotid fascia).
    3. **Zone III:** Buccomandibular; includes oral lining.
  B. **Muscular anatomy:** The superficial musculoaponeurotic system (SMAS) is a fibrous network that interlinks the muscles of facial expression, lies under the subcutaneous fat, and is continuous with the superficial temporal fascia superiorly and the platysma inferiorly.
  C. **Sensory innervation:** Primarily cranial nerves V2 and V3.
  D. **Blood supply:** Predominantly the facial artery. Traverses the mandible at the facial notch and courses under the muscles of facial expression, where it anastomoses with the infraorbital and supratrochlear arteries. The subdermal plexus is supplied by perforating vessels that arise from axially oriented branches of the facial artery.
II. **Functional considerations:** Ectropion can be caused by excess tension of a flap on the lower eyelid or by scar contracture, or both. It can be avoided by securing flaps to the inferior orbital rim periosteum or temporal fascia, or both, and avoiding STSGs when possible.
III. **Reconstructive options**
  A. **Primary closure:** The treatment of choice for small defects throughout the entire cheek. Adequate skin undermining is the key. Increased skin laxity in older individuals allows primary closure of larger defects. Closure lines should be placed within lines of relaxed skin tension when feasible.
  B. **Secondary healing:** Results are variable. Best if used in areas of concavity such as the medial canthal or lateral temple regions. Contractures can lead to distortion.
  C. **Skin grafts:** Simple and efficient, and can provide coverage after excision of large defects (i.e., aggressive or recurrent tumor), allowing for excellent surveillance of recurrence. More aesthetic options can be considered once the tumor site remains cancer free.
  D. **Local flaps** (see Chapter 4, "Flaps")
    1. **Transposition flaps:** Excellent coverage around the cheek and eyes for small to moderate-sized defects.
      a. Rhomboid flap (classic Limberg, circular, Webster, and Dufourmentel modifications): Best utilized for coverage of defects in the cheek, lateral nose, jawline, inferior orbital region, and lower lip.
      b. Bilobed flap: Best used for coverage of the lateral and inferior cheek and lower third of the nose.
      c. Nasolabial flap: Designed to include perforating branches of the facial and angular arteries that course through the underlying muscles of the nasolabial fold. The flap can be based superiorly (angular artery) or inferiorly (facial artery). Superiorly based flaps are best used to cover defects of the nasal ala, tip dorsum, and sidewall; inferiorly based flaps are best for the upper lip and oral cavity (which requires a deepithelialized tunneled flap).

2. **Cheek rotation flap:** Can be used anywhere on the face and based superiorly or inferiorly. The alar-facial sulci and the nasolabial fold should be used as the medial border of the flap, if possible. Carry the incision along the subciliary margin laterally into the periauricular area. Wide undermining is required in the subdermal fat plane.

3. **V-Y flap:** Best designed to cover defects involving the nasolabial fold, medial canthal area, glabellar region, cheek, and side of nose. Provides excellent coverage of lateral skin defects of the upper and lower lip when advanced superiorly along the nasolabial groove.

E. **Regional flaps**

1. **Cervicofacial flap:** Useful for moderate-sized defects. Carry dissection deep to the SMAS. Anchoring sutures to inferior orbital rim periosteum and temporary Frost sutures can help to prevent ectropion.

2. **Cervicopectoral flap:** For large defects. Can be based medially or laterally. Flap design should extend from the base of the defect to below the clavicle.

F. **Tissue expansion:** Can increase available tissue and be used in combination with other flaps. Normal skin of the lateral face and upper aspect of the neck can be expanded, providing tissue for a large inferior and medially based rotation advancement flap. Neck tissue can be used to cover defects in this region because neck skin is nearly identical in texture, color, and hair-bearing qualities.

G. **Free flaps** are reserved for extensive cheek defects.

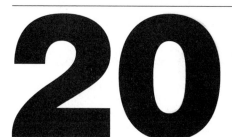

Ear Reconstruction

Jonathan S. Wilensky

I. **Ear anatomy**
   A. **Surface anatomy** (Fig. 20-1)
   B. **Vascular supply: Three main arteries**
      1. **Superficial temporal artery:** Supplies the lateral surface of the auricle. It is a terminal branch of the external carotid artery.
      2. **Posterior auricular artery:** Also a terminal branch of the external carotid artery; supplies the posterior auricle, lobule, and retroauricular skin.
      3. **Occipital artery:** Also supplies the posterior auricle, lobule, and retroauricular skin.
   C. **Innervation**
      1. **Great auricular nerve** (C2, C3): Innervates the lower half of the lateral surface of the ear and posterior auricle.
      2. **Auriculotemporal nerve** (V3): Innervates the superolateral surface of the ear and anterior and superior external auditory canal.
      3. **Lesser occipital nerve:** Innervates the superior cranial surface of the ear.
      4. **Auricular branch of the vagus nerve (Arnold's nerve):** Innervates the concha and posterior external auditory canal.
   D. **Size and position**
      1. The ear is normally 6 to 6.5 cm high and 3.5 cm wide.
      2. **Normal ear projection:** 17 to 21 mm from the temporal scalp.
   E. **Embryology**
      1. **Fourth week of gestation:** Ear development begins.
      2. **Sixth week of gestation:** Six ear hillocks (three anterior and three posterior) arise from the first and second branchial arches, respectively.
         a. **First branchial arch:** Forms the malleus and incus and the upper one-third of the ear.
         b. **Second branchial arch:** Forms the stapes and the lower two-thirds of the ear.
II. **Indications for reconstruction**
   A. **Congenital defects**
      1. **Microtia**
         a. Incidence of approximately 1 in 8,000 births.
         b. Right-sided predominance.
         c. 50% have associated hemifacial microsomia.
         d. The most appropriate age to start correction is around 6 to 7 years.
         e. Ear reconstruction for microtia is typically a three-stage procedure.
            (1) **First stage:** The cartilaginous framework is constructed from costal cartilage. A subcutaneous pocket is designed, and the cartilage framework is inserted.
            (2) **Second stage:** The cartilage framework is elevated off the head posteriorly, and a skin graft is used in the postauricular sulcus.
            (3) **Third stage:** Rotation of the lobule into its anatomic position.
      2. **Protruding or prominent ears**
         a. The two deformities responsible for prominent ears are the lack of an antihelical fold and conchal hypertrophy. Although one usually

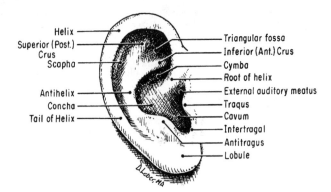

Fig. 20-1. External anatomy of the ear. (From Leber D. Ear reconstruction. In: Georgiade G, Riefkohl R, Levin S, (eds). *Plastic, Maxillofacial, and Reconstructive Surgery*, 3rd ed. Philadelphia: Williams & Wilkins, 1997, with permission.)

predominates in a given patient, both are usually present to some degree. Surgical planning depends on an accurate assessment.

- **(1) Conchomastoid (Mustarde) sutures** are used to reduce conchal projection by pulling the concha toward the head to reduce the prominence of the ear. A wedge of cartilage can also be excised from the concha to reduce its overall prominence.
- **(2) Conchoscaphal sutures** are used to recreate the antihelical fold.
  - b. Prominent or malformed ears can be treated in the newborn period with splinting. A customized splint or wire can be used to hold the ears in their desired position. The malleability of newborn cartilage persists for the first week due to circulating maternal estrogens.
- **3. Cryptotia**
  - a. In this deformity, the upper pole of the ear is buried under skin, with absence of the superior auriculocephalic sulcus.
  - b. Operative correction involves release of the helix and creation of the auriculocephalic sulcus with skin grafts, after the age of 5.
- **4. Stahl's ear**
  - a. This deformity results from the presence of an abnormal third crus that is oriented horizontally and extends from the antihelix to the helical rim.
  - b. Additionally, the superior crus is either hypoplastic or absent.
  - c. The scaphoid fossa is malformed, while the conchal fossa is normal.
- **B. Acquired defects**
  - **1. Malignancy**
    - a. Skin cancers of the ear account for 5% to 10% of head and neck cutaneous malignancies.
    - b. Squamous cell cancers are the most common type of cutaneous malignancy of the ear.
  - **2. Trauma**
    - a. The ear is quite susceptible to trauma because of its position on the head.
    - b. **Hematomas:** Must be evacuated and then the skin bolstered to prevent fluid reaccumulation between the perichondrium and the cartilage, which can result in a cartilaginous deformity known as cauliflower ear.
    - c. **Avulsions and amputations:** The size and condition of the amputated tissue and of the stump and surrounding tissue are key determinants in whether reapproximation will yield an aesthetically acceptable result.

Additionally, the location of the defect (either upper third, middle third, lower third, or total loss) will determine the course of treatment (see below).

    3. Thermal injury

        a. Frostbite: Management includes rapid rewarming and the use of a topical antimicrobial agent that penetrates cartilage, such as mafenide acetate.

        b. Burns: Management includes careful positioning and head dressings to prevent further injury and the use of mafenide acetate. Most ear burns heal well with conservative therapy, but large segments of exposed cartilage must be covered or excised.

III. Helical and upper-third defect reconstruction

    A. Wedge resection

        1. To prevent buckling, a star-shaped resection pattern can be designed.

        2. The upper size limit for wedge resection with direct closure is 1.5 cm.

    B. Antia-Buch technique

        1. Essentially a rim advancement, this flap is useful for helical rim defects.

        2. The rim is incised from the inferior portion of the defect to the upper part of the lobule, through the anterior skin, perichondrium, and cartilage. The posterior skin is left intact, is undermined, and is redraped following rim advancement and closure.

    C. Converse tunnel procedure

        1. This flap is useful for helical defects larger than 3 cm, where the Antia-Buch technique is limited by distortion.

        2. First stage: A cartilage strut is harvested and placed in a tunnel beneath the retroauricular skin, to which the margins of the helical rim defect are sewed.

        3. Second stage: The cartilage strut is elevated, along with the retroauricular skin that will be used to resurface the helical rim, and the reconstruction is completed. The retroauricular skin donor site is closed by advancement or is skin grafted.

    D. Tubed pedicle flap

        1. First stage: A thin tube of retroauricular skin is fashioned from a bipedicled skin flap, and the long edge is sewn to the helical rim.

        2. Second stage: One or both ends of the tube are elevated. Sometimes, the second end is elevated at a third stage.

IV. Middle-third defect reconstruction

    A. Postauricular (Dieffenbach) flap

        1. A postauricular flap based on the edge of the hairline is planned, with the width equal to that of the defect, and the length sufficient to reconstruct the anterior surface, rim, and posterior surface.

        2. First stage: The flap is raised down to the postauricular fascia, and the free margin of the flap is sutured to the anterior free skin edge of the ear defect.

        3. Second stage (14–21 days later): The flap is divided and used to resurface the posterior ear.

V. Lower-third defect reconstruction

    A. In this area, soft and flexible tissue is required. This is achieved with local flaps that can be folded over on themselves.

    B. To avoid skin-only reconstructions that have little support, contralateral conchal grafts can be used subcutaneously to provide support and contour.

VI. Total auricular reconstruction

    A. Microvascular replantation

        1. The vessels of the ear are extremely small, making microvascular reattachment technically difficult.

        2. If microvascular reattachment is attempted, an artery-only reattachment can be performed, with the subsequent use of leeches for venous drainage.

    B. Banking of the ear cartilage, or replantation of the auricle after removal of the postauricular skin and cartilage fenestration, although often discussed, is of uncertain clinical utility.

C. When a large portion of the ear cartilage is exposed, a temporoparietal fascia flap may be used to achieve cover, and is eventually covered with a skin graft.

D. Costal cartilage remains the gold standard for total auricular reconstruction.

Pearls

1. Patients with oropharyngeal cancers may complain of ear pain referred via Arnold's nerve, the auricular branch of the vagus.
2. For the burned ear, mafenide acetate is preferred because of its superior cartilage penetration.
3. Prominent ears can be treated nonoperatively in the first week of the newborn period with splinting techniques.
4. Microsurgical replantation attempts may sacrifice the superficial temporal artery, which would impair the use of the temporoparietal fascia in the future.

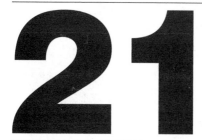

Scalp and Calvarial Reconstruction

Nicholas C. Watson

Scalp and Skull Anatomy

I. Anatomic layers of the scalp
   A. S = Skin
      1. The anterior and temporal thickness is 3 to 4 mm.
      2. The posterior thickness may be up to 8 mm.
   B. C = Subcutaneous tissue = Connective tissue
      1. Consists of fat, blood vessels, lymphatics, nerves, hair follicles, sebaceous glands, and sweat glands.
      2. The scalp bleeds easily when lacerated because the tough connective tissues inhibit blood vessel constriction (similar to the situation found in scar tissue).
   C. A = Aponeurosis epicranialis = Galea aponeurotica
      1. Consists of a fibrous sheet joining the frontalis muscle with the occipitalis muscle.
      2. Acts as a barrier to infection.
   D. L = Loose connective tissue = Loose areolar plane
      1. Creates the subaponeurotic space and enables the scalp to move on the cranium. It is the most common plane of scalp avulsion injuries.
      2. Contains the emissary veins.
   E. P = Pericranium = Periosteum
      1. Contains a generous vasculature.
      2. Loss of the pericranium is a contraindication to skin grafting.
II. Anatomic layers of the cranium
   A. External table
   B. Diploë
   C. Internal table
   D. Epidural space (a potential space)
   E. Endocranium = Dura mater. Contains the middle meningeal artery and vein.
   F. Subdural space
III. Blood supply of the scalp (Fig. 21-1)
   A. Anteriorly: Supraorbital and supratrochlear arteries and veins.
   B. Laterally: Superficial temporal arteries and veins.
   C. Posteriorly: Occipital and posterior auricular arteries and veins.
   D. The subcutaneous tissue contains a network of interconnecting vessels.
      1. Branches dive through the galea to supply the cortex.
      2. A single arterial system may maintain scalp viability through the rich vascular plexus (e.g., in cases of scalp replantation or revascularization).
   E. Scalp infection may spread via the emissary veins to the dural sinuses and the ophthalmic veins.
IV. Innervation of the scalp
   A. Motor
      1. Posterior auricular branch of the facial nerve: Auricular (anterior, posterior, superior), occipitalis muscles.
      2. Temporal branch of the facial nerve: Frontalis muscle.

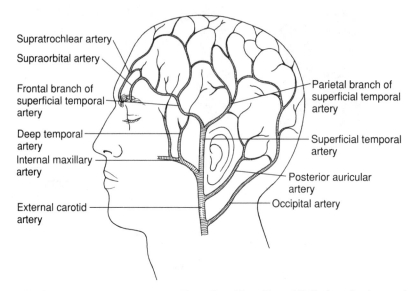

Fig. 21-1. Blood supply of the scalp. (Reproduced from Freund R. Scalp, calvarium, and forehead reconstruction. In *Grabb and Smith's Plastic Surgery*, 5th ed. Aston SJ, Beasley RW, Thorne CH, eds. Philadelphia, Lippincott-Raven, 1997. With permission.

B. **Sensory**
1. **Trigeminal nerve, ophthalmic division (V1):** Forehead and anterior scalp.
2. **Maxillary division (V2):** Forehead lateral to eye.
3. **Mandibular division (V3):** Temple and lateral scalp.
4. **Greater occipital nerve:** Posterior scalp.
5. **Lesser occipital nerve:** Posterior and superior to ear.

Scalp Reconstruction

I. **Principles of scalp reconstruction**
A. **The location, depth, and dimensions of the wound** are critical elements in reparative planning.
B. **All scalp reconstruction** is ideally based on a viable bony surface.
C. **The scalp's ample vascularity** confers a relative resistance to infection.
D. **Use hair-bearing skin** for reconstruction when possible.
II. **The reconstructive ladder in scalp reconstruction**
A. **Perform direct approximation** in wounds lacking tissue loss.
B. **Skin grafts**
1. **A split-thickness skin graft** is often an excellent choice for repair of partial-thickness wounds.
2. **The wound site** must have a good vascular supply and be without infection.
3. **A skin graft may be used as a temporary covering** for decorticated calvarial external table injuries prior to definitive repair.
C. **Local scalp flaps for repair** of full-thickness wounds
1. **Advancement flaps**
a. Posterior scalp advancement flaps may be advanced easily due to the loose neck skin.

      b. Advancement flaps in other areas of the scalp require galeal scoring to allow sufficient advancement.

      c. Bipedicle flaps and Gillies tripedicle flaps may be used to cover a central defect via direct advancement.

2. Rotation flaps

      a. Single scalp rotation flaps may be used to close wounds up to 6 cm in diameter.

      b. Double opposing rotation flaps utilizing peripheral bases may be used to close wounds of the scalp vertex.

      c. A rotation flap may require galeal scoring along the edges of the donor defect to increase scalp movement. If this does not provide sufficient mobility for closure, a split-thickness skin graft may be used to close the flap donor defect.

      d. A dog-ear normally occurs at the base of a rotation flap of the scalp and should not be altered at the primary operation because this may negatively affect blood flow in the flap. Dog-ears usually flatten out with time.

3. Periosteal flaps may be used as pedicle flaps to cover exposed cranium to create a base for skin grafting.

4. Multiple flaps

      a. Multiple flaps can be used to cover defects up to one-third the surface area of the scalp.

      b. Each flap must have its own vascular pedicle included in its base.

      c. The Orticochea method uses two flaps adjacent to the scalp wound to cover the defect, and a third larger flap (generally the rest of the scalp) to cover the donor defects after rotation of the other two flaps. This may also be performed as a four-flap technique.

D. Tissue expansion

1. Tissue expansion is indicated in the repair of large defects in which the time required for expansion is acceptable.

      a. Primary excision and repair of large scalp nevi are aided with tissue expansion.

      b. Scalp expansion may be used in secondary reconstruction to allow primary closure of the flap donor defect.

      c. A single course of expansion allows repair of defects as large as 50% of the scalp surface area.

      d. For larger defects, serial expansions may be necessary.

2. Benefits: Use of hair-bearing skin, total coverage of large wounds without disturbing hair growth, and absence of donor defect.

3. Disadvantages: Extended treatment time (2–5 months) and potential complication by hematoma, infection, or failure of the expander.

4. Tissue expanders are placed in the subgaleal plane at the edge of a scalp wound through an incision at a right angle to the wound edge.

5. Expanders are typically increased in volume by approximately 10% once weekly via sterile saline injection. Generally, the expander is inflated until the skin is tight but not painful.

E. Microvascular free tissue transfer

1. Indicated when a pedicled flap is not possible.

2. The best option for single-stage, acute coverage of large defects.

3. The relatively large size (thickness) and absence of hair-bearing tissue on free flaps makes them aesthetically limiting.

4. Common free flaps for the scalp include latissimus dorsi muscle with split-thickness skin graft, omentum, and radial forearm flaps.

III. Trauma reconstruction

A. Lacerations

1. Irrigation and debridement.

2. Meticulous hemostasis.

3. Closure of galea aponeurotica with further advancement of wound edges achieved by galeal scoring if necessary.

4. **Layered closure is usually unnecessary.** Typically, a single-layer closure with staples is adequate and provides excellent hemostasis.
5. **Healing by second intention** is acceptable in small wounds.

B. **Avulsions (amputation)**
1. **Repair depends** on the layers involved and the extent of injury.
2. **The loose connective tissue layer** is the most common plane of avulsion.
3. **Determine if the tissue has adequate perfusion** before performing local flap procedures during the acute phase.
4. **Microvascular anastomosis** is the standard of treatment for total and near-total scalp avulsions.
   a. Vessels on the side away from the avulsion defect are usually the most optimal for use in anastomosis.
   b. Vein grafts are almost always necessary to bypass the zone of injury.
   c. The whole scalp may survive on just one venous and one arterial connection. The superficial temporal system is preferred.
   d. The avulsed scalp may be stored and transported from the field in a plastic bag placed in an ice water bath.
   e. Contraindications to replantation include ischemia time greater than 30 hours, failure to identify a suitable vascular pedicle, and medical condition precluding prolonged operation.
5. **Skin grafting** may be used in the repair of avulsion injuries.
   a. Skin grafts work well on partial-thickness avulsions.
   b. Decorticated calvarial bones may be burred and have skin grafts placed on them as a temporary covering until definitive repair can be performed.

IV. **Burns**
A. **The mechanism of burn** is of marked importance in the treatment plan.
1. **Chemical, electrical, and grease burns** generally cause deeper burns.
2. **Scald and thermal burns** typically result in relatively superficial burns.
B. **The extent of a burn** injury may initially be difficult to assess.
C. **First-line treatment** is debridement of necrotic tissue and standard wound care.
D. **Escharotomy** may be done with tangential excision to preserve dermal appendages in skin with intact dermis.
E. **For burn alopecia,** skin grafting followed by tissue expansion and local flaps ultimately allows reconstruction with hair-bearing skin.
F. **The mainstay for burns with exposed calvarium** is free tissue transfer, not local flaps.

V. **Tumor excision**
A. **Multiple incisions** made during excision can complicate the repair by compromising the local vasculature.
B. **For nonurgent tumors,** tissue expansion followed by excision and local flap reconstruction affords the best opportunity for an aesthetically pleasing outcome.
C. **The vacuum-assisted closure (VAC) device** has been used to cover wounds as deep as through the outer table using delayed split-thickness skin grafting.

VI. **Radiation wounds**
A. **Split-thickness skin grafting** may be used for repair of partial-thickness radiation wounds.
B. **Full-thickness wounds** require more advanced reconstructive techniques such as local flaps or free flaps.

VII. **Congenital defects**
A. **Aplasia cutis congenita,** the partial or total absence of scalp tissue, is treated by wound management while the ulcers heal by secondary intention.

B. **Arteriovenous malformations** and hemangiomas are best assessed preoperatively by using magnetic resonance imaging (MRI) to identify the layers of the scalp involved.

C. **Craniopagus is a rare deformity** of twins connected at the head, requiring reconstructive techniques specific to each case.

Calvarial Reconstruction

I. **Principles of calvarial reconstruction**

A. **The goals of calvarial reconstruction** are protection of the brain and restoration of form.

B. **Definitive soft tissue coverage** of exposed calvarium is essential to prevent infection and damage.

II. **Operative planning**

A. **Determine the extent of the defect** (three-dimensional computed tomography is excellent).

B. **The surgical approach** is determined by the location and extent of the defect.

1. **Frontal region:** Reconstruction is necessary for protective and cosmetic purposes.

2. **Temporal region:** Defects less than 10 cm^2 seldom require cranioplasty, because the overlying temporalis muscle confers a degree of protection and contour.

3. **The parietal and occipital regions** require repair for protection of underlying structures; aesthetics in these areas are of less importance.

III. **Autogenous materials used in cranioplasty**

A. **Split cranial bone grafts**

1. **Advantages**

a. Minimal complications.

b. The donor site is often in the same field as the recipient site.

c. Cranial bone revascularizes quickly and can be readily positioned such that it undergoes minimal resorption.

d. Cranial bone can be contoured easily.

2. **The main disadvantage of utilizing cranial bone** is the risk of injury to the underlying structures during harvesting.

3. **Parietal calvarium is the optimum donor location** due to increased calvarial thickness.

B. **Split rib grafts**

1. **Split rib grafts** revascularize well and have minimal infectious complications.

2. **After harvest,** ribs with remaining periosteum will regenerate.

3. **Donor site morbidity** is moderate and the aesthetic result may be mediocre.

C. **Iliac bone graft**

1. **Iliac bone** is a good contour match for reconstruction of the frontal region.

2. **Unicortical grafts** are most successful due to their rapid revascularization.

3. **Donor site morbidity (pain)** can be significant.

D. **Bone paste**

1. **Bone dust can be harvested** from the cranium or ilium.

2. **Bone dust may be spread** over exposed dura and covered with a protective coating such as oxycellulose.

3. **The bone dust may also be combined** with an elastomer-coated mesh, such that new bone grows along the contour of the mesh scaffolding.

IV. **Alloplastic materials used in cranioplasty**

A. **Methylmethacrylate (acrylic)**

1. **Advantages:** Elimination of a harvesting procedure, durability, and low heat conduction.

2. **Disadvantages:** Increased risk of infection, risk of fracture, and the need for delay between the initial debridement operation and acrylic cranioplasty.
  B. **Stainless steel mesh:** Provides excellent protection and is easily contoured, but also carries a risk of infection

Hair Restoration

I. **Hair**
  A. **There are approximately 100,000 hairs on the adult scalp.**
  B. **Hair grows about 1 cm per month.**
  C. **Individual hair follicles** go through three growth phases.
    1. **Anagen phase:** Acute growth; duration 3 years; accounts for 90% of hair at any time.
    2. **Catagen phase:** Involution; duration 1 to 2 weeks.
    3. **Telogen phase:** No growth; duration 3 to 4 months.
II. **Alopecia**
  A. **Nonscarring hair loss.**
    1. **Male pattern baldness (MPB):** Male pattern androgenetic alopecia.
      a. Genetically determined individual hair follicle response to dihydrotestosterone.
      b. MPB results from mature hair falling out.
      c. Hair follicles remain, but only produce a fine hair shaft.
    2. **Female alopecia:** Less common than MPB.
    3. **May be drug induced.**
    4. **Often the result of various dermatologic diseases.**
  B. **Scarring hair loss** (cicatricial alopecia) can result from scalp injury, infection, and dermatologic disease.
III. **Treatment options for hair loss**
  A. **Toupee:** A nonpermanent solution.
  B. **Chemical treatment (shampoos)** or styling, producing the appearance of increased volume.
  C. **Pharmacologic interventions.**
    1. **Minoxidil:** Opens potassium channels and causes vasodilation.
    2. **Finasteride:** 5-alpha reductase inhibitor.
    3. **Medical interventions** must be continued in order to continue to derive benefits; otherwise, alopecia will recur.
    4. **Primary side effect:** Undesirable hair growth.
  D. **Surgical interventions.**
    1. **Hair transplantation (scalp grafts)**
      a. Micrografting (1–2 follicles per graft) and minigrafting (3–6 follicles per graft) for a total of 1,000 to 3,000 follicles are the most common procedures.
      b. Other procedures include standard, strip, and follicular unit grafts.
    2. **Scalp flaps**
      a. Small areas of alopecia can be treated with rotation flaps.
      b. Scalp reduction by excision of bald regions and advancement of adjacent tissue is best used on the vertex of the scalp.
      c. In extensive alopecia, transposition flaps such as Juri's temporoparietal-occipital flap, lateral scalp flaps, and temporal vertical flaps can be used to move hair from the donor site to the frontal area.

Pearls

1. **Exercise caution when performing galeal scoring** in order to avoid interrupting the blood supply to the scalp flap.
2. **Locate scalp vessels for replantation efforts** in the subcutaneous plane, and plan on using vein grafts from the outset. A single good arterial inflow (preferably the superficial temporal artery) is often sufficient.
3. **The mainstay for burns** with exposed calvarium is free tissue transfer, not local flaps.
4. When you think you have enough **expansion for a scalp flap,** expand some more.
5. **Use temporary coverage while awaiting definitive margin clearance** prior to performing flap reconstruction following tumor extirpation.

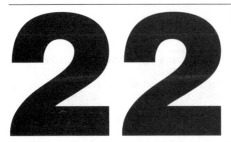

Facial Paralysis

Gregory H. Borschel

I. **Anatomy** (Table 22-1 and Fig. 22-1)
   A. **The facial nerve (cranial nerve VII)** contains sensory, parasympathetic, and motor fibers.
   B. **Sensory:** Somatic afferent fibers innervate the skin of the external auditory meatus; visceral afferent fibers (via the greater palatine nerve) innervate part of the palatal, nasal, and pharyngeal mucosa.
   C. **Parasympathetic** secretomotor fibers innervate the submandibular and sublingual glands (via the chorda tympani); the lacrimal, nasal, and palatine glands (via the greater superficial petrosal nerve); and the parotid gland (via the lesser superficial petrosal, which gives rise to the auriculotemporal nerve).
   D. **Afferent taste** fibers from the anterior two-thirds of the tongue are carried by the chorda tympani.
   E. **Motor function**
      1. **The facial motor nucleus** lies within the pons, and the facial nerve exits the brainstem and traverses the temporal bone, exiting through the **stylomastoid foramen.**
      2. **The extratemporal facial nerve** enters the parotid gland and divides into the upper and lower branches (two upper branch divisions: temporal and zygomatic; three lower branch divisions: buccal, mandibular, and cervical).
      3. Most **muscles of facial expression** can be classified as either constrictors or expanders of the ocular, nasal, or oral sphincters.
II. **Types of facial paralysis**
   A. **Facial paralysis** can occur within the central nervous system (i.e., motor cortex or brainstem), within the temporal bone, or distal to the temporal bone.
   B. The **classification of degree of paralysis** uses a nomenclature system that is not intuitive. Paralysis can be described as partial (in which some of the branches are affected) or complete (in which all five branches are affected). Individual branches can be described as having complete paralysis (the branch has no motor function) or incomplete paralysis (the branch has some motor activity remaining).
   C. **Various grading scales,** including the House-Brackman system, have been proposed. However, these are not universally applicable to all types of facial paralysis and are of limited value in planning treatment.
   D. **Neonatal (congenital) facial paralysis**
      1. **Möbius syndrome:** A defect in development of the facial nucleus; it is often associated with paralysis of the extraocular muscles. (Also see "Special Considerations in Pediatric Facial Paralysis," later in this chapter.)
      2. **Obstetrical facial paralysis** may result from forceps delivery. It is typically extratemporal, producing a neuropraxic or axonotmetic injury, resulting in a favorable prognosis with nonoperative management.
   E. **Acquired facial paralysis**
      1. **Trauma or surgery:** Acute trauma to the central nervous system (CNS), temporal bone, or distal facial nerve.
      2. **Infectious agents:** Herpes zoster viral infection of the intratemporal nerve can lead to edema and ischemia, producing facial paralysis. Other

Table 22-1. Principal structures innervated by the facial nerve and its branches

Branch	Structure	Function
Temporal	Frontalis muscle	Brow elevation
	Corrugator supercilii	Brow medialization/depression
	Procerus	Brow depression; production of transverse wrinkles of the nasal radix
Temporal/zygomatic	Orbicularis oculi	Eyelid closure
Zygomatic/buccal	Zygomaticus major	Lateral upper lip elevation (primary smile actuator)
Buccal	Zygomaticus minor	Upper lip elevation
	Levator labii superioris	Upper lip elevation; elevation of nasolabial fold
	Levator labii superioris alaeque nasi	Upper lip elevation; elevation of medial-most nasolabial fold
	Risorius	Oral commissure lateral retraction (additional smile actuator)
	Buccinator	Cheek compression
	Levator anguli oris	Oral commissure elevation and medialization
	Nasalis	Dilates and constricts nares (via transverse and alar heads)
Buccal/mandibular	Depressor anguli oris	Oral commissure depression
Mandibular	Depressor labii inferioris	Lower lip depression
	Mentalis	Chin soft tissue elevation
Cervical	Platysma	Oral commissure depression
Nerve to posterior digastric and stylohyoid muscle	Anterior belly of digastric muscle and stylohyoid muscle	Hyoid elevation
Somatic afferent fibers	Skin of external auditory meatus	Cutaneous sensibility
Greater palatine nerve	Palatal, nasal, and pharyngeal mucosa	Mucosal sensibility
Chorda tympani	Submandibular and sublingual glands	Parasympathetic secretomotor function
Nerve to stapedius	Stapedius	Dampening of loud noises
Greater superficial petrosal nerve	Lacrimal, nasal, and palatine glands	Parasympathetic secretomotor function
Chorda tympani	Taste buds of anterior two-thirds of tongue	Taste
Auriculotemporal nerve	Parotid gland	Parasympathetic secretomotor function

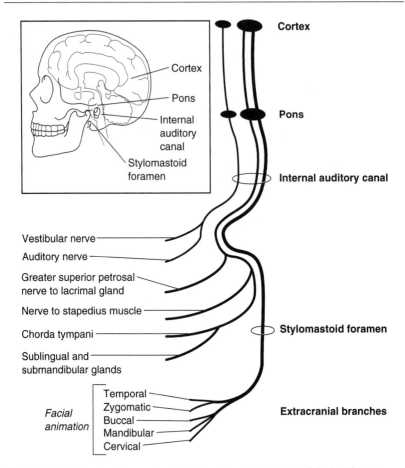

Fig. 22-1. The topognostic examination is based on the anatomy of the facial nerve.

infections, such as bacterial otitis externa or media, mastoiditis, parotitis, or varicella zoster infection, have been implicated.

3. **CNS masses:** Temporal bone or CNS masses typically present with an indolent course, whereas a cerebrovascular accident can cause rapid-onset facial paralysis.

4. **Extracranial masses**
   a. Parotid masses can cause encasement or invasion of the facial nerve as it traverses the parotid gland.
   b. Other masses may include cholesteatoma, sarcoma, schwannoma, neurofibroma, and fibrous dysplasia.

5. **Systemic conditions:** Pregnancy (paralysis is typically transient), diabetes mellitus, hypo- or hyperthyroidism, hypertension, and exposure to lead, tetanus, diphtheria, and carbon monoxide.

6. **Bell's palsy** (idiopathic facial nerve paralysis): The most common form of facial paralysis. Many cases are thought to be of viral origin. The pathophysiology consists of inflammation leading to a cycle of edema and ischemia. However, the clinical features of Bell's palsy are well described. It is usually of abrupt onset, and recovery may be rapid. The majority of patients with Bell's palsy (90%) recover nearly fully or at least partially, and

50% have total recovery. The maintenance of some motor activity (i.e., incomplete paralysis) is a good prognostic sign. In the setting of an otherwise normal physical examination and a normal audiogram, steroids (prednisone for 10 days) may be used. In the absence of signs of recovery within 3 months, other diagnoses must be sought (see "Diagnosis"). Some have advocated acute facial nerve decompression, but there is inadequate evidence of efficacy.

III. Diagnosis

A. **Facial paralysis** should be approached in the same manner as other neurologic conditions. The anatomic lesion is localized via a detailed history and physical examination, supplemented with select diagnostic studies. The history should ascertain the duration of paralysis, abruptness of onset, associated infections, history of trauma or surgery, past medical history, and medications.

B. **Topognostic physical examination** (Fig. 22-1): A thorough physical examination and documentation of deficits are essential.

  1. **Upper motor neuron (supranuclear) lesions** present with bilateral sparing of frontalis function because cortical fibers decussate prior to innervating the lower motor neuron.

  2. **Bell's phenomenon** (presence of superolateral duction of the eye on attempting lid closure) suggests a lower motor neuron lesion.

  3. **Lower motor neuron lesions** can be localized by testing the three intratemporal branches and the muscles of facial expression.

     a. The greater superficial petrosal nerve supplies the lacrimal gland, and can be tested with the Schirmer test of tear production, in which a filter paper strip is placed in the fornix; length of wetting that measures 10 mm or more in 5 minutes is considered normal. The test has predictive value in determining need for eye protection.

     b. The stapedial nerve innervates the stapedius muscle; loss of function results in intolerance to loud sounds. It can be definitively tested with an audiogram. If the audiogram is abnormal, a magnetic resonance imaging (MRI) scan is indicated to rule out central causes such as a mass lesion.

     c. The chorda tympani supplies taste to the anterior two-thirds of the tongue (tested with application of salt solution to the anterior tongue—highly subjective).

     d. Examination of (mimetic) muscles of facial expression includes evaluation of the following.

        (1) Brow elevation/forehead wrinkling (frontal division of temporal branch)

        (2) Forced eyelid closure and symmetry of smile (zygomatic branch)

        (3) Ability to pucker the lips (buccal branch)

        (4) Ability to bare the teeth, exposing the lower dentition (mandibular branch)

C. **Electrodiagnostic testing** is mainly of prognostic value in cases such as blunt trauma or viral infection.

  1. **Nerve excitability test (NET):** The facial nerve is transcutaneously stimulated, and the least stimulation required for muscle motion is recorded and compared with the normal opposite side (a difference of 3.0 milliamperes is considered abnormal). Easy to perform, but relatively subjective.

  2. **Maximum stimulation test (MST):** The facial nerve is transcutaneously stimulated using a maximal stimulation protocol. The degree of muscle motion is graded and compared with the normal opposite side. Also relatively subjective.

  3. **Electroneuronography (ENOG):** The facial nerve is transcutaneously stimulated, and the resulting muscle action potentials are recorded and compared with the normal opposite side. This test is the most predictive of recovery of all electrodiagnostic tests.

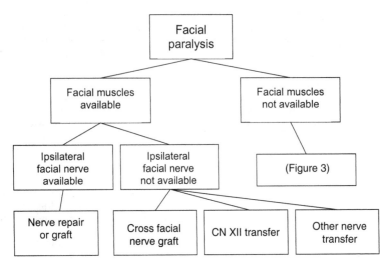

Fig. 22-2. Algorithm for treatment of facial paralysis.

4. **Electromyography (EMG):** Intramuscular electrodes record action potentials during rest and voluntary activity. The presence of fibrillation potentials indicates that the muscle has been denervated. Polyphasic reinnervation potentials (motor unit action potentials) indicate the presence of axonal regeneration. Testing must be delayed until 2 or 3 weeks after onset of paralysis in order to evaluate fibrillation potentials. A repeat EMG should be performed at 3 months to assess regeneration. If no reinnervation potentials are seen, then further workup and possible exploration should be considered.

IV. **Urgent priorities in facial paralysis**
   A. **Corneal protection:** Priority should be given to the eye in all cases of facial paralysis. An ophthalmologic consultation should be obtained, and a regimen of corneal protection with taping and lubrication should be instituted. Bell's phenomenon, when present, serves to partly protect the cornea. A tarsorrhaphy (suturing the lids together) should be considered in refractory cases.
   B. **Steroids:** The indications for steroids are controversial, but in some cases of acute-onset facial paralysis (e.g., Bell's palsy) steroids should be given to decrease edema of the facial nerve within the temporal bone.
   C. Definitive diagnosis should be prioritized in order to establish the best course of treatment.

V. **Surgical treatment of facial paralysis.** An algorithmic approach is helpful because of the variable deformities and the large number of operations available to the surgeon. It is most applicable to the patient with long-standing paralysis of lower motor neuron origin.
   A. **If facial muscles and the ipsilateral facial nerve are available** (e.g., with traumatic transection or resection during parotidectomy) (Fig. 22-2)
      1. Muscles can be reinnervated as long as 2 years after denervation, depending on patient age; reinnervation is best within 6 months postparalysis.
      2. **Early exploration and nerve repair** is performed when possible. If concomitant injuries prohibit immediate direct repair, the wound should be explored and nerve ends tagged for future exploration. Nerve injuries medial to the lateral canthus do not require repair because of extensive crossover.
      3. **If a nerve gap exists,** or the repair is under tension, then nerve grafting must be performed. Nerve grafting produces more synkinesis (voluntary mass

movement) than does nerve repair, because axons can become mismatched twice with the two coaptations required by a graft.

B. If facial muscles are available, but the ipsilateral facial nerve is not (e.g., with intratemporal or intracranial tumor ablation, infections, and trauma) (Fig. 22-2)

   1. Cross-facial nerve grafting is performed if the contralateral facial nerve is available. Branches from the normal side are coapted to the sural nerve grafts, which are tunneled subcutaneously to the opposite side, and coapted to the distal stumps of the affected facial nerve. Cross-facial nerve grafting provides the advantage of spontaneous animation, but synkinesis can be expected, and results are not uniform.

   2. Nerve transfers can be used as an alternative to cross-facial nerve grafting. Nerve transfers offer a potentially greater number of axons, but have the disadvantage of synkinesis and lack of spontaneous expression.

      a. Hypoglossal-facial (XII–VII) nerve transfer can be performed end to side, so that most cranial nerve (CN) XII function is retained. Advantages: Excellent tone, low donor site morbidity. Disadvantages: Synkinesis, lack of spontaneous expression, alteration of expression with

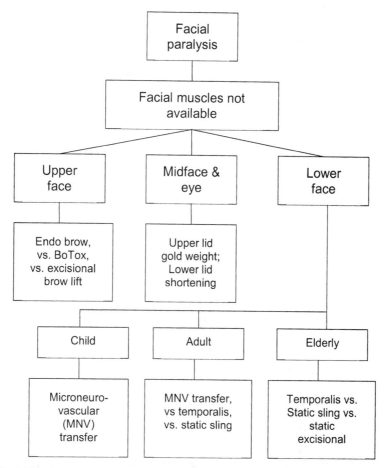

Fig. 22-3. Algorithm for treatment of facial paralysis if facial muscles are not available.

chewing. This procedure is sometimes used as a "babysitter" (to maintain muscle innervation) during the long period of axonal regeneration through a cross-facial graft.

    b. Other transfers: Spinal accessory–facial (XI–VII) transfer is rarely performed because of the resultant painful shoulder droop. Phrenic-facial transfer is rarely used because of hemidiaphragm paralysis.

C. If facial muscles are not available (e.g., long-standing paralysis and some congenital cases) (Fig. 22-3): Must address the lack of motors to the upper face (brow), midface and eye region, and lower face (smile) without the use of normal facial muscles. New motors must be introduced if dynamic function is sought; otherwise, static procedures are used.

  1. Treatment of the brow when facial muscles are unavailable: Endoscopic brow lift is usually sufficient to restore static symmetry. In cases of elderly patients with lax skin, a direct (excisional) unilateral brow lift may restore symmetry. In some cases, botulinum toxin may be used to decrease tone on the normal side, to match the paralyzed side.

  2. Treatment of the eye when facial muscles are unavailable

    a. The upper lid is best addressed with loading procedures. A gold (or platinum) weight is implanted anterior to the tarsus to provide lid closure with gravity. The lid must be taped when the patient is supine to achieve lid closure. Dynamic muscle transfers, such as the temporalis transfer, are not very effective for eyelid closure.

    b. Lower lid ectropion is addressed with a lateral canthoplasty (see Chapter 17, "Eyelid Reconstruction"). Eversion of a lax lid may produce epiphora (uncontrolled tearing) because the punctum is not in contact with the conjunctiva. This can be addressed with medial canthoplasty (partial excision and redraping of lid tissue).

  3. Treatment of the lower face when facial muscles are unavailable is highly dependent on patient age and motivation level. To be an optimal candidate for a microneurovascular muscle transfer, a patient must demonstrate the motivation to undergo lengthy procedures in multiple stages and to comply with physiotherapy (regimen of neuromuscular rehabilitation).

    a. Young or highly motivated patients: A microneurovascular transfer can provide a dynamic reconstruction of the lower face. The donor muscle of choice is typically the gracilis, innervated by either a cross-facial nerve graft, the masseteric branch of the trigeminal nerve, or a transfer from the hypoglossal nerve. Sometimes the gracilis is transferred with a long branch of the obturator nerve, obviating the need for a nerve graft.

    b. Adults, or patients with average motivation (Fig. 22-4).

      (1) Dynamic mouth motion can be achieved with a temporalis transfer. The Rubin procedure is a turndown of the temporalis with a fascial extension to secure it to the lips; the McLaughlin procedure involves transferring the insertion of the muscle from the coronoid process to the lips via fascial strip(s).

      (2) Static techniques (including static slings) use a fascial strip (such as fascia lata) that extends to the midline of the lips.

    c. Elderly patients.

      (1) Static slings establish oral symmetry in repose with temporalis fascia transfers or suspension with fascia lata grafts.

      (2) Static excisional procedures (e.g., unilateral facelifting) can be of considerable benefit.

  4. Treatment of the nose: Nasal airway collapse can be treated with fascial grafts to expand the nasal sphincter laterally. Septoplasty with spreader grafts may be of benefit if the patient has middle vault collapse.

VI. Adjunctive treatments

  A. Botulinum toxin injection can be used to improve facial symmetry. If significant synkinesis exists, toxin injections can be used to decrease the activity of

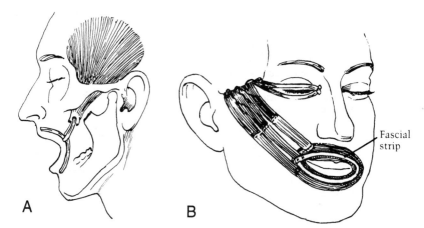

Fig. 22-4. Temporalis transfers for facial reanimation. **A:** The McLaughlin procedure transfers the coronoid attachment of the temporalis to the oral sphincter. **B:** The Rubin procedure consists of a turn-down of the temporalis over the zygoma, with connection to the oral sphincter via fascial strip(s). A separate slip can be directed to the orbicularis oculi, but this is not usually successful for improving lid closure. (From Baker D. Reconstruction of the paralyzed face. In *Grabb and Smith's Plastic Surgery*, 5th ed. Aston SJ, Beasley RW, Thorne CH, eds. Philadelphia, Lippincott-Raven, 1997. With permission.)

hypertonic muscles. As well, muscles on the normal side can be partially paralyzed to achieve a more balanced, aesthetic appearance.

B. Physical therapy (neuromuscular rehabilitation) is as essential to the management of facial paralysis as it is to the management of upper extremity tendon repairs. Stretching, vibration, biofeedback, and active exercises are used to rehabilitate the patient's control of facial expression. Specialized therapists can also advise patients on certain clothing and hairstyles that minimize the visual impact of facial asymmetry.

C. Patients often find **counseling** valuable. Depression is understandably common.

VII. Special considerations in pediatric facial paralysis

    A. Epidemiology

        1. Evidence of facial paralysis (usually transient) has been found to be present in up to 1% of live births in some studies.

        2. Most cases (70%–80%) result from obstetrical trauma.

    B. Causes and syndromes associated with pediatric (congenital) facial paralysis

        1. Trauma: Usually associated with forceps delivery, but pressure from the maternal sacrum can cause nerve injury; often managed with observation and steroids (controversial). Over 90% of cases resolve.

        2. Congenital unilateral lower lip paralysis (CULLP): Congenital absence or hypoplasia of the lower lip depressors.

        3. Velocardiofacial syndrome: Presents with CULLP, cardiac anomalies, and cleft palate.

        4. Intracranial hemorrhage can produce facial motor nucleus injury (supranuclear palsy).

        5. Hemifacial microsomia (oculoauriculovertebral dysplasia): Called Goldenhar's syndrome if vertebral anomalies and epibulbar dermoids are present; associated with congenital facial paralysis in some cases.

        6. Möbius syndrome: Consists of bilateral congenital facial paralysis resulting from a defect in development of the facial nucleus; it is often associated with paralysis of the abducens nerve (CN VI). Other nerves, including CN III, IV, IX, X, and XII, may be involved. Associated limb deformities may include club foot (most common), syndactyly, brachysyndactyly, absence of the sternal head of the pectoralis major (Poland's syndrome), and transverse or longitudinal arrest (see Chapter 42, "Congenital Anomalies of the Hand and Upper Extremity").

7. **Infectious causes** include otitis, mastoiditis, meningitis, and varicella infection.

8. **Teratogens:** Thalidomide and misoprostol.

C. **Key differences in management of pediatric patients** versus adult patients

1. **Evaluation** of congenital facial paralysis should involve a search for syndromic stigmata. Obtain input from a pediatric genetics team, especially with associated cardiac and CNS anomalies.

2. **Corneal protection** is usually best accomplished with corneal lubrication. Surgery is usually unnecessary, but when indicated, a lid loading procedure alone is usually sufficient.

3. **Feeding difficulties** may be present. Children should be monitored for appropriate growth, and, if needed, supplements or tube feeds should be used.

4. **Nerve transfers** in children should never include the phrenic nerve, since young children are obligate diaphragmatic breathers.

5. **Static slings** are rarely useful in children because soft tissue tone is usually preserved. In cases where facial muscles are not available, a microneurovascular transfer should always be considered.

Pearls

1. **Mnemonic device** for the motor branches of the facial nerve (temporal, zygomatic, buccal, mandibular, cervical): "**T**wo **z**ebras **b**it **m**y **c**at."

2. **The most common causes of adult facial paralysis are as follows.**
   a. Bell's palsy
   b. Trauma
   c. Ramsay Hunt syndrome (herpes zoster oticus, which presents with facial paralysis and ear pain)

3. **The facial nerve** innervates the posterior belly of the digastric muscle; the trigeminal nerve innervates the anterior belly.

4. **Facial paralysis** actually lessens the degree of age-related fine wrinkling on the affected side, because wrinkle-forming muscular activity is absent. However, the overall tissue laxity produced by aging is accentuated, leading to greater ptosis on the paralyzed side.

5. **The facial nerve** usually innervates mimetic muscles from their deep surfaces except in three cases: the mentalis, buccinator, and levator anguli oris.

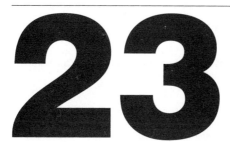

Cleft Lip

Lynn C. Jeffers

I. **Embryology**
  A. **The critical developmental period** of the lip and primary palate occurs during weeks 4 to 6 of gestation.
  B. **Failure of complete union** of the medial nasal prominence and the maxillary prominence leads to a variable extent of clefting of the primary palate, involving the upper lip, alveolus, and anterior hard palate anterior to the incisive foramen.
  C. **Cleft lip alone (CL) and cleft lip and palate (CLP)** are considered to be the same entity along a morphologic continuum. Cleft palate alone (CP), on the other hand, has different demographics.

II. **Epidemiology and genetics**
  A. **Incidence of cleft lip and of cleft lip and palate**
    1. The **overall** incidence is 1 in 1,000 live births.
    2. **White** ancestry: 1 in 750 live births.
    3. **Asian** ancestry: 1 in 500 live births.
    4. **African** ancestry: 1 in 2,000 live births.
  B. **Demographics**
    1. **Male-to-female** ratio of 2:1.
    2. The ratio of left (L) to right (R) to bilateral (B) clefts **(L:R:B):** 6:3:1.
    3. **The ratio of CLP to CL** is 2:1.
    4. **Three percent are syndromic.**
    5. **Risk factors**
      a. Medications: Phenytoin, methylprednisolone (Solu-Medrol), steroids, phenobarbital, diazepam, and isotretinoin.
      b. Smoking.
      c. Parental age, especially father's age, or both mother and father over 30 years old.
      d. Family history (see "Genetics").
  C. **Genetics**
    1. **The risk** of having a child with CLP (see Table 24-1 in Chapter 24, "Cleft Palate").
      a. If parents have one child with CLP: 4%.
      b. If one parent has CLP: 2% to 4%.
      c. If parents have two children with CLP: 9%.
      d. If one child and one parent have CLP: 14% to 17%.
    2. **Most cases are sporadic** (and multifactorial), but may be X-linked, autosomal dominant (Van der Woude's syndrome) or familial (see "Syndromes Associated with Cleft Lip and Palate," later in this chapter).

III. **Anatomy**
  A. **Normal lip anatomy**
    1. **Topographic landmarks**
      a. Nasal alae.
      b. Columella.
      c. Philtral columns.
      d. White roll: Well-defined mucocutaneous or vermilion-cutaneous border.

   e. Vermilion: Red portion of lip.
   f. Tubercle.
   g. Cupid's bow.
   h. Wet-dry border: The vermilion-mucosa junction is the border between keratinized and nonkeratinized mucosa.
  2. Musculature.
   a. Orbicularis oris.
      (1) Fibers cross (decussate) in the midline and create the opposite philtral columns.
      (2) Functions as a sphincter (deep fibers) and for speech (superficial fibers).
   b. Levator labii superioris.
      (1) Inserts into the dermis at the vermilion border and the lower edge of the philtral columns.
      (2) Elevates the upper lip.
   c. Nasalis or depressor septi nasi muscle: The fibers run from the alveolar bone into the medial crural footplates, skin of the columella and the tip of the nose, and into the opposite philtral columns.
  3. Normal measurements.
   a. Vertical length (height) of the upper lip.
      (1) Newborn: 10 mm.
      (2) Age 3 months: 13 mm.
      (3) Adult: 17 mm.
   b. The distance between the peaks of Cupid's bow: Approximately 3 mm at 3 months.
  4. Arterial blood supply: The labial artery, bilaterally.
  5. Sensory innervation: The trigeminal nerve, cranial nerve (CN) V, maxillary division (V2).
  6. Motor innervation: The facial nerve, CN VII, zygomatic and buccal branches.
 B. Cleft lip anatomy.
  1. Alterations in the orbicularis oris, levator labii, and nasalis result in disruption of continuity, orientation, and quality of the muscles.
   a. Fibers are disoriented and run parallel to the cleft margin.
   b. Fibers insert into the alar base on the cleft (lateral) segment and into the columella in the noncleft (medial) segment, as well as intradermally.
   c. Incomplete clefts.
      (1) Simonart's band consists of a skin bridge across the nasal sill. It does not usually contain any significant muscle mass.
      (2) Some fibers may cross the cleft, if the cleft is less than two-thirds of lip height.
   d. Bilateral complete clefts: No muscle tissue is present in the prolabium.
  2. Vertical lip length is decreased: Cupid's bow and the lip are rotated cephalad on both the lateral, cleft side as well as the medial side.
  3. Disrupted Cupid's bow.
  4. The alveolus and nostril floor are open in a complete cleft lip.
  5. The premaxilla is rotated and protruding, especially in bilateral cleft lip, often with collapse of the lateral segment of the cleft side(s).
  6. Associated cleft lip nasal abnormalities (Fig. 23-1).
   a. Hypoplastic, flattened alar dome on the affected side.
   b. Lack of upper lateral cartilage overlap of lower lateral cartilage.
   c. Subluxed lower lateral cartilage with alar base displaced cephalad and posteriorly.
   d. Hypoplastic bony foundation (maxilla).
   e. The caudal septum is pulled toward the noncleft side.
   f. Flattening of the nasal bones.
   g. Shortened columella, especially in bilateral cases.

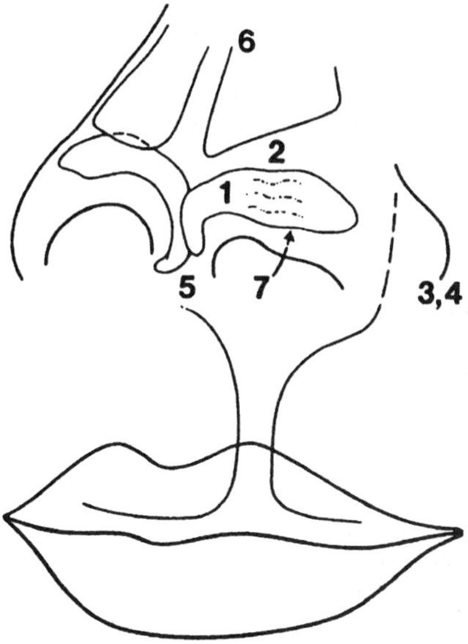

Fig. 23-1. Cleft lip nasal deformity. 1 and 7: Hypoplastic, flattened alar dome on the affected side. 2: Lack of upper lateral cartilage overlap of lower lateral cartilage. 3: Subluxed lower lateral cartilage with alar base displaced cephalad and posteriorly. 4: Hypoplastic bony foundation (maxilla). 5: The caudal septum is pulled toward the non-cleft side. 6: Flattening of the nasal bones. (From LaRossa D and Randall P Unilateral cleft lip. In *Plastic, Maxillofacial, and Reconstructive Surgery*, 3rd ed. Georgiade G, Riefkohl R, Levin S, eds. Philadelphia, Williams & Wilkins, 1997. With permission.)

IV. Classification
A. Extent of the cleft: Complete versus incomplete
 1. **Complete cleft lip**
  a. Complete disruption of the soft tissues to the nasal floor.
  b. Tends to be wider than incomplete clefts, with greater nasal deformities.
 2. **Incomplete cleft lip**
  a. Disruption of the soft tissues to varying degrees.
  b. The alveolus is usually intact, with less of a tendency for the premaxilla to protrude.
  c. Forme fruste: A very mild cleft.
   (1) May be difficult to detect.
   (2) May appear as vermilion notching or a scarlike line or depression.
B. Location of the cleft: Unilateral versus bilateral
 1. **Unilateral cleft lip**
 2. **Bilateral cleft lip**
  a. May have a complete or incomplete cleft on both sides, or a combination.
  b. More likely to be complete clefts and are often wide.
  c. The premaxillary segment may include tooth buds.
  d. In bilateral complete clefts, the prolabium lacks muscle tissue, and therefore lacks philtral columns.
C. Alveolar segments
 1. Narrow versus wide cleft
 2. Collapse versus no collapse

V. Syndromes associated with cleft lip and palate

A. Van der Woude's syndrome

1. **Autosomal dominant,** with variable penetrance.
2. **Associated with CLP or CP** (40%–50% penetrance).
3. **Associated with lip pits** (accessory salivary glands, 70%–80% penetrance).
4. May also have absent second molar, syndactyly, abnormal genitalia, and popliteal pterygia.

B. Waardenburg's syndrome

1. A group of anomalies arising from abnormal development and migration of neural crest cells.
2. Features may include cleft lip, cleft palate.

C. Down syndrome (trisomy 21)

D. Trisomy 13

E. Stickler's syndrome

1. **A group of anomalies** caused by connective tissue dysplasia.
2. **Typical features:** Cleft palate, progressive joint degeneration, and various ocular abnormalities that may lead to blindness.
3. **Autosomal dominant inheritance.**
4. **Other anomalies:** Cardiac, sensorineural, and learning disorders or mental retardation.

F. Pierre Robin sequence (*Note:* A *sequence* is a group of anomalies that result from a single disrupted event.)

1. Micrognathia or retrognathia prevents normal descent of the tongue. The tongue then interferes with fusion of the palatal shelves. As a result, typical features include micrognathia or retrognathia, glossoptosis (tongue falls back into the pharynx, causing airway obstruction), and a U-shaped cleft palate.
2. May be a part of multiple different syndromes or may be an isolated finding.
3. **Treatment.**
   a. Prone positioning to help move the tongue out of the airway; the most conservative approach.
   b. Supplemental oxygen.
   c. Tongue-lip adhesion.
   d. Mandibular distraction osteogenesis.
   e. Intubation/tracheostomy.
4. **Patients may show catch-up mandibular growth,** depending on their syndromic association.
5. **Polysomnogram:** Necessary to evaluate for desaturations as well as apneic events.

G. Velocardiofacial syndrome

1. **Autosomal dominant inheritance:** Fluorescent *in situ* hybridization (FISH) may show an abnormality in chromosome 22.
2. **Characteristic features** include the following.
   a. Cleft palate.
   b. Congenital heart disease.
   c. Broad nasal dorsum and elongated face.
   d. Narrow, down-slanting palpebral fissures.
   e. Velopharyngeal insufficiency is common, even with a submucous cleft palate.
   f. The carotid arteries may be displaced medially, placing them at high risk of injury during pharyngeal flap surgery or dynamic sphincter pharyngoplasty. Always palpate the posterior pharynx prior to making an incision; consider obtaining a preoperative angiogram.

H. Median cleft lip

1. **Rare.**
2. **A different entity** from the typical cleft lip; more accurately considered a median craniofacial cleft (Tessier type zero).
3. **Associated with a group of syndromes** (median cerebral facial dysgenesis) that involve more severe deformities of midline CNS and facial structures.

   4. Further workup is needed, including a formal CNS evaluation.
   5. May be associated with holoprosencephaly, pituitary problems, and a limited lifespan.
VI. Staging of intervention
   A. Initial evaluation
      1. Reassure the parents and family that they are not to blame.
      2. Explain the stages and operations that should be expected throughout the child's lifetime.
      3. Evaluate for associated anomalies.
      4. Consultations
         a. Genetics, for evaluation and possible counseling
         b. Social work
         c. Feeding/nutrition
            (1) The child may need special nipples or bottles (e.g., cross-cut nipple).
            (2) Monitor for appropriate weight gain.
         d. Otolaryngology: Children with cleft lip and palate have a high incidence of eustachian tube dysfunction, and therefore otitis media, requiring close follow-up.
            (1) The child may need myringotomy tubes.
            (2) If untreated, repeat otitis may affect hearing and speech development.
   B. Wide clefts (>1 cm)
      1. Goal: Bring the segments closer together to facilitate a tension-free repair.
         a. Has not been shown to change skeletal development in the anteroposterior direction.
         b. Does not seem to prevent future crossbite.
      2. Passive: Preoperative taping
         a. Steri-Strip tapes applied across both segments of the lip.
         b. Requires reliable parents who can reapply the tape and keep it on at all times.
      3. Passive: Lip adhesion operation
         a. Suturing the edges of the cleft together is performed under anesthesia.
         b. The definitive lip repair is performed once the segments have moved closer together.
         c. Variable success.
      4. Active: Latham-type device
         a. An orthodontic appliance that must be placed onto the palatal segments under anesthesia.
         b. Parents turn a screw daily, which slowly brings the palatal segments into better alignment.
         c. Removed at the time of definitive lip repair.
   C. Repair
      1. Timing (controversial)
         a. Repair at 3 months is generally accepted.
         b. Some argue for earlier repair in order to produce better scars.
      2. Rule of tens: For increased anesthetic safety, an infant should
         a. Be 10 weeks old.
         b. Weigh 10 pounds.
         c. Have a hemoglobin level of at least 10 mg/dL.
      3. Cleft palate repair and secondary alveolar grafting (see Chapter 24, "Cleft Palate").
      4. May also choose to address the cleft nasal deformity at time of lip repair.
VII. Intraoperative considerations
   A. Landmarks
      1. Tattooed with methylene blue, using a hypodermic needle or a quill pen.
         a. Alar bases.
         b. Columella.
         c. Philtral columns.

      d. Peak of Cupid's bow and midline on the medial segment. Measure the anticipated distance for the new Cupid's bow (approximately 3–4 mm).

      e. Peak of Cupid's bow on the lateral segment.

  2. Account for distortion from the uncountered pull of the orbicularis on the medial segment. The philtral columns are usually slightly C-shaped.

B. Mark lines for expected repair type.

C. Only *after* **marks are completed, infiltrate tissue with local anesthetic** to avoid distortion of anatomy and measurements.

D. Goals of repair

  1. Reconstitute Cupid's bow.

  2. Minimize scarring.

  3. Produce a slight pout of the tubercle.

  4. Produce functional continuity of the muscles.

  5. Recreate symmetry.

VIII. Types of repair

A. Straight-line repair

  1. Historically, the first cleft lip repairs relied on freshening the edges of the cleft and suturing them together. These have been largely replaced by various Z-plasty-based techniques.

  2. Rose-Thompson repair

    a. Modified straight-line repair that can be used for minor clefts with lip length nearly equal on both sides of cleft (e.g., forme fruste).

    b. Fusiform excision with straight-line closure.

B. Quadrangular flap

  1. Proposed by LeMesurier and Hagedorn.

  2. Cupid's bow is derived from the lateral lip.

  3. 90-degree Z-plasty.

  4. Violates Cupid's bow and philtral dimple.

  5. Has a tendency to produce a long lip.

C. Triangular flap

  1. Proposed by Tennison and Randall

    a. The Z-plasty is placed at the vermilion border.

    b. Produces a natural-appearing Cupid's bow.

    c. May be used for clefts of all widths.

    d. Violates Cupid's bow and the philtral dimple.

    e. May also have problem with a long lip.

  2. Skoog repair

    a. Consists of two Z-plasties.

    b. Violates Cupid's bow and the philtral dimple.

D. Rotation advancement (Fig. 23-2)

  1. Popularized by Millard

    a. Likely the most commonly used repair. Often described as the "cut-as-you-go" technique.

    b. The medial lip is rotated downward to fill the cleft defect.

    c. A small pennant-shaped C-flap can either be rotated to create the nasal sill or used to lengthen the columella.

    d. Does not violate Cupid's bow or the philtral dimple.

    e. Difficult for wider clefts.

    f. Common pitfall is inadequate flap rotation leading to notching and inadequate vertical lip length.

      (1) Repeat advancement or a small Z-plasty at the vermilion border can be performed.

      (2) Better results are obtained if adequate rotation is performed at the time of the original operation.

  2. Poole repair

    a. Preserves the integrity of the aesthetic unit at the columellar-labial junction.

    b. Allows lengthening of the lip without extending the advancement flap up on the ala or encroaching on horizontal lip length.

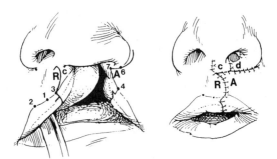

Fig. 23-2. Unilateral cleft lip rotation advancement repair. 1: The lowest point of cupid's bow. 2: The peak of the noncleft side cupid's bow. 3: Extrapolated by marking the same distance as from 1 to 2. 4: The point at which the white roll disappears on the cleft side. The flap R rotates down and laterally to provide height to the cleft side. The flap A advances into the defect created by the rotation flap, thus completing a modified plasty. (From Byrd S. Unilateral cleft lip. In the textbook, *Grabb and Smith's Plastic Surgery*, 5th ed. Aston SJ, Beasley RW, Thorne CH, eds. Philadelphia, Lippincott-Raven, 1997. With permission.)

E. Bilateral cleft lip repair
  1. The premaxillary segment is often a greater problem than in a unilateral cleft lip.
  2. Consider taping, lip adhesion, or presurgical orthodontics (see above).
  3. Most common techniques
    a. Dissect the prolabium to maintain a central skin flap to resemble the philtrum.
    b. Deepithelialize the remainder of the prolabium.
    c. Use the prolabial vermilion to create a labial sulcus, not for the final lip vermilion. The final lip vermilion is composed only of vermilion from the lateral lip segments, not from the prolabium.
    d. Columellar lengthening may be performed at the time of lip repair or as a secondary procedure.
IX. Postoperative care
  A. Orders
    1. Arm restraints ("no-no's") for 3 weeks to prevent disruption of repair.
    2. Specialized nipple/bottle to decrease sucking effort when bottle-feeding.
    3. Breast-feeding is controversial; based on surgeon preference.
  B. Leave Steri-Strips in place over the incision for reinforcement.
  C. Follow up in 1 week for suture removal if nonabsorbable skin sutures were used.

Pearls

Preoperative

1. Practice lip markings and cuts on foam first.
2. Do not forget to assess for an adequate bony platform and the need for orthognathic surgery when assessing cleft nasal deformities.

Intraoperative

1. Mark several times, cut once.
2. Beaver scalpel blades are helpful.

3. Line up the white roll first, placing a stitch above and below the white roll, then reapproximate the wet-dry border.
4. Bilateral cleft: Do not use the "vermilion" of the premaxillary segment in the final vermilion. It tends to look like an abnormal, dry patch postoperatively.

Postoperative

1. Instruct the parents to hold off feeding prior to the clinic appointment. In the clinic, the baby will stay quiet during feeding usually just long enough for suture removal.
2. Keep a Steri-Strip tape in place for 1 to 2 weeks for support.

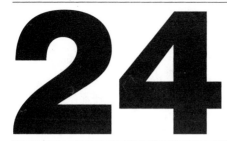

Cleft Palate

Douglas Sammer

I. **Normal anatomy**
  A. **Hard palate**
    1. **Primary (anterior) hard palate:** Formed by fusion of the bilateral palatine processes of the maxilla.
    2. **Secondary (posterior) hard palate:** Formed by fusion of the bilateral horizontal plates of the palatine bone.
    3. **Incisive foramen:** Separates the primary from the secondary hard palate.
    4. **Premaxilla:** The maxilla anterior to the incisive foramen, including the anterior hard palate and alveolus.
  B. **Soft palate (velum):** Contains the muscles involved in velopharyngeal closure
    1. Levator veli palatini.
    2. Tendon of the tensor veli palatini.
    3. Palatopharyngeus.
    4. Palatoglossus.
    5. Uvulae.
  C. **Vascular and nerve supply**
    1. **Hard palate:** The greater palatine artery and nerves, through the greater palatine foramen in the posterior lateral hard palate.
    2. **Soft palate:** The lesser palatine artery and nerves.
II. **Cleft anatomy**
  A. **Clefts of the secondary palate**
    1. **A variable degree of clefting can be seen.**
      a. Bifid uvula.
      b. Submucous cleft palate triad.
        (1) Bifid uvula.
        (2) Hard palate notching (palpable).
        (3) Zona pellucida: Midline white line, due to the anomalous insertion of the palatal musculature.
      c. Cleft velum.
      d. Cleft of the entire secondary palate.
    2. **Anomalous insertion** of the tensor veli palatini.
      a. The normal bilateral tensor veli palatini muscles interdigitate and insert transversely in the posterior part of the velum.
      b. With clefting, the tensor veli palatini muscles course anteriorly and insert onto the posterior edge of the hard palate.
      c. In this position, their ability to lift the soft palate is significantly impaired.
  B. **Clefts of the primary palate**
    1. **The lip, nostril sill, alveolus, and primary palate** are all considered derivatives of the primary palate.
    2. **Clefts of the primary palate** can involve the lip alone, extend into or through the alveolus and primary palate, or extend through the secondary palate.
  C. **Kernahan's striped Y** serves as a shorthand for recording cleft palate extent.
III. **Facial embryology**
  A. **Five facial prominences** (develop during week 4 of gestation)

   1. Midline frontonasal prominence: Mesenchyme ventral to the forebrain, not a branchial arch.
   2. Bilateral maxillary prominences: First branchial arch.
   3. Bilateral mandibular prominences: First branchial arch.
  B. **Bilateral nasal placodes**
   1. Appear on the inferior frontonasal prominence, late in week 4.
   2. The medial and lateral nasal prominences emerge on each side of the nasal placodes.
  C. **Fusion: week 5**
   1. The lateral nasal prominence fuses with the maxillary prominence, connecting the nose to the cheek.
   2. The medial nasal prominences fuse.
   3. The medial nasal prominence fuses with the maxillary prominence, connecting the nose and lip. Failure of this fusion results in a cleft lip.
IV. **Palatal embryology**
  A. **Primary palate and premaxilla**
   1. The medial nasal processes fuse to form the median palatine process in week 5.
   2. The median palatine process becomes the premaxilla.
  B. **Secondary palate: weeks 5 to 12**
   1. **The bilateral lateral palatine processes** develop from the medial portion of the maxillary process.
   2. **The lateral palatine processes** hang vertically, and then lift horizontally as the tongue drops.
   3. **Fusion starts at the incisive foramen** and moves posteriorly, forming the secondary palate.
V. **Epidemiology**
  A. **Racial distribution**
   1. **Isolated cleft palate**
     a. Incidence of about 0.5 per 1,000 births.
     b. Does not vary with race.
   2. **Cleft lip with or without cleft palate**
     a. Asians: 2 per 1,000 births.
     b. Whites: 1 per 1,000 births.
     c. Blacks: 0.4 per 1,000 births.
  B. **Gender distribution**
   1. Isolated cleft palate is more common in females.
   2. Cleft lip with cleft palate is more common in males.
  C. **Familial distribution** (Table 24-1)
   1. Cleft lip with or without cleft palate and isolated cleft palate appear to be genetically different.
   2. Isolated cleft palate is more common in relatives of cleft palate patients.

Table 24-1. Probability of subsequent children with isolated cleft palate or cleft lip with/without cleft palate

Family Members with Cleft Palate	Probability of Subsequent Child with Cleft Palate (%)	Probability of Subsequent Child with Cleft Lip +/− Cleft Palate (%)
One affected child only	2	4
One affected parent only	2–4	2–4
One affected child and a positive family history (with normal parents)	7	7
One affected parent and one affected child	15	14–17

3. Cleft lip/palate is more common in relatives of cleft lip/palate patients (see Chapter 23, "Cleft Lip").

VI. Etiology

A. Genetics

1. **An isolated cleft palate** is probably a single major gene autosomal recessive trait with other minor genes contributing.
2. **Cleft lip/palate** is probably polygenic with multiple major and minor genes contributing.

B. Environment

1. The exact role of any environmental factor is not clear.
2. **Alcohol** has not been conclusively shown to cause isolated cleft palate.
3. **Smoking:** Data are not conclusive.
4. **Many teratogens** (including alcohol, isotretinoin, and others) are known to cause multiple congenital malformations, which may include cleft palate as part of a series of malformations.
5. **Folic acid and vitamin B$_6$** intake during pregnancy may reduce cleft lip/palate.

VII. Surgical goals

A. Closure of the cleft

1. Closure of the cleft palate separates the oral and nasal cavities.
2. This prevents aerophagia and reflux of oral contents into the nasal cavity.

B. Speech and hearing

1. Cleft palate repair must be performed early in life to prevent irreparable speech defects.
2. However, "early" palate surgery is associated with impaired facial growth.
3. Because facial structures can be surgically repaired later in life, whereas speech patterns cannot, most surgeons feel that normal speech development is more important than normal facial growth and therefore favor early repair.

C. Otitis and hearing

1. **Otitis media**
   a. Secondary to eustachian tube dysfunction.
      (1) The levator veli palatini (LVP) originates along the eustachian tube.
      (2) An abnormal LVP insertion is thought to decrease "milking" action and therefore lead to poor venting of the middle ear.
   b. Occurs in almost all patients with cleft palate, and can lead to permanently impaired hearing.
2. **Hearing** in cleft palate patients generally improves after myringotomy.
3. **The earlier the myringotomy** is performed, the greater the improvement in hearing. Normal hearing is usually achieved with early bilateral tympanostomy.
4. It is not clear whether repair of cleft palate or repair of velopharyngeal incompetence (VPI) reduces otitis media or improves hearing.

D. Facial growth

1. Early palate surgery can adversely affect maxillary growth.
2. Repair of the primary palate and alveolus has more significant effects on maxillary growth than repair of the secondary palate alone.
3. Facial growth is less affected if palatoplasty is delayed until 1 year of age.
4. For these reasons, some surgeons close the soft palate early (around 3 months) and the hard palate later (ranging from 9 to 18 months).
5. Each case must be approached individually, carefully considering facial growth and speech development.

VIII. Surgical repair

A. Hard palate clefts

1. **Von Langenbeck repair** (Fig. 24-1)
   a. Bilateral, bipedicled mucoperiosteal flaps.
   b. Lateral relaxing incisions are made bilaterally.
   c. The flaps are closed at the midline, nasal mucosa first and oral mucosa last.

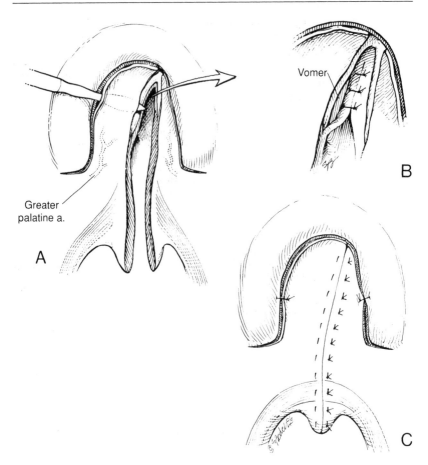

Fig. 24-1. Von Langenbeck palatoplasty technique. **A:** Bilateral, unipedicled mucoperiosteal flaps are elevated, based on the greater palatine arteries. **B:** Anteriorly, the nasal floor is repaired by suturing the vomerine mucosa to the nasal mucosa on the cleft side. **C:** The oral mucosa is reapproximated in the midline with interrupted horizontal mattress sutures. (From Hobar C., Johns D., and Flood J. Cleft palate repair and velopharyngeal insufficiency. In the textbook, *Grabb and Smith's Plastic Surgery*, 5th ed. Aston SJ, Beasley RW, Thorne CH, eds. Philadelphia, Lippincott-Raven, 1997. With permission.)

      d. Many modifications exist.
      e. This repair may result in a short palate and contribute to VPI.
   2. V-Y pushback (Veau-Wardill-Kilner)
      a. Bilateral mucoperiosteal flaps, unipedicled posteriorly.
      b. V-Y advancement posteriorly is performed.
      c. Anterior exposed areas are left open to granulate and mucosalize.
      d. Improves velopharyngeal closure by lengthening the palate; may improve speech.
B. Soft palate clefts
   1. Straight-line repair: Separate nasal and oral mucosal flaps are raised and approximated.

2. **Double Z-plasty (Furlow)**
   a. Z-plasty flaps of oral and nasal mucosa (with LVP muscle included) are used in opposing directions.
   b. Z-plasties are performed in layers, with nasal mucosal flaps transposed and closed, followed by transposition and closure of oral mucosal flaps.
   c. Lengthens the soft palate.
   d. Reorients the levator veli palatini muscles.
   e. Can be used along with hard palate closure in one operation, or as veloplasty to be followed later by hard palate closure (see above).
C. **Vomer flap**
   1. Flaps may be based inferiorly or superiorly, and may be unilateral or bilateral.
   2. Helps provide tissue for closure of wide clefts.
   3. Superiorly based flaps are used more commonly.
   4. Inferiorly based flaps are useful for wider clefts.
   5. May or may not impair maxillary growth (controversial).
D. **Alveolar repair**
   1. **Mucoperiosteal flaps** are raised and inset as advancement flaps.
   2. **Bone grafting** is performed if necessary.
   3. **Some perform grafting early** (primarily), although most prefer secondary bone grafting before the permanent cleft canine emerges, during the period of early mixed dentition, around 8 years of age.
   4. **For primary grafting,** a mucosal flap is raised in the vestibule of the lip anterior to the cleft, and a rib graft is commonly used.
   5. **For secondary grafting,** gingival mucoperiosteal flaps are raised on both sides of the cleft, with the incision at the gingival sulcus of the teeth, and cancellous bone from the ilium is used.

IX. **Complications**
A. **Fistulae**
   1. Occur in up to 50% of procedures depending on the preoperative anatomy and the repair technique.
   2. More common in wide or bilateral clefts.
   3. Most occur in the hard palate, posterior to the alveolus.
   4. More common with a single-layer closure.
B. **Midfacial growth problems**
   1. Multifactorial.
   2. Cleft palate patients have inherent facial growth impairment.
   3. Lip and alveolar repair significantly affect facial growth.
   4. The extent and timing of palate repair can affect facial growth (see above).
C. **Airway obstruction**
   1. May occur secondary to postoperative bleeding.
   2. More common in operations that include pharyngeal flaps.
   3. Patients should be monitored closely postoperatively.

X. **Velopharyngeal incompetence**
A. **Definition:** Inappropriate incomplete closure of the velum against the posterior pharynx during speech
B. **Etiology**
   1. **In cleft palate patients,** the levator veli palatini inserts anteriorly onto the hard palate, and loses its ability to lift the soft palate to achieve velopharyngeal closure.
   2. **Approximately 20% of patients** acquire clinical VPI following palate repair.
   3. **Some cleft palate operations greatly improve palate length and levator orientation,** whereas others do so to a lesser extent.
      a. The Von Langenbeck procedure tends to cause a short palate because no length is added in the procedure.
      b. The V-Y pushback techniques improve palate length.
      c. The Furlow double Z-plasty soft palate repair lengthens the palate and corrects muscle insertion on the palate.

C. Speech and velopharyngeal insufficiency

1. **Air escapes from the oropharynx** up through the nasopharynx.
2. **This results in hypernasal speech** and escape of excess air from the nose during speech (nasal emission), causing difficulty with consonants.
3. **The patient adjusts** to these problems by developing alternative methods for creating certain vocal sounds (pharyngeal fricatives and glottal stops). Plosives: /p/, /b/, /t/, /d/, /k/, /g/; fricatives: /f/, /v/, /th/, /s/, /z/, /sh/, /zh/.

D. Treatment of VPI

1. **Pharyngeal flaps**
   a. Best for patients with adequate lateral pharyngeal wall movement (good medial excursion) based on nasal endoscopy or videofluoroscopy.
   b. A myomucosal flap from the posterior pharyngeal wall is elevated.
   c. The flap contains mucosa and pharyngeal constrictor muscle, exposing the prevertebral fascia.
   d. May be based superiorly or inferiorly.
   e. The flap is then sutured to the posterior soft palate.
   f. This creates a tissue bridge between the soft palate and the posterior pharynx, allowing the lateral pharyngeal walls to close in and cause velopharyngeal closure.
   g. This is a static repair (the flap does not move to cause port closure).
   h. The difficulty is in adjusting the port/opening size correctly; too wide an opening leaves the patient hypernasal, whereas limiting air flow too much induces a state of hyponasality.

2. **Pharyngoplasty (dynamic sphincter pharyngoplasty)**
   a. Best for patients with inadequate lateral pharyngeal wall medial excursion.
   b. Superiorly based bilateral flaps that include the posterior tonsillar pillars and the palatopharyngeus muscles are elevated and are set in overlapping positions into a horizontal incision in the posterior pharyngeal wall.
   c. This is a potentially dynamic repair. The sphincter created may have some movement to help achieve port closure.

3. **Complications**
   a. Airway obstruction in the acute postoperative period can be life-threatening, and patients should have apnea monitors.
   b. Obstructive sleep apnea is not uncommon in the early postoperative period.
   c. Dehiscence, bleeding, and infection are other complications.
   d. Patients with velocardiofacial syndrome often have midline or medially deviated internal carotids, increasing the risk of carotid injury during flap elevation. Consider preoperative angiogram and/or magnetic resonance angiogram. Palpate intraoperatively for medialized carotid pulsations.

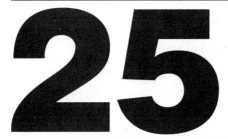

Craniosynostosis and Craniofacial Syndromes

Christi M. Cavaliere

I. Cranial vault development

A. Tissues that form the skull are derived from mesenchyme and develop through both intramembranous and endochondral ossification (Table 25-1).

1. **Some of the skull develops through intramembranous ossification** (direct ossification of mesenchyme).

   a. Flat calvarial bones (frontal and parietal).

   (1) Cranial sutures are fibrous connections between individual calvarial bones. Fontanelles ("soft spots") are sites where multiple sutures meet.

   (2) Soft cranial bones with fibrous connections allow deformation of the cranium during birth.

   (3) Growth occurs at bone edges along the sutures. Ossification begins centrally and proceeds radially within a given bone.

   b. Facial bones are derived from the first pharyngeal arch through intramembranous ossification.

   (1) Maxillary prominence of first arch develops into the premaxilla, maxilla, and zygoma.

   (2) Mandibular prominence becomes the mandible.

2. **Some bones form through endochondral ossification** (ossification of a cartilaginous precursor).

   a. The skull base, including the sphenoid, squamous temporal, and occipital bones.

   b. The first pharyngeal arch (Meckel's cartilage) forms the malleus and incus.

   c. The second pharyngeal arch (Reichert's cartilage) forms the stapes, styloid, and the hyoid (lesser cornu and superior body).

   d. The third pharyngeal arch cartilage forms the greater cornu and the inferior body of the hyoid.

B. Skull growth

1. **The period of most rapid postnatal skull growth** occurs concurrently with rapid brain growth (0–24 months).

2. **The brain is approximately 25% of adult size at birth,** 50% at 6 months, 75% at 1 year, and nearly 100% by 2 years.

3. **Skull growth ceases** around the mid-teen years.

4. **Sinus development** proceeds in a stepwise fashion (Table 25-2).

II. Craniosynostosis

A. Consists of premature fusion of one or more cranial sutures, limiting brain growth in the direction perpendicular to the affected suture. Compensatory growth occurs parallel to the affected suture (Virchow's law).

B. Primary craniosynostosis (nonsyndromic) occurs due to an abnormality of the suture, with no identifiable underlying cause.

C. Craniosynostosis syndromes are primarily due to genetic mutations (see below).

D. Secondary craniosynostosis occurs in the setting of other abnormalities.

1. **Microcephaly**

2. **Hyperthyroidism**

Table 25-1. Pharyngeal arch derivatives

Arch	Cranial Nerve	Skeletal Structures (Mode of Ossification)	Musculature
First arch	V2	Arch mesenchyme (intramembranous)	Mastication
	V3	Maxillary prominence	Temporalis
		Premaxilla	Masseter
		Maxilla	Medial pterygoid
		Zygoma	Lateral pterygoid
		Mandibular prominence	Mylohyoid
		Mandible	Anterior belly digastric
		Mandibular cartilage (Meckel's) (endochondral)	Tensor tympani
		Malleus	Tensor veli palatini
		Maxillary cartilage (endochondral)	
		Incus	
Second arch	VII	Reichert's cartilage (endochondral)	Muscles of facial expression
		Stapes	Posterior belly digastric
		Styloid	Stapedius
		Hyoid (lesser cornu, superior body)	Stylohyoid
Third arch	IX	(Endochondral)	Stylopharyngeus
		Hyoid (greater cornu, superior body)	
Fourth arch	X (superior laryngeal)	Laryngeal cartilages	Pharyngeal constrictors
			Cricothyroid
			Levator veli palatini
Fifth arch	X (recurrent laryngeal)	Laryngeal cartilages	Intrinsic muscles of larynx

    3. **Rickets.**
    4. **Mucopolysaccharidoses.**
    5. **Hematologic disorders,** including thalassemia and sickle cell.
  E. Diagnosis
    1. **Clinical history:** An irregular head shape that worsens with time.
    2. **Craniofacial abnormalities** are typically more severe with earlier fusion.
    3. **Cranial as well as facial asymmetries.**
    4. **Ridging** along synostosed suture.
    5. **Fontanelle** may be poorly defined, and infant cranial bones may fail to move relative to one another as they normally do.
    6. **Measure head circumference** and compare with growth chart-predicted values.
    7. **Plain cephalic radiographs** may show sclerosis of suture or absent suture. Computed tomography (CT) is necessary if plain films poorly visualize suture.
    8. **Genetic evaluation** may be performed for patients with a potentially syndromic synostosis; refer family for genetic counseling.
    9. **Evaluate for elevated intracranial pressure (ICP):** Present in approximately 10% of patients with single-suture synostosis and 40% with multiple-suture involvement. Signs may include the following.
      a. Irritability, difficult to console.
      b. Vomiting.

Table 25-2. Sinus development

Sinus	Age of First Appearance	Age When Sinus Development Is Completed
Maxillary	3 months' gestation	Childhood
Sphenoid	5 months' gestation	Childhood
Ethmoid	5 months' gestation	Puberty
Frontal	5 years old (only sinus to appear postnatally)	Adolescence

      c. Papilledema.
      d. Bulging fontanelles.
      e. Copper-beaten appearance of skull on radiographs.
  F. Craniosynostosis versus positional head deformity (positional or deformational plagiocephaly, PHD) (Table 25-3)
    1. PHD results from deformation of the pliable fetal or infant skull in response to external pressure.
    2. Causes of PHD
      a. Sleeping predominantly in the supine position.
      b. *In utero* compression.
      c. Congenital muscular torticollis.
      d. Abnormal neck range of motion due to skeletal deformity. Evaluate with cervical spine radiographs.
      e. Abnormal vision leading to preferred head position.
    3. Treatment of the underlying cause
      a. Physical therapy with active and passive stretching of sternocleidomastoid for torticollis. Muscular release if needed.
      b. Encourage head and neck rotation while feeding.
    4. Shaping helmet treatment can improve contour.
      a. Passive process with helmet fitted to widest skull dimension. Room is left in the helmet for compensatory growth/expansion in areas that are relatively recessed.

Table 25-3. Features that distinguish positional head deformity from craniosynostosis

Structure	Synostotic Plagiocephaly	Plagiocephaly Due to Positional Head Deformity*
Forehead	Affected forehead flat	Affected forehead flat
Orbit	Affected side with elevated brow, harlequin orbit	Orbit lower on affected side
Ear	Affected side with ear displaced anterior and superior	Affected side with ear displaced posterior and inferior
Face	C-shaped facial deformity with nose and chin deviated toward contralateral side	C-shaped facial deformity with nose and chin deviated toward affected side

*For *left* occipital flattening, the affected side includes the *right* forehead and facial structures.

   b. Effective if used for 23 hours or more per day.
   c. Effective if worn for at least 2 months.
   d. Loses efficacy after 18 months of age.
   e. Repeated helmet fittings are needed as the head shape improves.
G. Phenotypic effects of synostosis
   1. Sagittal synostosis
      a. Most common form of craniosynostosis.
      b. Scaphocephaly: Cranial growth is restricted in the biparietal dimension and elongated in the anteroposterior (AP) direction.
   2. Coronal synostosis
      a. Unilateral: Frontal plagiocephaly (asymmetric skull with shortened AP dimension on one side).
      b. Bilateral: Brachycephaly (skull with shortened AP dimension and wide transverse dimension).
   3. Metopic synostosis
      a. Premature fusion of vertical forehead suture, between frontal bones.
      b. Suture normally patent and functional until 24 months.
      c. Occurs with very low frequency.
      d. Trigonocephaly: Keel-shaped skull with pointed forehead; may appear to have hypotelorism and bitemporal constriction.
   4. Lambdoid synostosis
      a. Posterior plagiocephaly.
      b. Rare. The overwhelming majority of cases of posterior plagiocephaly are caused by PHD.
      c. May be unilateral or bilateral.
   5. Kleeblattschädel deformity ("cloverleaf skull")
      a. Multiple-suture synostoses or pansynostosis.
      b. Trilobe (cloverleaf) shape results from bulging of sagittal and squamosal sutures.
      c. Surgical decompression is necessary immediately after birth due to elevated ICP and severe exorbitism.
      d. Usually requires cerebrospinal fluid (CSF) shunting.
      e. Evaluation for associated cervical spine abnormalities is mandatory.
III. Craniosynostosis syndromes (Different sutures may be affected in patients with the same syndrome.)
   A. Crouzon's syndrome
      1. Inheritance.
         a. Autosomal dominant; most cases sporadic.
         b. Mutation in fibroblast growth factor receptor 2 gene (FGFR2, chromosome 10).
      2. Physical features: Characteristic triad includes craniosynostosis, midfacial hypoplasia, and exophthalmos. Other features include the following.
         a. Turribrachycephaly (short AP skull dimension, wide transverse dimension, increased projection of superior skull).
         b. Orbital hypertelorism, class III malocclusion, beaklike nose, high-arched palate.
      3. Mental status: Variable.
   B. Apert's syndrome (acrocephalosyndactyly)
      1. Inheritance.
         a. Autosomal dominant; most cases sporadic.
         b. Mutation in FGFR2.
      2. Physical features.
         a. Craniosynostosis, turribrachycephaly.
         b. Midface hypoplasia, class III malocclusion, orbital hypertelorism, acne, syndactyly of hands and feet, occasional cleft palate.
      3. Mental status: Variable.
   C. Saethre-Chotzen syndrome
      1. Inheritance.
         a. Autosomal dominant.

   b. Mutation in TWIST gene
  2. Physical features.
   a. Craniosynostosis.
   b. Shallow orbits, telecanthus, deviated nasal septum, low hairline; may have partial soft tissue syndactyly.
  3. Mental status: Often normal.
 D. Carpenter's syndrome
  1. Inheritance: Autosomal recessive. (*Note:* Most other craniosynostosis syndromes are dominant.).
  2. Physical features.
   a. Craniosynostosis.
   b. Flat nasal bridge, low-set ears, abnormal globe and canthi, brachydactyly, variable soft tissue syndactyly of hands and feet, short stature.
 E. Pfeiffer's syndrome
  1. Inheritance.
   a. Autosomal dominant.
   b. Mutation in FGFR1, FGFR2, or FGFR3.
  2. Physical features.
   a. Craniosynostosis, turribrachycephaly.
   b. Broad thumbs and great toes, may have partial soft tissue syndactyly, may have other facial abnormalities.
  3. Mental status: Intelligence variable.
 F. Jackson-Weiss syndrome
  1. Inheritance.
   a. Autosomal dominant.
   b. Mutation in FGFR2.
  2. Physical features.
   a. Craniosynostosis.
   b. Mild midfacial hypoplasia, broad great toes, may have syndactyly of toes.
 G. Boston-type craniosynostosis
  1. Inheritance.
   a. Autosomal dominant.
   b. Mutation in MSX2 gene.
  2. Physical features.
   a. Craniosynostosis.
   b. Cleft of the soft palate, short first metatarsal, triphalangeal thumb.
IV. Functional problems associated with craniosynostosis
 A. Central nervous system
  1. All patients require formal neurosurgical evaluation.
  2. Abnormal CSF circulation leads to hydrocephalus.
  3. Risk of chronic herniation of cerebellar tonsils (Chiari malformation). Signs include cranial nerve palsy, and dysfunctional swallowing or difficulty feeding. May require occipital decompression.
 B. Airway
  1. Midfacial hypoplasia may compromise airway.
  2. Mental status may diminish ability to protect airway.
  3. Consider risk of perioperative airway compromise.
 C. Abnormal speech and hearing
  1. May require speech therapy.
  2. Consider early hearing evaluation.
 D. Early dental and orthodontic involvement should be obtained.
 E. Ocular
  1. Corneal exposure may result from exorbitism.
  2. Strabismus.
  3. Orbital and ocular abnormalities may compromise vision and result in deprivation amblyopia.
  4. Formal ophthalmology evaluation should be performed for signs of ocular impairment.

V. Treatment

A. **Multidisciplinary team** approach includes plastic surgeon, neurosurgeon, otolaryngologist, geneticist, pediatrician, pediatric dentist, orthodontist, psychologist for developmental evaluation, speech therapist, social worker, and dietitian.

B. **Preoperative considerations**

1. **Extensive discussion of risks,** benefits, and anticipated postoperative course with parents/caregivers. Craniofacial edema, ecchymosis, and inability to open eyes can be very distressing to parents. Typical hospital stay is 5 to 7 days. Postoperative fevers are common and usually are not a result of infection.

2. **Type and crossmatch.**

3. **Intensive care unit (ICU) bed for at least 24 to 48 hours.**

4. **Preoperative antibiotics are used,** due to dural exposure intraoperatively.

5. **Some surgeons may give a loading dose of dexamethasone and maintenance** for approximately 48 hours.

6. **Two large-bore peripheral intravenous lines,** possibly central venous catheter; urinary catheter and arterial line.

7. **Scalp is rarely shaved.**

8. **Ophthalmic ointment.**

9. **Careful positioning** based on surgical plan (prone vs. supine).
   a. Avoid any pressure on eyes.
   b. Specific headrest may be necessary.

10. **Warming blanket or other warming device.**

C. **Operative interventions** (Table 25-4)

1. **Surgery before 6 months old** takes advantage of rapid brain growth on reshaping skull and may lead to a more normal head shape.

2. **Early surgery prevents secondary deformities** from arising.

3. **Elevated ICP** is an indication for urgent intervention.

D. **Postoperative considerations**

1. **ICU admission.**

2. **ICP monitoring** per neurosurgeon preference.

3. **Regular neurologic checks.**

4. **Hematocrit** should be checked frequently.

5. **Serum electrolyte abnormalities** are common due to disruption of the hypothalamic-pituitary axis. The clinical picture may be similar to diabetes insipidus (high serum sodium, increased urine output) or syndrome of inappropriate ADH secretion (SIADH; low serum sodium).
   a. SIADH: Treat with fluid restriction or increase sodium in intravenous fluid.
   b. Diabetes insipidus: Risk of dehydration; therefore, treat with fluid replacement.

6. **Dressing is left in place approximately 48 hours** (some surgeons prefer antibiotic ointment only). Remove dressing sooner if concerned about infection or potential source of fever.

7. **Postoperative fever is common.** Although postoperative infection is rare, all fevers must be carefully evaluated.
   a. Consider incision site, i.v. line sites, urinary tract infection, respiratory infection, CNS infection, osteomyelitis.
   b. Blood and urine analysis based on clinical judgment.

8. **Postoperative antibiotics.**

VI. Craniofacial clefts

A. **Bony and soft tissue clefts** occur along lines of embryonic fusion of craniofacial structures.

B. **Incidence is roughly 1.5 to 5 per 100,000 births,** and is usually nonfamilial.

C. **Tessier classification is most commonly used** (Fig. 25-1).

1. **Lines extending superiorly from lid margin** indicate cranial clefts.

2. **Lines extending inferiorly from lid margin** indicate facial clefts.

3. **Cranial and facial clefts** often occur together, with corresponding numbers adding up to 14 (e.g., 1 and 14, 4 and 10).

Table 25-4. Surgical interventions in craniosynostosis

Type of Synostosis	Surgical Intervention	Other Considerations
Unilateral coronal	Frontoorbital advancement. Unilateral or bilateral depending on extent of deformity.	
Bilateral coronal	Bilateral frontoorbital advancement. For more severe brachycephaly, abnormal contour of both the frontal and occipital region may require total cranial vault reshaping.	
Metopic	Forehead reshaping involves removal of the supraorbital bar with a posterior corticotomy along the synostosed metopic suture. The bone is then flattened to restore forehead contour. Correction of hypotelorism may be necessary.	
Sagittal	Procedures range from strip craniectomy to total calvarial reshaping. Strip craniectomy often fails to fully correct the deformity. Biparietal diameter may be widened with barrel-stave osteotomies.	Sagittal sinus lies immediately deep to the sagittal suture. Injury to the sinus may result inuncontrollable hemorrhage, CNS infarction, or death.
Lambdoid	Early intervention may require only strip craniectomy. If older than 6 months, will likely require reshaping of the posterior cranial vault.	
Kleeblattschädel	Total cranial vault expansion usually performed on emergent basis within the first few days of life.	Secondary reshaping often necessary before 1 year due to repeated need for CNS decompression.
Syndromic synostoses	Extensive surgical intervention necessary. If elevated intracranial pressure, early cranial decompression. Frontoorbital advancement with later LeFort III osteotomy may be performed. Alternatively, monobloc advancement may be performed at a later age.	Distraction osteogenesis is increasingly applied to the craniofacial skeleton and may be used for midfacial advancement.

    D. Soft tissue abnormalities may predict underlying bony clefts.
        1. Abnormal tufts of hair.
        2. Irregular hairline, brow line, lashes.
        3. Irregular lid margin.
    E. Clefts involving the orbit may affect globe and extraocular muscles.

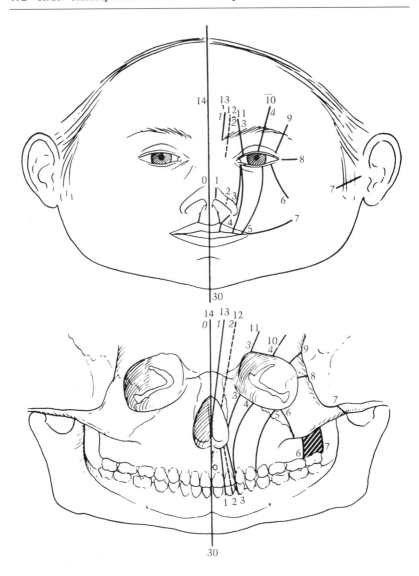

Fig. 25-1. The Tessier classification of craniofacial clefts. **A:** Path of various clefts on the face. **B:** Location of the clefts on the facial skeleton. (Courtesy of Dr. P. Tessier.) Reproduced from Kawamoto H. Craniofacial clefts. In *Grabb and Smith's Plastic Surgery*, 5th ed. Aston SJ, Beasley RW, Thorne CH, eds. Philadelphia, Lippincott-Raven, 1997. With permission.

VII. **Craniofacial microsomias/branchial arch syndromes:** Treacher-Collins-Franceschetti complex, hemifacial microsomia, and Goldenhar's syndrome are often classified together despite heterogeneous etiologies. All involve combinations of Tessier clefts 6, 7, or 8. Proposed causes include vascular disruption during embryonic development, exposure to teratogens such as thalidomide and retinoic acid, and maternal diabetes.

A. **Treacher-Collins-Franceschetti complex (mandibulofacial dysostosis)**

1. **Inheritance**
   a. Autosomal dominant.
   b. Mutation in TCOF1 gene.
   c. Variable penetrance.
2. **Physical features**
   a. Absent or hypoplastic superior/lateral/inferior orbital rim, absent or hypoplastic zygomas, hypoplastic mandible, downward-slanting palpebral fissures, lateral canthal dystopia, lower lid colobomas (congenital cleft of the eyelid), medial lower eyelash deficiency.
   b. Other associated deformities.
      (1) Microtia, ear deformities.
      (2) Conductive hearing impairment.
      (3) Abnormal pneumatization of mastoid air cells.
      (4) Macrostomia.
      (5) Cleft palate.
3. **Mental status:** Generally normal
B. **Hemifacial microsomia (HFM, craniofacial microsomia, branchial arch syndrome)**
   1. **Inheritance**
      a. Sporadic, occasional family clustering.
      b. Affects 1 in 3,500 to 5,600 births.
      c. Males are more often affected.
      d. Right side is more commonly affected than the left.
   2. **Physical features**
      a. The majority of HFM cases are unilateral.
      b. The mandibular deformity usually is the defining characteristic, ranging from mild hypoplasia to complete absence of the ramus, condyle, or temporomandibular joint.
      c. Maxillary hypoplasia; orbital dystopia is often present; upper lid colobomas; macrostomia; hypoplasia and weakness of facial musculature.
      d. Abnormal occlusion includes crossbite, open bite, and an occlusal cant.
      e. External ear malformations vary from mild deformity, such as preauricular skin tags or mild microtia, to complete anotia.
      f. Auditory canal, ossicles, and temporal bone may be underdeveloped or absent.
      g. Major anomalies occur at a higher rate than in the general population, and further workup is warranted.
   3. **Mental status:** Mental deficiency occurs in approximately 10% of cases.
   4. **Treatment**
      a. Mandibular deformity.
         (1) Very mild cases may not require treatment.
         (2) Rib graft for mandible reconstruction was previously the standard of care and remains a viable option.
         (3) Mandibular distraction osteogenesis is becoming the preferred treatment option.
      b. External ear reconstruction.
      c. Reconstruction of other facial features as needed.
      d. Audiologic evaluation and treatment by otolaryngologist; often no intervention is needed if contralateral hearing is normal.
C. **Goldenhar's syndrome (oculoauriculovertebral dysplasia)**
   1. **Inheritance unknown.** Majority of cases are sporadic.
   2. **Considered a severe form of hemifacial microsomia.**
   3. **Physical features.**
      a. Hemifacial microsomia (features as above).
      b. Hypoplastic facial musculature, facial nerve weakness, epibulbar dermoids, ear tags and ear pits, conductive hearing impairment, vertebral abnormalities.

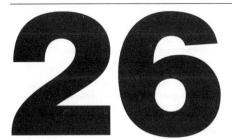

Facial Trauma

Sean P. Edwards

Facial trauma is a multidisciplinary arena that requires the cooperation of the trauma surgeon, neurosurgeon, ophthalmologist, anesthesiologist, and maxillofacial surgeon to achieve optimal results. Facial injuries often look impressive but are rarely an immediate threat to life. Treatment of abdominal, thoracic, and neurologic injuries will, in general, take precedence. Remember the ABCs.

Evaluation and Emergency Department Care

I. History
   A. **Mechanism of injury and witness reports** can help one judge the severity of injury and the potential for multiple injuries.
   B. **Classic mechanisms** are associated with characteristic patterns of injury (e.g., trauma to the chin resulting in bilateral condylar fractures).
   C. It is important to **determine the degree and type of wound** contamination, because it predicts the potential for foreign body implantation and chance of infection.
II. Clinical examination
   A. **Develop your own regimented,** organized system to ensure complete examination of all structures and systems (like reading a chest x-ray). Assessing from top to bottom works well.
   B. **Begin with an overall inspection,** noting any facial asymmetries, hemorrhage, and ecchymoses.
   C. **Remove crusted blood** with saline-soaked gauze to enhance evaluation.
   D. **Perform a neck exam,** maintaining cervical spine precautions (palpate for tenderness, bony step-offs, and crepitus).
   E. **The neurologic examination** of the head and neck is as important as it is in the hand.
      1. **Test the 12 cranial nerves.** Recall the cranial foramina from which the nerves emanate (Table 26-1).
      2. **Sensory examination,** usually performed by testing light touch in the regions of the three sensory branches of the trigeminal nerve (ophthalmic, maxillary, and mandibular).
   F. Scalp examination
      1. **Palpate the entire scalp** for depressions and lacerations.
      2. **Inspect lacerations** for calvarial defects.
   G. Orbital examination
      1. **Bilateral periorbital ecchymoses** (raccoon eyes) suggest a skull base fracture.
      2. **Subconjunctival hemorrhage** suggests fracture of the bony orbit.
      3. **Assess globe position.**
         a. Fractures of the orbital wall increase orbital volume and change the position of the globe.
         b. Inspect from patient's front for vertical dystopia or hypoglobus.

Table 26-1. Cranial nerves and their foramina

Number	Name	Foramen
I	Olfactory	Cribriform plate
II	Optic	Optic foramen
III	Oculomotor	Superior orbital fissure
IV	Trochlear	Superior orbital fissure
V	Trigeminal: Ophthalmic division (V1)	Superior orbital fissure
	Trigeminal: Maxillary division (V2)	Foramen rotundum
	Trigeminal: Mandibular division (V3)	Foramen ovale
VI	Abducens	Superior orbital fissure
VII	Facial	Internal acoustic meatus and stylomastoid foramen
VIII	Auditory	Internal acoustic meatus
IX	Glossopharyngeal	Jugular foramen
X	Vagus	Jugular foramen
XI	Accessory	Jugular foramen
XII	Hypoglossal	Hypoglossal canal

    c. Inspect from patient's side (using exophthalmometer) or looking down over top of patient's head for exophthalmos or enophthalmos.

  4. Assess ocular range of motion.

    a. Limited upward gaze indicates entrapment after orbital floor fracture.

    b. Limited lateral gaze suggests medial orbital wall injury.

    c. Ophthalmoplegia in multiple vectors is suggestive of cranial nerve injury or compression.

    d. Edema can also result in ophthalmoplegia.

    e. Forced duction test is useful if examination is equivocal or the patient is unconscious; it differentiates mechanical entrapment from neural injury or edema. Anesthetize eye with topical anesthetic and grasp conjunctiva (away from cornea) with Adson forceps; manually assess globe mobility.

  5. Pupillary response: Pupils should be round, equal in size, and equally reactive to light and accommodation.

  6. Swinging flashlight test: Pupillary dilation with illumination denotes the presence of a relative afferent papillary defect (suggests damage to optic nerve or retina).

  7. Visual acuity: Test grossly with pocket card; note baseline vision correction.

  8. Palpate the orbital rim.

  9. Measure intercanthal distance.

    a. Normal intercanthal distance is 30 to 32 mm.

    b. In traumatic telecanthus, intercanthal distance is 35 mm or greater.

  10. Medial canthal tendon stability: Palpate with index finger and distract lids laterally with the other hand (if unstable, suggests nasoorbital ethmoidal fracture).

H. Otologic examination

  1. Inspect external ear, including posterior surface, for lacerations. Examine for perichondral hematoma and exposed cartilage. Drain hematomas and splint to avoid "cauliflower ear" (scarring of ear caused by fibroblastic proliferation in response to organized hematoma).

  2. Inspect for Battle's sign: Bruising of the mastoid process; suggests cranial base fracture.

  3. Otoscopy: Otorrhea, bruising in the external auditory canal (suggests condylar fracture) perforation of the tympanic membrane, and hemotympanum (suggests skull base fracture).

I. Nose
1. **Inspect and palpate for septal deviation** and bony deformities.
2. **Inspect for septal hematoma.** See "Emergency Department Care" for treatment.

J. Midface
1. **Look for malar flattening and downsloping** of the palpebral fissure. The lateral canthal tendon can be inferiorly displaced with the fractured malar bone.
2. **Cheek/lateral nasal/upper lip paresthesia** is often caused by impingement of the infraorbital nerve within the infraorbital canal.
3. **Assess maxillary stability.** Attempt to manipulate the maxilla while stabilizing the nasofrontal and zygomaticofrontal sutures with the other hand.

K. Mandible, oral cavity, and occlusion
1. **Swelling and bruising** indicate points of impact.
2. **Palpate for tenderness and step-offs.**
3. **Palpate the temporomandibular joint (TMJ) for tenderness,** crepitus, and range of motion. Place a finger in the external auditory canal and have patient open and close mouth slowly. A fractured condyle will often rotate but will not translate well.
4. **Oral cavity:** Evaluate for malocclusion; subluxed, fractured, or avulsed teeth; and ecchymoses.
   a. Ask patient if teeth fit together normally.
   b. Ask patient if teeth are numb.
   c. Bruising generally indicates torn periosteum from a fracture.
   d. Palatal ecchymosis may indicate a LeFort I fracture or palatal split.
   e. Bruising and tenderness at the zygomatic buttresses are sensitive indicators of zygomaticomaxillary complex (ZMC) fractures.
5. **Lower lip paresthesias** from trauma to the inferior alveolar nerve with mandible fractures should be documented preoperatively.
6. **Examine for oral lacerations.**
7. **Note level of oral hygiene** and state of dentition: Carious teeth may serve as a source of infection.

III. Radiologic evaluation
A. **Radiographs** should augment the clinical examination, not replace it.
B. **Plain films** have a limited role in the radiographic evaluation of facial trauma, with two notable exceptions.
   1. **Panoramic radiographs (Panorex):** The gold standard for evaluation of the mandible.
   2. **Submentovertex view:** Good for evaluation of the zygomatic arch.
C. **Maxillofacial computed tomography (CT):** The study of choice for evaluating most facial injuries (both axial and coronal cuts).
   1. **Coronal views:** Essential for evaluating orbital trauma and the extent of herniation of orbital contents through the floor. Axial images alone are insufficient for delineating LeFort fractures.
      a. Require hyperextension of the neck, and should be avoided when C-spine injury is suspected.
      b. In these cases, a fine-cut axial CT with coronal reconstruction images will provide a reasonable alternative.
   2. **Three-dimensional reformats:** Useful in treatment planning for complex, panfacial injuries.

IV. Emergency department care
A. **Wounds:** Cover with saline-soaked gauze to avoid tissue desiccation while awaiting definitive repair.
B. **Mandible fractures:** Can be stabilized with a bridle wire (25-gauge wire passed around two teeth on either side of the fracture).
   1. **Stabilization increases patient comfort.**
   2. **A bridle wire will help stabilize** a prolapsed bilateral mandible fracture that could compromise the airway.

      3. In cases of bilateral parasymphyseal fractures, pulling the tongue anterior with a towel clamp or a suture can also be an airway-preserving maneuver.

  C. Nasal septal hematomas: Should be drained, and a pressure dressing applied to prevent nasal septal perforation.

      1. Drain using an 18-gauge needle or a small caudal incision.

      2. Apply dressing consisting of strip gauze impregnated with antibiotic ointment, or septal splints.

  D. Auricular hematomas: Must be drained to prevent cauliflower ear.

      1. Drain as with a septal hematoma.

      2. After drainage, a pressure dressing is applied by bolstering the area with dental cotton rolls sewn through and through with 2-0 nylon, or by packing convolutions of cartilage with Xeroform gauze.

V. Treatment sequence and timing

  A. Attention to most facial injuries can be delayed until the patient has been stabilized.

  B. If possible, **bony repair** is best done immediately (prior to formation of significant edema) or within 10 days to 2 weeks of injury.

  C. Soft tissue injuries should be closed as soon as possible, usually within 8 hours.

      1. Closure does not always need to be definitive, because it may be revised at the time of fracture repair.

      2. Exposed cartilage should be covered with mafenide acetate (Sulfamylon dressings).

Treatment of Specific Injuries

I. Soft tissue abrasions and lacerations

  A. The face is "high-priced real estate," both aesthetically and functionally; therefore, debridement of wounds should be conservative.

  B. Local anesthetic with vasoconstrictor may be used on the face, with the possible exception of the nasal tip (although routinely safe).

      1. Use sparingly: Anesthetic infiltration will distort important anatomic landmarks.

      2. Mark structures such as the vermilion border before infiltration, particularly when using epinephrine.

      3. The face lends itself well to **regional anesthesia** (nerve blocks; see Chapter 8, "Local Anesthetics").

  C. Cleanse the wound with normal saline.

      1. For **irrigation,** consider using an 18-gauge needle and 60-mL syringe.

      2. Mechanical debridement may require a surgical scrub brush: Remove all debris to prevent traumatic tattooing.

  D. Explore the injury to its full depth.

  E. Cheek and temporal region: High risk for injury to the facial nerve and parotid gland and duct. Do not forget their evaluation before infiltration and repair!

  F. Layered closure

      1. Muscle and dermis: 4-0 and 5-0 undyed absorbable sutures, such as polyglycolides (e.g., Vicryl), work well.

      2. Skin: 5-0 or 6-0.

         a. Monofilamentous nonresorbable sutures (such as nylon) are commonly used; remove in 4 to 7 days.

         b. Fast-absorbing gut suture can be used when suture removal is undesirable (e.g., young children), but increased scar potential must be balanced with the minor trauma associated with removal of permanent sutures.

      3. Scalp lacerations: Staples can be used for skin closure; remove in 10 to 14 days.

4. **Eyelid lacerations:** Require precise alignment of the tarsal plate and lid margin (line these up first with interrupted sutures).
5. **Lip lacerations:** Align the white roll and vermillion border first (do not forget to mark prior to infiltration).

II. **Dental injuries**
   A. **Fractures:** Ellis classification is based upon the layer of tooth that has been violated.
      1. **Class I:** Through enamel only. No urgent care required; treated by elective composite resin buildup or simply by smoothing rough edges.
      2. **Class II:** Through enamel and dentin. Very sensitive to hot and cold; will need resin buildup.
      3. **Class III:** Exposed pulp. Can be temporized with a pulp cap; will probably need root canal therapy.
   B. **Avulsions:** Need to be reimplanted within 90 *minutes*; goal is to minimize extraalveolar time.
      1. **Transport in *milk* or a balanced salt solution;** alternatively, the buccal vestibule may be used.
      2. **Gently cleanse tooth** without touching the root surface, and replace in the socket.
      3. **Stabilize** with a passive light wire splint bonded to adjacent teeth.
      4. **Follow up with dentist** in 1 to 2 weeks for root canal therapy.
   C. **Luxated teeth:** First rule out root fracture with periapical radiographs.
      1. **Tooth is manually repositioned** and fixated with a passive light wire splint.
      2. **An adult tooth impacted** into the alveolus may be left to reerupt on its own.
      3. **Primary teeth:** An avulsed or luxated primary tooth should not be repositioned or reimplanted for fear of damaging the developing permanent tooth.
   D. **Dentoalveolar fractures**
      1. **Manually reduce and stabilize** with a segmental arch bar or a bonded wire splint.
      2. **Dental exam within 2 weeks** to evaluate the need for root canal therapy.

III. **Fractures of the mandibular condyle**
   A. **Presentation and physical examination**
      1. **Contralateral open bite** with deviation toward the injured side due to loss of vertical height at the fracture site.
      2. **Condyle** will not translate; therefore, opening is limited, and the chin is deviated toward the fractured side.
      3. **Bilateral fractures** result in an anterior open bite deformity.
   B. **Fractures may be low on the neck of the condyle** or even intracapsular (especially in children), but the treatment is similar.
   C. **If stable occlusion:** Conservative management is used, consisting of a soft diet for 4 to 6 weeks.
   D. **If malocclusion present:** Placement of arch bars with heavy elastic or wire intermaxillary fixation (IMF; also called MMF, maxillomandibular fixation) will be required.
      1. **IMF for 2 weeks.**
      2. **After 2 weeks,** IMF should be released in favor of guiding elastics (pulling the mandible forward) to distract the posterior segment and permit TMJ physiotherapy. A class I vector (straight up and down) may be employed if the occlusion is as desired without premature contacts to maximum intercuspation.
      3. **Jaw range-of-motion exercises** are key in preventing ankylosis; of paramount concern in the pediatric population.
   E. **Consider open reduction of a condylar fracture if the following conditions exist.**
      1. **Open fracture.**
      2. **Severely dislocated.**

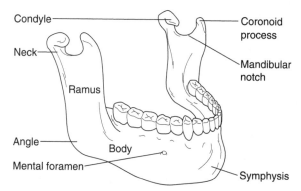

Fig. 26-1. Anatomy of the mandible.

      3. **Translocated** into the middle cranial fossa (very rare due to strong horizontal fibers of the lateral TMJ capsular ligament).

      4. **Part of a complex panfacial fracture;** useful to reestablish posterior vertical dimension.

IV. **Fractures of the mandible excluding the condyle**

  A. **Includes the angle, body, parasymphysis, and symphysis** (Fig. 26-1)

  B. **Key physical exam findings**

    1. **Steps in the occlusions**

    2. **Gingival tears**

    3. **Inferior alveolar nerve paresthesia**

    4. **Hematomas in the floor of the mouth**

  C. **Classified as favorable or unfavorable** based on whether the vectors of muscle pull tend to displace the fracture.

  D. **Almost all fractures** can in principle be managed via closed reduction with IMF.

    1. **Ivy loops,** or arch bars and intermaxillary wiring, can be used.

    2. **Intermaxillary fixation screws** are quick and simple to use but are generally less stable than arch bars and do not permit use of elastics to guide the occlusion during healing.

    3. **IMF** is generally maintained for 4 weeks and replaced with light guiding elastics for another 2 weeks; the arch bars are removed at 6 weeks.

  E. **Open reduction and internal fixation (ORIF)** of the mandible

    1. **Allows for early mobilization, allowing the following.**

      a. Decreased stiffness at TMJ.

      b. Improved caloric intake and therefore improved healing.

      c. No interruption in speech.

    2. **IMF** is established prior to plating to aid in reestablishing preinjury occlusion.

    3. **Transoral application** of miniplates along lines of tension is commonly used.

  F. **If teeth are involved** in the line of the fracture

    1. **Management is controversial.**

    2. In general, **maintain healthy teeth** and manage them expectantly (eventually may need root canal therapy).

    3. **If the tooth is grossly carious** or has suffered a root fracture, it needs to be extracted to prevent infection of the fracture.

V. **Fractures of the zygomaticomaxillary complex**

  A. **Key physical exam findings**

    1. **Malar flattening**

    2. **Downsloping palpebral fissure**

    3. **Infraorbital nerve paresthesias**

    4. **Tenderness and bruising at the zygomatic buttress**

  B. ZMC fracture disrupts **four** bony buttresses: zygomaticomaxillary, frontozygomatic, zygomatic arch, and orbital rim (frequently mistakenly called a "tripod" fracture).

  C. ZMC fractures vary in stability and occasionally do not require fixation after reduction.

   1. Zygomatic buttress: May require miniplate fixation through an intraoral incision.

   2. Frontozygomatic process and orbital rim: Can be accessed through a variety of incisions. A transconjunctival incision with a lateral canthotomy will provide access to both sites.

VI. Isolated zygomatic arch fractures

 A. Key physical exam findings

  1. Flattening of the arch.

  2. Limitation of mandibular range of motion (lateral excursion toward the affected side; due to the depressed arch impinging on the coronoid process).

 B. Arch is elevated via a Gillies approach using a Rowe forceps (transtemporal, sliding down along temporalis muscle), or via a transoral approach using a periosteal elevator.

 C. Fixation is not always necessary because the periosteum will sometimes maintain reduction.

 D. Check a postreduction submentovertex film and caution the patient against putting pressure on the area.

VII. Fractures of the bony orbit

 A. Key physical exam findings

  1. Subconjunctival hemorrhage.

  2. Diplopia due to a lack of coordinated eye movements (muscle or nerve injury), gaze restrictions, enophthalmos, and/or hypoglobus.

 B. Inferior and medial walls are most frequently involved.

 C. Goals of surgery

  1. Restore orbital volume, and thereby restore the position of the globe.

  2. Correct any soft tissue entrapment.

 D. Multiple approaches to the orbit exist. The transconjunctival (with or without lateral canthotomy) and subciliary approaches are the most common.

 E. After reduction of herniated orbital contents, the orbital walls (floor) are reconstructed with autogenous or alloplastic materials.

  1. Autogenous: Calvarial bone, coronoid process. Autogenous materials are generally preferred because they experience superior incorporation and fewer infections. However, they require harvest from a donor site, thus incurring additional morbidity.

  2. Alloplastic: Titanium mesh, Medpor, and Supramid alloplasts are commonly used.

 F. Following repair, use forced duction test to confirm full range of globe movement.

VIII. Fractures of the nasal bones

 A. Key physical exam findings.

  1. Nasal deviation, crepitus, nasal airway obstruction.

  2. Septal deviation, fractures, and hematomas.

 B. Septal hematomas: See "Emergency Department Care," earlier

 C. Nasal fractures: Bimodal timing of repair.

  1. Immediately, before significant edema develops.

  2. More typically, wait for 3 to 5 days for swelling to subside.

 D. Corticosteroids are often used to minimize edema and facilitate evaluation of fracture reduction.

 E. Asch forceps are used to align the nasal bones and septum.

 F. Doyle splints are used to support the septum, if necessary. These are soft silicone splints, placed on either side of the septum and sewn through the membranous columella.

G. **Internal packing** (alternative to septal splints).
   1. **Merocel packing,** petrolatum gauze, etc.
   2. **Packs should be removed** on day 3 to prevent septic shock and sinusitis.
H. **External splinting.**
   1. **Layer of skin tapes.**
   2. **Thermoplastic splint, heated in a water bath.**
   3. **Patients should avoid getting the splint wet.**
IX. **Fractures of the nasoorbital ethmoidal complex**
   A. **Can be some of the most challenging fractures** in facial trauma.
   B. **Key physical exam** findings (see "Clinical Examination," earlier).
      1. **Saddle nose deformity.**
      2. **Traumatic telecanthus.**
      3. **Avulsion of medial canthal ligaments.**
   C. **Many surgical approaches** have been described. The most useful in terms of exposure and aesthetics is the coronal incision.
   D. **Classified based on condition of the canthi.**
      1. **Type I:** Medial canthal ligament attached to a large central fragment of bone.
      2. **Type II:** Medial canthal ligament attached to a smaller piece of bone in a more comminuted fracture.
      3. **Type III:** Medial canthal ligament avulsed/detached.
   E. **Bones are first reduced** and secured with 1.0-mm or 1.5-mm plating systems.
   F. **Transnasal wires** are used if canthal ligaments are not adequately repositioned with fracture reduction.
   G. **For severe nasal bone comminution,** cranial bone graft may be used as a dorsal strut to prevent saddle nose deformity.
X. **Fractures of the frontal sinus**
   A. **Fractures of the frontal sinus** are high-energy injuries. Therefore, the presence of other injuries, such as cervical spine fractures, should be evaluated.
   B. **Posterior table injuries** require neurosurgical collaboration for potential cranialization (posterior table is removed).
   C. **Displaced anterior table injuries:** ORIF of bony fragments, through coronal incision (to address the cosmetic deformity).
   D. **Sinus obliteration** is frequently necessary to prevent mucocele formation. If the nasofrontal ducts do not drain methylene blue dye into the nose intraoperatively:
      1. **Sinus mucosa** is removed with a burr, and nasofrontal ducts are plugged.
      2. **The sinus cavity** is obliterated with abdominal fat or hydroxyapatite cement.
XI. **LeFort fractures**
   A. **Maxillary fracture patterns** first described by anatomist René Le Fort in 1901 (Fig. 26-2).
      1. **LeFort I:** Movement palpated at the pyriform rim.
      2. **LeFort II:** Movement at the nasal root (nasofrontal suture).
      3. **LeFort III** (craniofacial disarticulation): Movement at the zygomaticofrontal suture.
   B. **Key physical exam findings:** Anterior open bite and mobility of the maxilla when manipulated at the anterior maxillary alveolus.
   C. **If severely impacted,** the maxilla may be mobilized with Rowe disimpaction forceps.
   D. **Occlusion is reestablished** with arch bars and IMF.
   E. **Internal fixation** is achieved with 1.5-mm or 2.0-mm plating systems.
XII. **Complex panfacial/craniofacial fractures**
   A. **Diligent preoperative planning** is critical (Fig. 26-3).
   B. **In general, an outside-in, top-down approach** is employed to recapitulate correct height and width (i.e., lateral components are stabilized first). If, however, the mandible is a stable template, a bottom-up approach may be preferred.

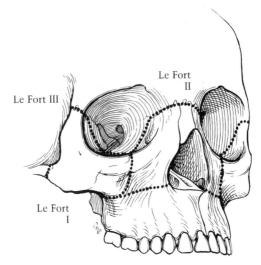

Fig. 26-2. LeFort fracture patterns. (From Manson P. Facial fractures. In *Grabb and Smith's Plastic Surgery*, 5th edition. Aston SJ, Beasley RW, Thorne CH, eds. Philadelphia, Lippincott-Raven, 1997. With permission.)

C. **Wide exposure of all fractures is the first step.**
D. **The goal is to first reestablish sagittal projection** (sometimes called facial height or projection), then the vertical dimension, and lastly the transverse dimension.
E. **1.5-mm and 2.0-mm fixation** are adequate for the midface.

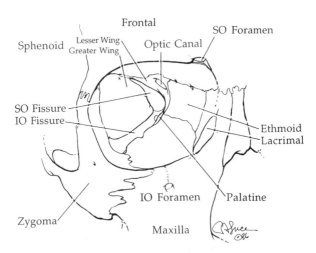

Fig. 26-3. Skeletal orbital anatomy and the relationship of the superior and inferior orbital fissures and optic foramen. (From Turk A. Deformities of the orbit—dystopia, exorbitism, and posttraumatic enophthalmos. In *Grabb and Smith's Plastic Surgery*, 5th ed. Aston SJ, Beasley RW, Thorne CH, eds. Philadelphia, Lippincott-Raven, 1997. With permission.)

    F. Bony gaps in the midfacial buttresses greater than 3 mm due to comminution should be primarily bone grafted to improve skeletal stability.

    G. Reestablish sagittal dimension and midface projection.

        1. Restore the continuity of zygomatic arches and the occlusion.

        2. Open reduction of a subcondylar fracture as an initial step may be essential to reestablishing the mandible as a template for this dimension.

    H. Next, fixation of the frontozygomatic process is accomplished, and the remainder of the midface is reduced and fixed with 1.5-mm or 2.0-mm hardware.

    I. Lastly, the mandible is fixed while the patient is still in IMF.

XIII. Injuries to the extracranial facial nerve: See Chapter 22, "Facial Paralysis."

XIV. Injuries to the parotid gland and Stensen's duct

    A. Injuries along a line running from the tragus to the midpoint of the upper lip should be considered for injury to Stensen's duct.

        1. The duct opens to the oral cavity adjacent to the maxillary second molar.

        2. Saline, dilute hydrogen peroxide, or *small* amounts of methylene blue are injected through the cannulated duct (use Angiocath).

        3. Dye or bubbles expressed in the wound confirm injury.

    B. Dyes may impair facial nerve exploration efforts if they flood the wound.

    C. Duct is repaired over a polyethylene tube, which is sutured in place intraorally for 2 weeks to prevent stricture.

    D. Isolated parotid parenchymal injury without duct injury requires capsular repair to prevent sialocele and salivary fistula.

        1. Pressure dressings such as a Jobst face bra.

        2. Antisialagogues such as glycopyrrolate are used selectively.

XV. Injuries to the lacrimal system

    A. Ophthalmologic consultation is warranted if such an injury is suspected.

    B. Delicate lacrimal system is at risk for injury with nasoorbital ethmoidal fractures and lid lacerations.

    C. Jones I test: Integrity of the system is examined with fluorescein dye applied to the inferior conjunctival fornix, and flow is confirmed into the inferior meatus.

    D. Jones II test: If Jones I test is unsuccessful, the canaliculus is cannulated and saline is injected to diagnose a partial obstruction overcome by the force of injection.

    E. Lacerated canaliculus should be explored under magnification and repaired over polyethylene tubing.

    F. Dacryocystorhinostomy may be required to treat epiphora (excessive tear production, bothersome to the patient).

XVI. Considerations in pediatric fractures

    A. Facial fractures are less common in the pediatric population.

    B. Greenstick fractures are relatively common.

    C. Rigid fixation must be applied selectively and with great care to avoid injury to developing teeth.

    D. Arch bars can be difficult to place with deciduous teeth; custom-made acrylic splints and suspension wires are often used.

    E. Fractures, particularly those of the mandibular condyle, can significantly impair facial growth.

XVII. Considerations in geriatric and edentulous patients

    A. Atrophic mandibular fractures are difficult problems and are not well managed with miniplate fixation.

    B. Reconstruction plates or primary bone grafting with cranial bone struts are the best methods of internal fixation.

    C. Closed reductions may be accomplished using the patient's dentures as splints (drill holes for wiring fracture fragments). Gunning splints and suspension wiring techniques are also useful.

XVIII. Airway management

    A. Should always be a consideration when planning reconstruction of the facial skeleton.

B. **Nasoendotracheal intubation** is preferred for most cases, since it permits establishment of the occlusion intraoperatively with IMF.

C. Other options include placing an **armored endotracheal tube** in an edentulous space or in a retromolar position, or tracheostomy.

D. **Tracheostomy** may be the preferred route when prolonged ventilation is anticipated.

Pearls

1. **Patients leaving the operating room in IMF** should have wire cutters near them at all times, in case of urgent need for oral intubation. Tape them to the patient's chest or the head of the bed.
2. **Oral hygiene** can be maintained with twice daily chlorhexidine mouth rinse in patients who cannot brush their teeth.
3. **Preinjury facial photos** are helpful in surgical planning.
4. **Dental impressions,** plaster models, and preoperative model surgery for splint fabrication are valuable in helping reestablish proper occlusion where fractures are grossly displaced and patients have poor preinjury occlusion. Molds can easily be made, even in ventilated intensive care unit patients.
5. **The mandible is like a pretzel;** it is hard to break in only one place. With suspected isolated mandibular fractures, look hard to rule out the presence of others.

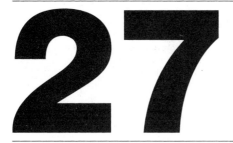

Orthognathic Surgery and Temporomandibular Joint Dysfunction

Gregory H. Borschel

Orthognathic Surgery

I. **Teeth**
   A. **Pediatric (also known as primary or deciduous) dentition:** 20 teeth.
      1. **Eruption sequence** (the mandibular set leads the maxillary set by 1 to 4 months).
         a. Incisors: 6 months.
         b. Canines: 16 months.
         c. First molars: 12 months.
         d. Second molars: 20 months.
      2. **Naming system** (Table 27-1): Use the letters *A* to *P*. Mnemonic: "**A**ll **J**ust **K**ids **T**eeth"; A, right maxillary second molar; J, left maxillary second molar; K, left mandibular second molar; T, right mandibular second molar.
   B. **Mixed dentition:** Primary and secondary teeth present, between 6 and 9 years.
   C. **Adult (secondary or permanent) dentition.**
      1. **Eruption sequence** (the mandibular set leads the maxillary set by 0 to 1 year)
         a. Incisors: 6 to 9 years.
         b. Canines: 9 to 10 years.
         c. First premolars: 10 to 12 years.
         d. Second premolars: 11 to 12 years.
         e. First molars: 6 to 7 years (usually the first adult teeth).
         f. Second molars: 11 to 13 years.
         g. Third molars: 17 to 21 years.
      2. **Numbering system (international standard,** Table 27-2): Numbers 1 to 32. 1, right maxillary third molar; 32, right mandibular third molar.
II. **Standard dental terms**
   A. **Mesial:** Toward the midline.
   B. **Distal:** Away from the midline. (The incisors are mesial to the molars.)
   C. **Buccal (labial):** Facing the lip or cheek.
   D. **Lingual:** Facing the tongue.
   E. **Overbite:** Amount of vertical overlap of apices of teeth.
   F. **Overjet:** Amount of horizontal overlap of apices of teeth.
   G. **Proclination:** The crown of the tooth is labially angulated.

Table 27-1. Nomenclature system for pediatric dentition

	Right					Left				
Maxillary	A	B	C	D	E	F	G	H	I	J
Mandibular	T	S	R	Q	P	O	N	M	L	K

Table 27-2. International nomenclature system for adult dentition

	Right								Left							
Maxillary	1	2	3	4	5	6	7	8	9	10	11	12	13	14	15	16
Mandibular	32	31	30	29	28	27	26	25	24	23	22	21	20	19	18	17

   H. Retroclination: The crown is inclined toward the tongue.
   I. Angle class: Describes occlusion, usually relating the maxillary first molar to the mandibular first molar (Fig. 27-1). However, occlusion can be determined at any tooth, including the canines. Named for orthodontist Edward Hartley Angle.
      1. Class I (normal) occlusion: The mesial buccal cusp of the maxillary first molar lies in the buccal groove of the mandibular first molar.
      2. Class II malocclusion: The mesial buccal cusp of the first maxillary molar lies mesial to the buccal groove of the mandibular first molar.
         a. Division I: There is excessive overjet, with a normal angulation of the maxillary incisor.

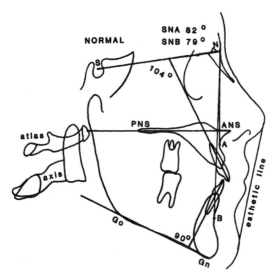

Fig. 27-1. Selected radiographic landmarks and angles express the position of maxilla and mandible compared with the base of the skull. This allows 1:1 measurements of distances between key landmarks of the facial skeleton. Common cephalometric landmarks: S: sella, the bony housing of the pituitary gland; N: nasion, the most posterior point of the nasal radix; A point: the most posterior point on the anterior maxilla; B point: the most posterior point on the anterior mandible; PNS: posterior nasal spine; ANS: anterior nasal spine; Go: gonion; Gn: gnathion. The SNA angle expresses the horizontal position of the maxilla. The SNB angle expresses the horizontal position of the mandible. ANS-PNS shows the palatal plane, which is typically at the same vertical level as the atlas. (From Mason R. Orthodontics and cephalometrics. In *Georgiade Plastic, Maxillofacial, and Reconstructive Surgery,* 3rd ed. Georgiade G, Riefkohl R, Levin S, eds. Philadelphia, Williams & Wilkins, 1997. With permission.)

b. Division II: The angle of the maxillary incisor is more upright, reducing overjet and increasing overbite; usually with associated retroclination of the mandibular incisor.

    3. Class III malocclusion: The mesial buccal cusp of the first maxillary molar lies distal to the buccal groove of the mandibular first molar.

J. Open bite: Part of the dentition does not make contact (can be anywhere along the dental arch).

K. Deep bite: A pronounced overbite.

L. Crossbite: Horizontal malalignment of the teeth, especially the molars. A crossbite can be buccal (maxillary molar lies buccal to the mandibular molar) or lingual.

M. Incisor show: The amount of vertical show of the maxillary central incisor in repose. Incisor show is ideally 2 to 4 mm in women and 0 to 2 mm in men.

N. Centric occlusion: Occlusion resulting in the maximal intercuspation of the teeth.

O. Centric relation: The position of the mandible relative to the maxilla in which the condyles are fully seated in the temporomandibular joint (TMJ).

III. Evaluation of candidates for orthognathic surgery

A. Complete medical and dental history, including a psychosocial evaluation, should be performed. Document functional (chewing, breathing, speaking) as well as aesthetic problems.

B. Experienced orthodontic and dental consultation and cooperation are essential.

C. Oral examination: Occlusion, dental restoration, general oral health, and the status of the TMJ.

D. Aesthetic evaluation: Be systematic and use 1:1 photographs.

    1. Note skin thickness and the proportions of the face.

    2. See also Chapter 29, "Evaluation and Surgical Management of Facial Aging."

    3. Note the proportion of the midface to the lower face and the positions of the mandible and chin.

    4. The midfacial height (MFH, distance from the soft tissue glabella to the alar base plane) should be equal to the lower facial height (LFH, distance from the alar base plane to the soft tissue menton).

    5. Inequality of MFH and LFH can result in aesthetically displeasing facial imbalance, which is often amenable to surgical improvement.

E. Cephalometric evaluation (Fig. 27-2): Standard radiographic measurements

    1. Posteroanterior and lateral cephalometrograms allow 1:1 measurements of distances between key landmarks of the facial skeleton. A Panorex is also obtained to evaluate the dentition. Common cephalometric landmarks include the following (angles subtended by these points are clinically significant).

        a. Sella (S): The bony housing of the pituitary.

        b. Nasion (N): The most posterior point of the nasal radix.

        c. A point: The most posterior point on the anterior maxilla.

        d. B point: The most posterior point on the anterior mandible.

    2. Allow comparison of the patient's facial skeleton with population norms.

    3. Can be useful in planning operations.

    4. Do not strive to correct isolated cephalometric abnormalities without a defined aesthetic or functional goal.

    5. Exercise caution when applying cephalometric norms (which are derived largely from white populations) to nonwhite populations.

IV. Treatment sequence

A. Tracing analysis: Project the optimal or desired result and determine required movements of the maxilla and/or mandible.

B. Define objectives. These must be coordinated with the orthodontist.

C. Model surgery: Plaster casts are made of the maxillary and mandibular arches.

D. The orthodontist places arch bars and moves the teeth such that class I occlusion will be obtained postoperatively.

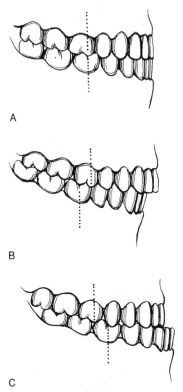

Fig. 27-2. A: Class I, normal occlusion. **B:** Class II, retrooclusion or mandibular deficiency. **C:** Class III, prognathic occlusion (maxillary deficiency or mandibular excess). The key relationships to be discerned are the relationship of the first molars, the cuspids, and the incisors. (From Manson P. Facial fractures. In *Grabb and Smith's Plastic Surgery*, 5th ed. Aston SJ, Beasley RW, Thorne CH, eds. Philadelphia, Lippincott-Raven, 1997. With permission.)

   E. Postsurgical care: Maxillomandibular fixation (MMF) with wires or elastics is maintained for 1 to 6 weeks. TMJ physiotherapy is begun as soon as possible.
V. Common pathologic orthognathic conditions
   A. Vertical maxillary excess, also known as "long face" or "gummy smile".
      1. Features: Incisor show of more than 4 mm, mentalis strain, flattened midface, class II malocclusion, decreased SNA and SNB angles (<82 and <80 degrees, respectively), and increased ANB angle (>3 degrees).
      2. Etiology: A chronically open mouth during development. Oral breathing, nasal obstruction, myotonic dystrophy, and large adenoids are associated with vertical maxillary excess.
      3. Surgical goals: Class I occlusion and reduction of maxillary height.
      4. Treatment: Usually LeFort I maxillary impaction; may need mandibular advancement and/or genioplasty if posterior movement of the maxilla would be indicated by the projection tracing.
      5. Complications: Relapse, tooth damage, gingival anesthesia, and bleeding.
   B. Vertical maxillary deficiency, also known as "short face".
      1. Features: Little or no incisor show in repose. The chin may appear to be excessively prominent anteriorly. Prominent jowling may be pres-

ent. Class II malocclusion and increased SNA and SNB angles are frequent.

2. **Surgical goals:** Class I occlusion and 2 to 3 mm of incisor show.
3. **Treatment:** LeFort I downfracture (with bone grafting for >5 mm lengthening). Mandibular surgery is also needed for significant class II malocclusion.
4. **Complications:** Similar to correction of vertical maxillary excess.

C. **Maxillary retrusion (sagittal deficiency)**
1. **Features:** Flattened or "dished-in" face, malar hypoplasia, depressed nasal tip and alar base, short upper lip, and class III malocclusion with or without an anterior open bite.
2. **Surgical goals:** Class I occlusion; maxillary advancement.

D. **Mandibular retrusion**
1. **Features:** Posterior recession of the lower facial third, lower lip eversion, obtuse cervicomental angle with excess soft tissue, often angle class II and increased ANB angle with decreased SNB angle.
2. **Surgical goals:** Class I occlusion, restoration of facial balance between the midface and the lower face, and correction of a chin projection deficit, when present.
3. **Complications:** Relapse, limited mouth opening, and mental nerve dysfunction (usually a neuropraxic injury that resolves within 6 months).

E. **Mandibular prognathism**
1. **Features:** Prominence of the mandible, midfacial retrusion, mandibular overrotation and class III malocclusion, sometimes with anterior open bite, increased SNB with negative ANB angles and a negative overjet.
2. **Surgical goals:** Class I occlusion, balance of the profiles of the midface and lower face. In mild cases, maxillary advancement alone can be used. In more severe cases, double jaw surgery (maxillary advancement and mandibular setback) is required.
3. **Treatment**
   a. Sagittal split ramus osteotomy or intraoral vertical ramus osteotomy for setbacks greater than 1 cm.
   b. If necessary, a genioplasty is performed.

F. **Types of relapse**
1. **Surgical:** Loss of plate fixation (malunion).
2. **Dental:** Correct jaw repositioning with malpositioned teeth, causing the jaws to move back to their presurgical state (i.e., the orthodontic "setup" was not optimal).
3. **Condylar:** Resorption of bone at the TMJ results in changes in occlusion, leading to relapse.
4. **Soft tissue forces:** Recoil forces from the soft tissues can cause changes in bone morphology, leading to relapse.

Temporomandibular Joint Dysfunction

The diagnosis and treatment of TMJ dysfunction is not well understood. Plastic surgeons are usually well advised to refer suspected cases of TMJ dysfunction to experienced oral surgeons.

I. **Anatomy**
A. Diarthrodial synovial joint.
B. Condyles measure 15 to 20 mm medial to lateral and 8 to 10 mm anteroposteriorly.
C. Both joints function as a single unit.
D. Lined with fibrocartilage, not hyaline cartilage as in other synovial joints.
E. A biconcave disk separates the two joint spaces.
   1. The disc is anchored to the superior head of the lateral pterygoid muscle.

2. The main function of the disk is to distribute the load evenly.
3. A retrodiskal pad may be one of the main causes of pain in TMJ dysfunction.

II. Temporomandibular joint motion
A. The first 20 to 25 mm of interincisor opening: **Hinge** motion via the inferior space.
B. The last 15 to 20 mm: **Sliding** motion via the superior space.

III. Demographics
A. 75% of TMJ patients are female.
B. 30% of the general population may have some form of TMJ dysfunction.

IV. Symptoms, signs, and patient history
A. History of trauma: Occasional.
B. Three cardinal symptoms: Facial pain, TMJ click, and limited jaw opening.
   1. Facial pain
      a. Early morning: Suggests bruxism (nighttime teeth grinding).
      b. Late in the day: Suggests intracapsular origin.
      c. Joint pain: Aggravated by chewing; tends to be constant.
      d. Muscle pain: Influenced by stress; may be intermittent.
   2. TMJ click
      a. Solitary clicks are "innocent"; occur in 40% of the general population.
      b. Reciprocal clicking is pathologic. The sound results from subluxation and recapture of the disk.
   3. Limited jaw opening
      a. Nonreducing anterior disk displacement.
      b. Ankylosis.
      c. Coronoid impingement.
C. Tinnitus: From spasm of the tensor tympani muscle. It is unlikely to be relieved by TMJ surgery.

V. Physical examination
A. Note psychologic disorders or stress.
B. Facial asymmetry.
C. Occlusion, dentition, and the presence of mucosal lesions.
D. Tympanic membrane and external auditory canal.
E. Cranial nerves II to XII.
F. Clicking or crepitus from the TMJ with motion. Test jaw opening with the examiner's fingers in the patient's external auditory canals during opening and closing.
G. Maximal interincisor opening. Normal is greater than 40 mm.
H. Lateral jaw excursion. Normal is greater than 10 mm on each side.
I. Inject local anesthetic into the joint and test for relief. If successful, this suggests internal joint derangement.

VI. Imaging
A. Magnetic resonance imaging (MRI) is the modality of choice for internal derangement.
B. Computed tomography is best for suspected bony abnormalities.

VII. Types of temporomandibular joint disorders
A. Myofascial pain dysfunction syndrome
   1. Pain without anatomic abnormalities.
   2. Multifactorial: Includes dental and psychologic causes. Bruxism is a major factor.
   3. Treatment: Breaking the cycle of muscle spasm using splints to relieve premature dental contacts, thus relaxing muscles; nonsteroidal anti-inflammatory agents (NSAIDs); biofeedback; and a soft diet.
      a. If pain increases with splint therapy, get an MRI to rule out internal derangement.
      b. Dental occlusal adjustment: Reshaping the contact points of the teeth to reduce muscle stress.
B. Internal derangement
   1. An abnormal relationship between the disk and the condyle.

2. Most commonly results from trauma.
3. The disk displaces anteriorly, trapping highly innervated retrodiskal tissue in the joint fossa, leading to cartilage wear and possible perforation.
4. MRI is helpful.
5. **Operative management**
   a. Lavage: Can reduce symptoms in early-stage disease.
   b. Arthroscopy: Long-term benefits have yet to be determined.
   c. Arthrotomy.
      (1) Disk displacement requires repositioning.
      (2) Osteophytes are shaved.
      (3) If the disk is atrophied, diskectomy is performed. A temporalis flap may be used to aid in joint unloading.
   d. Implants and rib arthroplasty: Use as a salvage procedure only.

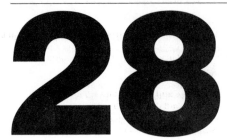

Rhinoplasty

Richard D. Klein

I. Nasal anatomy

A. Skin: Skin thickness determination is important in planning any rhinoplasty.
1. The upper half of the nose has thinner and more mobile skin.
2. The skin thickens and becomes more adherent and sebaceous caudally, yet remains thin along the alar margin and the columella.

B. Muscle: There are four nasal muscle subgroups.
1. **Elevators:** Shorten the nose and dilate the nostrils.
   a. Procerus.
   b. Levator labii superioris alaeque nasi.
   c. Anomalous nasi.
2. **Depressors:** Lengthen the nose and dilate the nostrils.
   a. Dilator naris posterior: The alar portion of the nasalis muscle.
   b. Depressor septi.
3. **Minor dilator:** Dilator naris anterior.
4. **Compressors:** Lengthen the nose and narrow the nostrils.
   a. Nasalis (transverse portion).
   b. Compressor narium minor.

C. Blood supply to the external structures of the nose.
1. **The ophthalmic artery via the internal carotid artery:** The dorsal nasal artery perforates the orbital septum above the medial palpebral ligament. It runs down onto the nasal sidewall to anastomose with the lateral nasal branch of the angular artery.
2. **The facial and the internal maxillary arteries.**
   a. The angular artery supplies the lateral caudal surface.
   b. The superior labial artery supplies the nostril sill and the base of the columella.
   c. The columellar artery, which is a substantial branch, ascends in the columella just superficial to the medial crura.
   d. The nasal tip is supplied by both the angular artery in the ala and by branches of the external nasal branch of the anterior ethmoidal artery.
3. **The venous drainage** accompanies the arteries and has the same names.

D. External sensory innervation: External nasal sensation is supplied by branches of cranial nerve V.
1. **Ophthalmic division (V1):** Sensibility at the radix, the rhinion, and the cephalic portion of the nasal side walls is supplied by the following:
   a. Supratrochlear branches of the ophthalmic nerve.
   b. Infratrochlear branches of the ophthalmic nerve.
2. **Maxillary division (V2).**
   a. Sensibility over the distal dorsum and nasal tip is supplied by the external nasal branch of the anterior ethmoidal nerve emerging from between the nasal bone and the upper lateral cartilage.
   b. Sensibility to the lower half of the nasal sidewall, columella, and vestibule is supplied by the infraorbital branches of the maxillary nerve.

E. The nostril.
    1. Alar bases: The ideal shape of the nasal base should resemble an equilateral triangle.
    2. Vestibule: The cavity located just inside the external naris.
F. Supporting structures (Fig. 28-1).
    1. Alar cartilages.
        a. The medial crus: Footplate and columellar segments.
        b. The middle crus: Lobular and domal segments.
        c. The lateral crus: The largest component of the nasal lobule. Lateral to the lateral crus lies a series of accessory cartilages.
    2. Cartilaginous vault.
        a. The upper cartilaginous vault consists of paired upper lateral nasal cartilages as well as the cartilaginous septum.
        b. The caudal ends of the upper lateral cartilages lie posterior to the cephalic ends of the lower lateral cartilages.

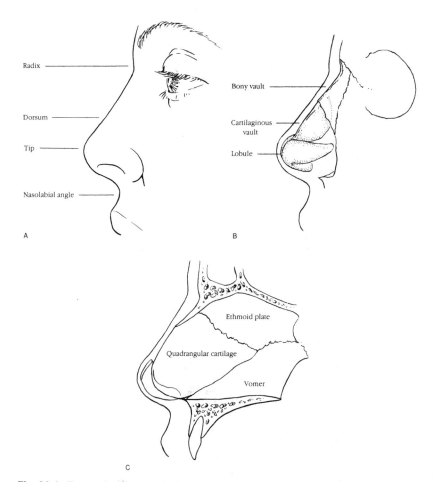

Fig. 28-1. External anatomy and supporting structures of the nose. (From Daniel R. Rhinoplasty. In the textbook, *Grabb and Smith's Plastic Surgery*, 5th edition. Aston SJ, Beasley RW, Thorne CH, eds. Philadelphia, Lippincott-Raven, 1997. With permission.)

3. **The bony vault** is composed of the paired nasal bones and the paired ascending processes of the maxilla.
   a. It is pyramidal in shape, except for the most cephalad portion, which flares out toward the nasofrontal suture.
   b. The intercanthal line marks the narrowest part of the bony pyramid and of the nasal dorsum.
4. **Septum.**
   a. Bony component: From the perpendicular plate of the ethmoid.
   b. Cartilaginous component: Caudal to the bony component.

II. Nasal aesthetics
A. Radix
1. **Frontal view:** The root of the nose, or radix, should be part of an unbroken curved line that starts at the superior orbital ridge and continues along the lateral nasal wall.
2. **Lateral view**
   a. The nasofacial angle is formed by the intersection of the facial plane and the dorsal nasal plane, usually measuring about 30 degrees.
   b. By lowering the radix, the nasofacial angle will increase. This will lead to an apparent increase in nasal tip projection.

B. Dorsum
1. The dorsum is characterized by two divergent concave lines starting at the superior orbital ridge, passing through the radix, and ending at the tip-defining points of the nasal lobule.
2. On frontal view the nasal dorsum should be sufficiently prominent to provide the appearance of an anatomic convexity separating the eyes.

C. Nasal tip
1. The nasal tip determines the degree of nasal refinement.
2. Four landmarks make up a refined nasal tip.
   a. Lateral projection of the left dome.
   b. Lateral projection of the right dome.
   c. Point of tip differentiation from the dorsum.
   d. Columellar-lobular junction.
3. On oblique view these points should form two equilateral triangles with a common base.
4. The apex of the superior triangle is the point of tip differentiation from the dorsum.
5. The apex of the inferior triangle is the point of the columellar-lobular junction.
6. The highest projecting part of the nose on lateral view should be the apogee of the curved line that connects the two domes of the alar cartilages.
7. The nasal tip, on lateral view, influences the refinement, inclination, length, and width of the nose.
8. Changing the nasal tip contour will change both the apparent nasal length and dorsal height.

D. Columellar-alar complex
1. There is a bend in the line that extends from the tip to the base of the columella. This bend is at the area of the columellar-lobular junction and differentiates the tip lobule from the columella.
2. The columella must be sufficiently long to provide for necessary nasal tip projection above the dorsal line.
3. The nasolabial angle should be between 90 and 110 degrees.

III. Nasal physiology
A. Septum: Three components (Fig. 28-1, c)
1. Perpendicular plate of the ethmoid bone.
2. Quadrangular cartilage.
3. Vomer.

B. Internal nasal valve
1. The junction between the septum and the caudal border of the upper lateral cartilage.

    2. Narrows on inspiration and widens on expiration.

    3. Normal angle: 10 to 15 degrees.

    4. An angle of less than 10 degrees will lead to difficulty with airflow on inspiration.

    5. This angle can be altered (increased) by placement of spreader grafts.

C. Turbinates

    1. Superior: Not involved in nasal obstruction.

    2. Middle

        a. Main function is mucus secretion.

        b. Maxillary sinus and frontal sinus drain via ostia located underneath the middle turbinates.

        c. Not involved in nasal obstruction.

    3. Inferior

        a. Hypertrophy occurs when stimulated or irritated.

        b. The nasolacrimal ducts drain into openings located below the inferior meatus.

        c. Inferior turbinate hypertrophy is the most common cause of functional airway obstruction.

IV. Facial analysis

A. An attractive face has certain proportions.

B. Frontal facial analysis (Fig. 28-2)

    1. The face is divided into vertical fifths by lines drawn adjacent to

        a. The most lateral projection of the head

        b. The lateral canthi

        c. The medial canthi

    2. The face is divided into thirds by horizontal lines drawn adjacent to

        a. The menton

        b. Alar base

        c. Brows

        d. Hairline

    3. The lower third is divided into an upper third and lower two-thirds by a line drawn through the oral commissures.

    4. Additionally, the lower one-third of the face can be divided in half by a horizontal line through the lower lip vermilion border.

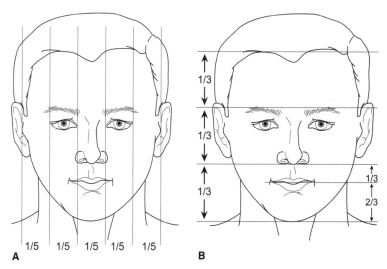

Fig. 28-2. Facial analysis, frontal view.

     5. The distance from stomion to menton can be divided into a 1:2 ratio by a horizontal line through the labial-mental groove.

  C. Lateral facial analysis

     1. The natural horizontal facial plane (NHFP): A line perpendicular to a vertical line superimposed over a head with the eyes in straight-forward position. The NHFP may not correspond to the Frankfort horizontal, which is a cephalometric coordinate.

     2. The face in lateral view can be divided into thirds by lines drawn at the hairline, the brow line at the level of the glabella, the alar base, and the menton. The lower third may be further divided into an upper third and lower two-thirds by a line drawn at the stomion.

V. Nasal analysis (Byrd's analysis)

  A. The aesthetic appearance of the face can be significantly altered by dimensional changes in the nose and chin.

  B. Patients seeking rhinoplasty often have dimensional abnormalities such as the following.

     1. Excessive or inadequate nasal length.

     2. Excessive or inadequate radix projection.

     3. Excessive or inadequate nasal tip projection.

     4. Excessive or inadequate chin projection.

     5. Excessive or inadequate chin vertical height.

  C. Anatomic landmarks for analysis (Figs. 28-3 and 28-4).

     1. Gs (soft tissue glabella): The clinically palpable and visible anatomic midline point in the lower forehead where the nasofrontal inclination begins.

     2. R (nasal root or radix): A point on the midline nasal dorsum at the level of the supratarsal folds. If a supratarsal fold is not present, then the radix can be reliably measured in the midline 6 mm above the inner canthus.

     3. T (nasal tip): The midline point of the nasal tip taken at the level of the dome-projecting points of the lower cartilages.

     4. S (stomion): The midline point at the junction of the upper and lower lips.

     5. Me (menton): The lowermost midline point on the inferior border of the chin.

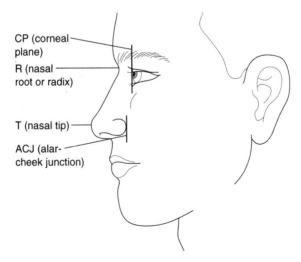

Fig. 28-3. Anatomic landmarks of the nose.

6. **ABP (alar base plane):** Runs horizontally through the alar bases. It is the most consistent vertical division between the midface and the lower face.
7. **CP (corneal plane):** A coronal plane tangential to the surface of the cornea. The CP is used as a reference from which the radix projection is measured.
8. **RP (radix plane):** A coronal plane tangential to the deepest point of the radix.
9. **ACJ (alar-cheek junction):** A coronal plane that passes through the junction of the nasal alae and the cheek.
10. **TP (nasal tip plane):** A coronal plane that passes through the anteriormost projecting point of the nose.
11. **NLCP (nose-lip-chin plane):** Ideally extends from a point one-half the distance of the ideal nasal length through the upper and lower lip vermilion and anteriormost projecting soft tissue of the chin.

D. **From these landmarks and reference planes,** the critical measurements for the nose, face, and chin can be obtained (Fig. 28-4).
   1. **MFH (midfacial height):** Gs to ABP.
   2. **LFH (lower facial height):** ABP to Me.
   3. **RT (nasal length):** R to T.
   4. **SMe:** S to Me.
   5. **Radix projection:** CP to RP.
   6. **Tip projection:** ACJ to TP.
   7. **Chin projection:** From the anteriormost projecting point of the chin to NLCP.

E. **Clinical analysis** and surgical planning
   1. **Determine the vertical height** of the midface and lower face.
      a. MFH should be equal to or slightly less (3 mm) than LFH.
      b. If it is not, reestablish correct occlusion and look specifically for the presence of a long or short face syndrome or microgenia.
   2. **The ideal nasal length** is determined by selecting the midface or lower face subunit as the standard (as above).
      a. When the mandible is normal and the midface and lower face are nearly equal, nasal length should be planned on the basis of chin vertical length: RTi = SMe.

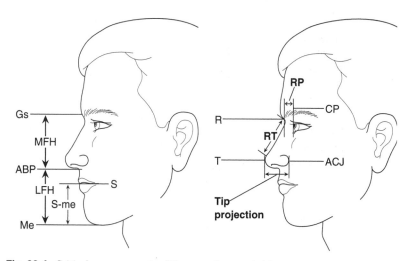

Fig. 28-4. Critical measurements of the nose, face, and chin.

      b. In cases of maldevelopment of the mandible or with microgenia, the ideal nasal length is determined from the midfacial height: RTi = 0.67 × MFH.

      c. Similarly, when the midface is overdeveloped and is not to be corrected orthognathically, the nose should be proportional to the midface rather than to the smaller mandibular segment: RTi = 0.67 × MFH.

  3. Determine the ideal tip projection: 0.67 × RTi.

  4. Determine the ideal radix projection: RTi × 0.28 (typically 9–14 mm).

  5. Chin projection is measured by dropping a vertical line from a point located at one-half the ideal nasal length. In women, the tip of the chin should be about 3 mm behind this line: Chin projection = −3 mm NLCP. In men the chin is more anterior.

VI. Anesthesia

  A. Topical anesthesia

    1. Neurosurgical pledgets soaked in 4% cocaine solution are placed along the nasal floor.

    2. The dose limit in most healthy adults is less than 5 mL (200 mg, or 2–3 mg/kg).

  B. Infiltrative anesthesia

    1. 1% to 2% lidocaine with 1:100,000 to 1:200,000 of epinephrine is used.

    2. For a complete septorhinoplasty, the following nerves are blocked.

      a. Supraorbital nerves, bilaterally

      b. Infraorbital nerves, bilaterally

      c. Anterior ethmoid nerves (endonasally), bilaterally

      d. Nasopalatine nerve

    3. The nasal soft tissues are infiltrated for hemostasis at different plane levels.

      a. Supraperiosteal nasal dorsum

      b. Supraperichondrial upper lateral cartilage

      c. Submucosal intranasal incision line

      d. Submucoperichondrial and submucoperiosteal nasal septum

VII. Basic rhinoplasty technique

  A. Incision and approach: Different approaches are available to gain access to the nasal skeleton.

    1. Intercartilaginous: The standard entrance route to the nasal dorsum.

    2. Intracartilaginous: Can allow better exposure for tip procedures.

    3. Infracartilaginous ("rim incision"): Useful if domal suturing or scoring is planned.

    4. Transcolumellar

      a. Open rhinoplasty approach.

      b. Best used for particular problems, including the following.

        (1) Difficult revision rhinoplasty.

        (2) Complicated asymmetric nasal tip.

        (3) Cleft nose corrections.

        (4) Difficult deviated nose.

        (5) Voluminous nose with thick overlying skin.

    5. A transfixion incision allows elevation of the soft tissue of the columella from the cartilaginous septum.

  B. Generalized technique to address specific issues.

    1. Reducing the nasal dorsum

      a. In a male nose the dorsum has a straight profile, whereas in a female profile the dorsum has a lower line with a supratip break.

      b. The dorsal skin is elevated subperiosteally.

      c. A bone rasp is used to take down the bony dorsum.

      d. The dorsal edges of the septal cartilage and upper lateral cartilages are resected with a no. 15 blade until the appropriate level is achieved.

      e. Excessive reduction will result in an "open roof deformity."

      f. If the nose appears flat and wide, then a narrowing procedure is required.

    2. Narrowing the nasal dorsum

warned that the effect on wrinkling is accompanied by a loss of facial expression in the involved muscles.

    d. The onset of paralysis may take 24 to 48 hours or more. The effect persists for 4 to 6 months, at which time reinjection is required to continue the effect.

  2. Fat injection

    a. Fat can be injected subcutaneously with a large-gauge needle.

    b. It can be used to camouflage forehead rhytids by filling out the tissues underneath.

    c. Fat injection can be an unpredictable adjunct to other therapies.

  3. Fat grafting

    a. Used to fill in glabellar frown lines.

    b. Used adjunctively with other facial procedures such as blepharoplasty or facial rhytidectomy.

  4. Transpalpebral corrugator resection

    a. Indicated in patients who exhibit significant glabellar frown lines and corrugator hyperactivity, but no brow ptosis.

    b. Used as an adjunct to blepharoplasty or alone in patients who do not need or desire full forehead rejuvenation.

    c. The procerus and corrugator supercilii are resected. A fat graft can be placed to fill in the depression left by this maneuver.

  5. Endoscopic brow lift

    a. This procedure is rapidly replacing open techniques as the standard for forehead rejuvenation. Preoperative markings consist of placing marks on the eyebrows directly above the medial canthus, midpupil, and lateral canthus, as well as the anterior hairline directly above the medial canthus and midpupil.

    b. Brow height at the midpupil level should be approximately 22 to 25 mm.

    c. The peak of the brow in women should lie at the junction of the middle and lateral thirds.

  6. Open brow lift: Indications are narrowing for the open procedure, as endoscopic brow lift techniques have become more popular. An open brow lift is indicated if the patient has a superiorly displaced (high) frontal hairline. A transcoronal or hairline incision is used to resect skin either posterior to or at the anterior hairline.

VI. Facial rejuvenation

  A. Anatomy

    1. Layers of the face: Skin, subcutaneous fat, superficial fascia, mimetic muscle, deep facial fascia (parotidomasseteric fascia, which is the plane containing the facial nerve), parotid duct, and buccal fat pad.

    2. SMAS (superficial musculoaponeurotic system).

      a. The SMAS is a thin fascial layer that separates the overlying subcutaneous fat from the underlying parotidomasseteric fascia and the facial nerve. It is continuous with the superficial cervical fascia.

      b. The SMAS thickens and becomes dense over the parotid and within the temporal region, where it is termed the temporoparietal fascia.

    3. Mimetic muscles.

      a. Superficial muscles include the orbicularis oculi, platysma, zygomaticus major and minor, and the risorius.

      b. Deep muscles are the buccinator and mentalis.

    4. Parotidomasseteric fascia.

      a. The parotidomasseteric fascia is continuous with the deep layer of cervical fascia.

      b. Facial nerve branches within the cheek lie deep to this layer laterally and become more superficial medially.

    5. Facial nerve.

      a. Cranial nerve VII.

      b. Separates the deep and superficial lobes of the parotid gland.

    a. Nasal osteotomies are crucial for narrowing the nasal bony vault and closing an open roof deformity.

    b. Best performed at the end of a procedure, since bleeding and swelling will ensue.

    c. Two osteotomies are used; digital pressure is used to shift the bony sidewall inward.

      (1) Transverse osteotomy: Percutaneous, just above the medial canthus. Use a 2-mm osteotome, and point upward toward the nasal dorsum.

      (2) Lateral osteotomy: Along the pyriform aperture, carried cephalad to join the transverse osteotomy; use a straight, guarded osteotome.

  3. Sculpturing the nasal tip

    a. Nasal tip volume reduction

      (1) Excess nasal tip volume is often due to the convexity of the lateral crus of the lower lateral cartilage.

      (2) Resection of the cranial edge of the lateral crus will lead to an aesthetically pleasing reduction in volume.

    b. Interdomal distance reduction

      (1) Reducing the interdomal distance will narrow the nasal tip.

      (2) This can be achieved by weakening the dome at the genu by performing interdigitating partial-thickness incisions.

      (3) Interdomal suturing and grafting are alternative techniques.

    c. Cranial rotation

      (1) Reducing the cranial edge of the lateral crus allows some degree of cranial tip rotation.

      (2) Additional rotation can be achieved by shortening the caudal septal edge or by severing the basal third of the lateral crus.

    d. Increasing tip projection

      (1) Placing an onlay graft overlying the alar domes.

      (2) Recruiting the lateral crura to elongate the medial crura.

      (3) Columellar graft if significant projection is required.

    e. Decreasing tip projection

      (1) Interrupting the tip cartilage support structures (attachments to the upper lateral cartilage and caudal septum) leading to retropositioning.

      (2) Excision of a segment of the domal cartilage or medial crura.

VIII. Adjunctive techniques

  A. Cartilage grafts

    1. Spreader grafts

      a. Used to restore the vault shape support between the upper lateral cartilage and the septum after dorsal reduction.

      b. Avoid the "inverted V" deformity.

    2. Columellar grafts

      a. Used to reinforce the medial crus.

      b. Increase nasal tip projection.

      c. Used to correct the retrusive columella.

    3. Tip grafts

      a. Increase nasal tip projection.

      b. Formation of two tip-defining points.

      c. Lower triangle surface contouring.

      d. Correction of the proportion between the nostril and the nasal tip.

  B. Alar reduction

    1. More often used in Asians and African Americans.

    2. Used for narrowing the nostrils and the alar base and shortening the length of the alar edge.

IX. Postoperative care

  A. An external nasal dorsal splint is applied for nasal dorsum protection.

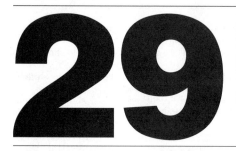

29

Evaluation and Surgical Management of Facial Aging

Salvatore J. Pacella

I. Facial aesthetics
A. **The face can be divided into three equal lengths.** (see Fig 28-2)
   1. **Upper facial height:** Browline to glabella.
   2. **Midfacial height:** Glabella to nasal base.
   3. **Lower facial height:** Nasal base to chin.
B. **Optimal facial dimensions** are approximately 8 "eye widths" high and 5 eye widths wide, similar to the "golden ratio" of 1:1.6 described by Fibonacci and others.
C. Facial features are proportional and symmetric in the aesthetically pleasing face.
D. **Eyes.**
   1. The eyes are essentially one eye width apart.
   2. The lateral canthus is slightly superior to the medial canthus.
   3. The distance from the lash line to the primary lid crease is 7 to 10 mm.
   4. The upper lid margin covers a portion of the iris but not the pupil. The lower lid margin is within 1 to 2 mm of the lower limbus of the iris.
   5. The ideal female brow position is 1 cm above the supraorbital rim.

II. Factors contributing to facial aging
A. Sun damage or "photoaging": Atrophy and loss of skin tone.
B. History of large weight gain or loss.
C. Chronic use of alcohol or cigarettes or both.
D. Chronic medical conditions, such as diabetes and renal failure.
E. History of facial trauma.
F. Facial paralysis. The paralyzed side develops fewer deep wrinkles, but becomes more ptotic.

III. Changes in facial appearance produced by aging
A. **Generalized skin changes**
   1. Fine wrinkles and lines develop, with loss of skin elasticity.
   2. Hyperpigmentation, keratoses, and papules.
   3. Decreased amount of subcutaneous adipose tissue.
B. **Perioral changes**
   1. Vertical rhytids, extending radially out from the upper and lower lip margins.
   2. Decreased fullness and flattening of the upper lip.
   3. Downturning of the oral commissures.
   4. Deepening of the nasolabial creases, also known as marionette lines.
C. **Cervical changes**
   1. Skin laxity and wrinkling.
   2. Formation of vertical platysmal bands.
   3. More obtuse cervicomental angle.
   4. Ptosis of the submandibular glands.
D. **Periocular changes**
   1. Dermatochalasis: Laxity of skin of the eyelids.
   2. Excessive eyelid edema and pigmentation.
   3. Protrusion of the periorbital fat.
   4. Ptosis of the lacrimal glands.

E. **Facial skeletal changes**
   1. Decreased mid and lower facial height.
   2. Laxity of support ligaments.
   3. Increased chin prominence.
   4. Increased prominence of the supraorbital rim.
   5. Increased prominence of the zygomatic arch.

IV. Initial aesthetic evaluation
A. **Determine the patient's *specific* desires:** "What concerns you the r
B. Perform a full history and physical examination.
C. Obtain appropriate laboratory and diagnostic tests, with preoperative eval by the patient's primary physician or cardiologist, as appropriate.
D. Visual examination, including acuity and visual fields.
E. **Photographic documentation** of preoperative characteristics, noti preoperative asymmetries and abnormalities.
F. **Patient education**
   1. Explanation of the procedure, the anticipated outcome, and po risks.
   2. Preoperative teaching (e.g., bandages, drains) and arrangements for
   3. Repeat preoperative visit 1 month after the initial presentation. Th ond visit" allows the patient to think about the procedure and as tional questions that may have arisen since the first visit.
G. **Informed consent**
   1. Must be clearly documented.
   2. Consent forms should be personalized and exhaustive.
   3. Consider mailing a copy of the consent form to the patient prioi preoperative visit.
   4. Consider line-by-line initialing of the form by the patient.
   5. Clearly document that consent is not a guarantee of the outcome.

V. Forehead rejuvenation
A. **Anatomy**
   1. **The frontalis muscle** elevates the brow and causes transverse w of the forehead skin. It has no bony origins. It traverses subcutaneou the eyebrows and the root of the nose to insert into the galea apone
   2. **The galea aponeurotica** spans from the frontalis muscle anterior occipitalis muscle posteriorly.
   3. **The corrugator supercilii** muscle is a triangular muscle locate medial end of the eyebrow deep to the frontalis and orbicula muscles. It causes vertical creases called "glabellar frown lines."
   4. **The procerus muscle** originates from the nasal bones and insert orly into the skin between the eyebrows, causing transverse creas radix.
B. **Patient assessment**
   1. The height of the forehead should be measured (see "Periocula nation").
   2. Glabellar and forehead rhytids should be noted.
   3. Brow ptosis should be documented.
   4. Upper lid ptosis should be assessed and specifically distinguisł brow ptosis by manually elevating the patient's brow.
   5. Upper lid dermatochalasis should be reevaluated with manual ele the brow.
C. **Operations**
   1. **Botulinum toxin (Botox) injections** (see chapter 30, Nonsurgi agement of Facial Aging.)
      a. By inducing paralysis of underlying musculature that attach skin, the pull on the skin is relaxed, thus alleviating wrinkling.
      b. Botox can be used to attenuate glabellar and forehead rhytids
      c. It is injected into the corrugator supercilii, procerus, and muscles, resulting in their temporary paralysis. Patients

      c. The nerve exits the parotid medially and travels along the superficial surface of the masseter muscle, deep to the parotidomasseteric fascia.

      d. Medial to the masseter, the nerve lies over the buccal fat pad.

      e. Branches penetrate the parotidomasseteric fascia to innervate the overlying mimetic muscles.

      f. Unlike the other branches, which lie deep to the deep facial fascia, once the frontal branch crosses the zygomatic arch, it comes to lie within the SMAS.

      g. Most of the facial muscles lie superficial to the plane of the facial nerve and receive their innervation from their deep surfaces. Muscles innervated from their superficial surface include the buccinator, levator anguli oris, and mentalis (these muscles are deep to the plane of the facial nerve).

      h. The SMAS invests the superficial muscles: the orbicularis oculi, platysma, zygomaticus major and minor, and risorius.

B. Indications and patient assessment

    1. The surgeon should address the specific complaints of each patient and tailor the operative plan individually.

    2. The preoperative evaluation also includes assessment and documentation of facial asymmetries as well as skin redundancy, abnormal fat accumulations, platysma laxity, and salivary gland abnormality.

    3. The contour of the jawline and neckline and the status of the nasolabial folds are evaluated.

C. Operations and approaches

    1. Subcutaneous rhytidectomy with SMAS plication or resection

      a. Thought to be the standard facelift by many authors.

      b. The incision is begun 1 cm posterior to the temporal hairline, continued down in front of the ear (either pretragally or retrotragally), around the base of the lobule, and then upward and posterior around the back of the ear, to finish in the postauricular scalp.

      c. Skin flap dissection is performed in a medial direction, leaving a small layer of fat on the flap. Dissection ends just lateral to the nasolabial folds.

      d. The SMAS is either plicated or a narrow (2 cm) ellipse is excised. The direction of pull is superior and lateral across the midface.

    2. Deep-plane rhytidectomy

      a. A reliable technique to specifically address redundant nasolabial folds.

      b. A sub-SMAS dissection is extended superiorly over the zygomaticus muscles and medially beyond the nasolabial folds, totally releasing all SMAS attachments and creating a thick flap composed of skin, subcutaneous fat, and platysma.

      c. The total release of the SMAS allows the components of the flap to be lifted and advanced back to their original position.

      d. The deep-plane technique is associated with a slightly higher risk of facial nerve injury.

    3. Minimal-incision rhytidectomy with lateral SMASectomy

      a. Facial rejuvenation is accomplished with less retroauricular scarring. The attempt is to avoid retroauricular skin flap ischemia.

      b. Ideal candidates are usually in their 40s with aging primarily in the mid and lower face, with moderate jowls.

      c. A standard incision is utilized with a truncated postauricular extension.

      d. Skin flaps are elevated in the standard fashion. The SMAS flap is created by incising along the medial edge of the parotid. A sling of inferiorly based SMAS is created and sutured to the mastoid fascia to achieve the desired pull (perpendicular to the nasolabial folds).

      e. This procedure can be combined with submental liposuction.

    4. Subperiosteal rhytidectomy

      a. Developed by Tessier, this extensive approach can specifically address structural laxity in the midface.

      b. Complications include an increased incidence of facial nerve injuries as well as prolonged facial edema.

      c. Indications: Patients with significant aging and ptosis of the central oval of the face, including the eyebrows, nasoglabellar soft tissue, nose, nasolabial folds, cheeks, angle of the mouth, and jowls.

      d. Operative technique: Extensive upper and midface degloving is interconnected with deep-plane undermining.

D. Complications of rhytidectomy

  1. Hematoma: Particularly under the mastoid skin flaps.

  2. Flap loss and/or ischemia: Most common in smokers.

  3. Infection.

  4. Asymmetry.

  5. Great auricular nerve injury.

  6. Facial nerve palsy or injury. The most commonly injured (but frequently unrecognized due to overlap of innervation) branch of the facial nerve is the buccal branch.

  7. Recurrence.

  8. Excessive scarring or temporal alopecia.

  9. Pixie ear deformity.

VII. Periocular rejuvenation

A. Anatomy

  1. Surface anatomy (ideal aesthetic values)

      a. Palpebral fissure: 12 to 14 mm vertically, 28 to 30 mm horizontally.

      b. Anterior hairline to brow distance: Approximately 5 to 6 cm at the midpupillary line.

      c. Brow to supratarsal crease distance: Approximately 1.5 cm.

      d. Supratarsal crease: Ideally 8 to 10 mm above the upper lid margin.

      e. Lateral canthus: 1 to 2 mm superior to medial canthus.

      f. In women, the brow usually peaks at the lateral limbus, corresponding to the junction of the middle third with the lateral third of the brow.

  2. Layers of the eyelid

      a. Anterior lamella: Skin (0.5–0.7 mm thick), subcutaneous fat, and orbicularis oculi muscle (divided into pretarsal and preseptal components).

      b. Middle lamella.

        (1) Upper lid: Septum, tarsus, and retractors.

        (2) Lower lid: Septum and tarsus.

        (3) The orbital septum originates from the arcus marginalis and is contiguous with the orbital periosteum.

        (4) Upper lid retractors include the levator palpebrae muscle (inserting into the upper eyelid crease) and Müller's muscle (sympathetically innervated, inserting on the superior edge of the tarsus).

      c. Posterior lamella: The conjunctiva and lower lid retractors. The lower lid analogue to the upper lid retractors is the capsulopalpebral fascia.

      d. Fat.

        (1) Preseptal fat: Suborbicularis oculi fat (SOOF).

        (2) Postseptal fat: Contiguous with intraorbital fat.

        (3) The upper lid has central and nasal fat compartments, separated by the superior oblique tendon. Laterally, the lacrimal gland takes the space of what would be the lateral fat pad.

        (4) The lower lid has lateral, central, and nasal fat pads. The nasal and central pads are separated by the inferior oblique tendon, which is the most commonly injured structure in a blepharoplasty.

B. Indications and patient assessment

  1. Particular attention is paid to a history of smoking, diabetes, myasthenia gravis, Graves' disease, bleeding disorders, abnormal scarring, dry eyes, glaucoma, cataracts, and visual impairment.

  2. Specific exams to document prior to blepharoplasty.

    a. Schirmer's test: A quantitative assessment of tear production, used to judge the postoperative protection of the eye. It consists of placing a piece of special filter paper in the fornix and measuring the length of wetting of the paper over a specified time.

    b. Lid symmetry and ptosis.

    c. Brow position and effect of manual brow elevation on the upper lids.

    d. Evaluation for compensated brow ptosis.

    e. Documentation of Bell's phenomenon (upward rolling of the globe with eye closing, which serves to protect the cornea in the event of lagophthalmos).

    f. Skin excess and lid excursion.

    g. Amounts of upper and lower lid fat, by compartment.

    h. Lower lid tone: Via the "snap" test.

    i. Scleral show.

    j. Tear trough deformity.

    k. Presence of excessive edema or pigmentation or both, which may be indicators of increased risk for excessive postoperative swelling.

C. Operations and approaches

  1. Upper lid blepharoplasty

    a. Preoperative markings: Made prior to injection with the patient awake. The lower incision is usually made 8 to 10 mm above the ciliary margin at the level of the superior edge of the tarsal plate. The upper incision is determined by gathering the lid skin with broad-tipped (Green) forceps until lagophthalmos occurs.

    b. The minimal distance from the brow to the upper incision line is usually 10 to 12 mm.

    c. The medial and lateral ends of the incisions can be altered with Z-plasties, W-plasties, or Y-V plasties.

    d. Muscle excision is variably recommended.

    e. The globe is gently depressed to aid in the identification of postseptal fat. The septum is incised high to avoid injury to the levator mechanism. Only fat that extends beyond the globe without pressure is excised, because overresection leads to a "hollowed-out" look.

    f. The superior oblique muscle may be identified between the nasal and central fat pads.

    g. The dermis and orbicularis may be sutured to the levator in order to recreate a distinct supratarsal fold.

    h. Lateral fullness may be corrected by a concomitant brow lift, suspension of the lacrimal gland, or partial SOOF resection.

  2. Lower lid blepharoplasty

    a. A conservative, skin-only resection via a subciliary incision may be coupled with retroorbital fat resection. This is recommended for patients with excess skin and good orbicularis tone.

    b. Skin and muscle may be resected together via a subciliary incision if poor orbicularis tone is present. Retroorbital fat is excised similarly to upper lid blepharoplasty, with care not to injure the inferior oblique muscle.

    c. After the orbital septum is incised along the arcus marginalis, it may be redraped to a more anterior and inferior position in an effort to diminish a prominent tear trough.

    d. The orbicularis may be repositioned laterally and superiorly to raise the lateral canthus.

    e. Transconjunctival approach: The orbital septum is left intact, and fat is removed via an incision through the conjunctiva. This technique can be combined with a separate skin incision or with a chemical or trichloroacetic acid peel. Disadvantages include a more limited exposure and the potential for inadequate fat removal.

  3. Ancillary procedures in case of lower lid laxity

    a. Temporary external support of the lower lid margin with tape or a tarsorrhaphy

        b. Wedge resection to shorten the lid
        c. Suspension or tightening of the lower lid muscle to create a suspensory sling
        d. Tarsal suspension
        e. Lateral canthopexy

D. Complications
    1. Blindness: 3 to 40 instances in 100,000 procedures, primarily from retrobulbar hematoma.
        a. Requires immediate decompression; a surgical emergency.
        b. Mannitol and/or acetazolamide administration.
        c. Emergent ophthalmologic consultation.
    2. Dry eyes (common temporarily postoperatively; managed with application of "artificial tears").
    3. Scarring.
    4. Asymmetry.
    5. Infection, orbital cellulitis.
    6. Ptosis.
    7. Diplopia.
    8. Enophthalmos.
    9. Lagophthalmos.
    10. Lash atrophy.
    11. Ectropion.
    12. Epiphora.

VIII. Facial augmentation and facial implants
  A. The chin is the most common site, followed by the malar region.
  B. Alloplastic materials
    1. Silicone: The most commonly used material because it is biocompatible, stable, and the shape can be easily modified. Silicone implants become encased by a tissue capsule and can be easily removed if necessary.
    2. Polyethylene (Medpor): Used less commonly than silicone. Uses include ear reconstruction, nasal augmentation, and orbital floor reconstruction. Polyethylene allows tissue ingrowth and is much more difficult to remove than silicone.
    3. Hydroxyapatite: Used for cranial reconstruction, alveolar ridges, and other bony facial structures.
  C. The ratio of soft tissue response to facial skeletal change is approximately 0.66 (an implant with 1 cm of projection will usually result in 0.66 cm of soft tissue augmentation). In general, chin implants usually provide sharper projection than malar implants due to their location and surrounding soft tissue contour.
  D. Chin implants are placed subperiosteally, via intraoral or submental approaches.
  E. Common complications include hematoma, infection, extrusion, malposition, and sensory nerve dysfunction.

IX. Diseases of premature aging
  A. Ehlers-Danlos syndrome: A rare, genetically transmitted disease of connective tissue with variable inheritance (autosomal dominant or recessive) caused by a genetic defect in collagen production. It is characterized by thin, friable, hyperextensible skin, unstable and hypermobile joints, and subcutaneous hemorrhage. Surgical rejuvenation is contraindicated.
  B. Cutis laxa: An extremely rare genetically transmitted disease with variable inheritance (autosomal dominant, recessive, or X-linked). It is characterized by a degeneration of elastic fibers in the dermis, resulting in coarsely textured, drooping skin. It is associated with mild mental retardation, chronic obstructive pulmonary disease, pulmonary infections, diverticula, and hernias. Surgical rejuvenation procedures may be performed provided the patient's overall health is satisfactory.
  C. Progeria: A rare autosomal recessive disorder marked by premature aging and a shortened lifespan. It is characterized by skin laxity, loss of subcutaneous fat, generalized atherosclerosis, craniofacial disproportion, growth retardation,

Nonsurgical Management of Facial Aging

Richard D. Klein and
Marlene S. Calderon

Fitzpatrick Classification of Skin Type

Patients with higher Fitzpatrick classifications (i.e., darker skin) have greater resistance to photoaging. However, they have a higher incidence of adverse pigmentation changes (darkening or lightening) following chemical peels or laser skin resurfacing.

I. **Type I**
   A. Color: White
   B. UV sensitivity: Very sensitive
   C. Sunburn history: Always burns and never tans
II. **Type II**
   A. Color: White
   B. UV sensitivity: Very sensitive
   C. Sunburn history: Always burns and sometimes tans
III. **Type III**
   A. Color: White
   B. UV sensitivity: Sensitive
   C. Sunburn history: Sometimes burns and gradually tans
IV. **Type IV**
   A. Color: Light brown
   B. UV sensitivity: Moderate
   C. Sunburn history: Minimal burn and tans well
V. **Type V**
   A. Color: Brown
   B. UV sensitivity: Minimal
   C. Sunburn history: Never burns and tans to deep brown
VI. **Type VI**
   A. Color: Black
   B. UV sensitivity: Insensitive
   C. Sunburn history: Never burns and deeply tans

Skin Preconditioning

Preconditioning regimens are often used before laser and chemical peel therapy.

I. **Retinoic acid preparations**
   A. **Tretinoin 0.05% (Renova):** Used for photodamaged skin and mottled pigmentation.
   B. **Tretinoin 0.025% (Retin-A):** Used for acne treatment.
   C. **Isotretinoin 5-mg capsules (Roaccutane):** Used for acne treatment; an isomer of tretinoin.
II. **Pretreatment with retinoids**
   A. Thins the stratum corneum and promotes angiogenesis.
   B. Increases dermal collagen.

    C. May help reduce post-treatment hyperpigmentation.

    D. May contribute to postoperative erythema.

    E. Has a rejuvenating effect, partially due to generating dermal edema.

    F. Contraindicated in early pregnancy.

III. Roaccutane

    A. Roaccutane use increases the risk of delayed healing and atypical scarring.

    B. If used, it should be stopped 1–2 years before any resurfacing therapy.

    C. Roaccutane inhibits reepithelialization from adnexal structures.

IV. Hydroquinone therapy

    A. Suppresses melanocyte activity.

    B. Helps prevent hyperpigmentation.

Chemical Peels

I. Histology

    A. There is a chemically induced injury to the epidermis and the superficial dermis. Elastotic skin is removed and replaced with a neocollagen-rich layer.

    B. Healing occurs via epithelial advancement from skin appendages. Epidermal regeneration begins by 48 hours and is usually complete by day 7. Dermal changes take longer to reach the full effect.

    C. Epidermal changes: Cellular uniformity, return of vertical polarity, and less lentiginous downgrowth. There is a mild possible increase in the number of melanocytes, but a decrease in the amount of melanin granules in the basal layer of the epidermis.

    D. Dermal changes: A homogenization of dermal collagen occurs, with dense parallel collagen bundles and a dense network of fine elastic fibers that parallel the collagen. There is less ground substance with evidence of chronic inflammation.

II. Complications: Can include hypopigmentation, milia, prolonged erythema, hypertrophic scarring, ectropion, and blotchy hyperpigmentation

III. Phenol peel

    A. Advantages

        1. Typically safe and effective, with long-lasting results.

        2. Produces a controlled and predictable partial-thickness chemical burn, with a consistent depth of penetration into the upper reticular dermis.

        3. Hypertrophic scarring is rare.

    B. Disadvantages

        1. Associated with a prolonged recovery period.

        2. There is a potential for significant bleaching action.

        3. The line of demarcation between treated and untreated areas may be obvious.

    C. Indications

        1. Best for coarse wrinkles and significant perioral rhytids.

        2. Irregular facial hyperpigmentation.

        3. Actinic keratoses.

        4. Spot treatment of individual lentigines of the dorsal hand and/or fingers.

        5. Ideal for types I to III skin.

    D. Patient selection

        1. Phenol peels work less well with thick and oily skin. There is a higher tendency to get areas of hyperpigmentation in these patients.

        2. Patients with darker complexions need full-face treatment; otherwise, the lines of demarcation can be obvious.

        3. Men are usually poor candidates because their thicker skin does not respond as well.

        4. Not suitable for patients with the following conditions:

            a. Acne scarring.

            b. Hemangioma or facial telangiectasia.

            c. Hyperpigmented skin grafts.

            d. History of cardiac disease.

E. Mechanism of action

1. Penetration extends past basement membrane of the epidermis and into the underlying papillary dermis.
2. Changes occur in the epidermis and superficial dermis.
3. Damaged elastotic skin is rejuvenated by neocollagen deposition in rigid compact parallel bundles.
4. **Early changes**
   a. Keratocoagulation necrosis of the epidermis extending into papillary dermis.
   b. Marked inflammatory reaction.
5. **After 48 hours**
   a. Epidermal regeneration.
   b. Usually complete by 7 days.
6. **Dermal regeneration lags.** There is only partial reconstitution of the dermis with attempts at reformation of rete pegs, dermal thickening, fibroblastic proliferation, and deposition of collagen at 2 weeks.
7. **At 3 months,** a majority of the healing is complete.

F. Toxicology

1. The phenol is absorbed through the skin, metabolized in the liver, and renally excreted.
2. It may be toxic to the liver and kidney, and may depress the respiratory center and myocardium.
3. Blood levels are low after topical full-face peeling.
4. There is a higher risk for cardiac dysrhythmia if more than 50% of the face is surfaced in less than 30 minutes. Therefore, the application must be performed over 1 hour.

G. Requirements for therapy

1. Electrocardiography, pulse oximetry, and intravenous access are mandatory because of possible cardiac dysrhythmias.
2. Have sterile water available for eye irrigation in case of accidental eye exposure.
3. Have appropriate medications and personnel available in case of a cardiac emergency.
4. Sedation is required for full-face peels.
5. Monitor patient closely for 1 to 2 days for eyelid edema.

H. Pretreatment

1. No pretreatment is performed with Retin-A or hydroquinone.
2. A patient history of herpes mandates antiviral therapy.
   a. Acyclovir 400 mg three times daily 24 hours preoperatively.
   b. Continue for 5 days postoperatively.
   c. If herpetic flare-up occurs, treat with 800 mg acyclovir three times daily until resolved.
3. Thoroughly clean and remove all makeup the night before.
4. Clean with liquid soap and thoroughly dry just prior to treatment.
5. Degrease the skin with either acetone or isopropyl alcohol to prevent an uneven peel.

I. Baker-Gordon formula

1. 3 mL phenol (88%).
2. 2 mL tap water.
3. 8 drops liquid soap.
4. 3 drops croton oil: A vesicant; enhances the mixture's keratolytic and penetrating actions.

J. Application

1. Apply with a damp cotton swab; do not drip or streak into nonpeel areas.
2. With eyelids, the cotton swab should be almost dry to avoid corneal or conjunctival contact. On the upper lids, stop at the upper border of the tarsal plate to minimize eyelid edema. For the lower lid, stop within 3 mm of the lid margin.
3. Paint on evenly and achieve complete coverage.

4. Turns frosty grayish-white immediately.
5. A burning sensation may last a few minutes until the local anesthetic property of phenol is realized.
6. Apply slowly to minimize burning and to avoid rapid absorption.
7. For full face: Apply over a 1- to 2-hour period.
8. Change applicators often to minimize facial oil accumulation.
9. Do one aesthetic unit at a time. Wait 15 minutes between units for renal excretion.
10. Stop below the mandibular border to avoid a noticeable transition from treated to untreated skin.

K. Postoperative care
1. Prophylactic antibiotic therapy is instituted for 7 days.
2. Occlusive dressings may be used for 24 hours.
    a. Tape: May lead to deeper penetration and is painful to remove.
    b. Petroleum jelly (Vaseline) is helpful.
3. Maximal edema occurs within 6 to 12 hours. The eyes may swell for 48 hours.
4. Wash with peroxide and water, and then use a petroleum-based ointment.
5. Reepithelialization is expected in 7 to 10 days.
6. Usually patients can use makeup within 10 to 15 days.
7. Start sunscreen in 12 to 14 days.
8. Erythema persists for 12 weeks, and possibly for up to 6 months.
9. Avoid sun exposure. The skin will never tan normally again and may blotch.

IV. Trichloroacetic acid peel
A. Advantages
1. Less morbidity than a phenol peel.
2. Less systemic toxicity.
3. The concentration can be varied.
4. A broader range of skin types can be treated.
5. There is less hypertrophic scarring in the neck, thorax, and extremities.
6. Less bleaching. Better for dark complexions and for regional peels.

B. Disadvantages
1. Less effective than phenol, with half the degree of dermis penetration than phenol and half the amount of neocollagen produced.
2. There is a less profound effect on coarse facial wrinkles, especially periorally.
3. Less effective on severe sun-damaged skin.
4. Less predictable than phenol.

C. Mode of action
1. The depth of the peel injury is controlled by varying its concentration.
    a. 10% to 25% for light peels; barely penetrates the epidermis.
    b. 30% to 35% for intermediate peels; into the papillary dermis.
    c. 50% to 60% for deep peels; associated with a higher risk of scarring.
2. There is less effect on melanocyte metabolism, compared with phenol.

D. Pretreatment
1. Pretreat with Retin-A and 4% hydroquinone for 4 to 6 weeks before peel is performed.
2. Retin-A increases the permeability of the epidermis to trichloroacetic acid (TCA).
3. Antiviral therapy for a history of herpes (see above).

E. Technique
1. **Increased depth of penetration** can by achieved by the following:
    a. Pretreatment with retinoids.
    b. Application of additional coats.
    c. Pretreatment with keratolytic agents, such as Jessner's solution: salicylic acid, lactic acid, and resorcinol.
    d. Mechanically abrading the skin with gauze.
2. **Judge the depth of penetration and injury** by the appearance of the skin after the solution is applied.
    a. Superficial depth: Erythema.

  b. Intermediate depth: Sparse, irregular, light, pink-white frosted skin.
  c. Deeper: More uniform, denser, white-colored frosted skin.
  d. Too deep: Grayish-white color.
 3. Application
  a. Wash and degrease the skin with either acetone or isopropyl alcohol.
  b. Stretch the skin to flatten out wrinkles.
  c. Apply the solution with cotton gauze, using even strokes, by aesthetic units.
  d. Leave in place for 30 seconds to 2 minutes. Wait for frosting to appear before rubbing off with a dry gauze pad.
  e. The solution is neutralized by washing the skin thoroughly with ice water.
  f. Cover generously with 1% hydrocortisone or petroleum-based ointment.

F. Postpeel care
 1. Very light peels: Symptoms are slight; minimal erythema; light makeup may be used immediately.
 2. Intermediate-depth peels
  a. Initial erythema.
  b. 48 hours: Desquamation, brown appearance of keratocoagulated epithelium; use moisturizer or hydrocortisone-based ointment; avoid makeup; peaks at 72 hours.
  c. 4 to 7 days: Healing and peeling skin; wash face several times per day to avoid crusting; resume makeup when peeling has subsided.
  d. Within 7 to 10 days: Start tretinoin and hydroquinone when peeling has stopped; use sunscreen daily to avoid hyperpigmentation.
 3. Deep peels
  a. Significant desquamation followed by erythema.
  b. Wash face at least four times per day with water followed by ointment.
  c. Expect reepithelization in 4 to 7 days.
  d. Tretinoin and hydroquinone are used when healing is complete.
  e. Wait at least 3 months before performing repeat peels.

V. Glycolic acid peels
 A. Alpha-hydroxy acids include glycolic acid from sugar cane, lactic acid from soured milk, citric acid from citrus fruits, tartaric acid from grapes, and malic acid from apples. They may be found in many cosmetics in low concentrations.
  1. May be used as pretreatment for chemical peels and laser therapy.
  2. May be used as skin peels at concentrations of 30% to 70%.
  3. Rejuvenate the stratum corneum in a manner similar to tretinoin.
  4. The depth of their penetration is related to the concentration and duration of therapy.
  5. Usually used as a superficial peel.
 B. Application
  1. Produces initial erythema followed by a white eschar, due to epidermolysis.
  2. Do not wait for full frosting as in TCA peels, because frosting indicates dermal destruction with a glycolic acid peel.
  3. Dilute with water or neutralize with sodium bicarbonate once the application is complete.

Dermabrasion

I. Histology
 A. Reepithelialization occurs from dermal appendages in 7 days.
 B. The removal of a partial thickness of dermis is permanent.
 C. Changes are less severe than after chemical peels.

      1. No flattening of dermal collagen.
      2. Less change in pigmentation.
      3. No increase in elastic fibers.
      4. Less neocollagen deposition.

II. Advantages compared with peeling.
    A. Less significant bleaching effect than phenol.
    B. Better for darker skin because it leads to less significant demarcation.
    C. Depth more controllable than with chemical peel.
    D. Better for acne scars.

III. Disadvantages
    A. Not recommended for periorbital wrinkles.
    B. Less efficacious for wrinkles than peels.
    C. Often additional dermabrasion is needed.

IV. Indications
    A. Acne scars: Depressed or raised scars do not respond as well.
    B. Coarse facial wrinkles.
    C. Highly effective in the perioral region, lower lip, and chin.
    D. The best results are obtained in thick skin with many adnexal structures.
    E. Not as effective on the back, medial arms, and low anterior neck.
    F. Can be used to remove tattoos, although a laser is usually more effective.

V. Action: An abrasive process is used to remove the epidermis and a superficial layer of the dermis.

VI. Technique
    A. Institute antiviral therapy, as above, for a history of herpes.
    B. Local or general anesthesia is required.
    C. A motor-driven abrader, coarse brush, or drywall sanding screen is used.
    D. Stretch the skin and apply the abrader parallel to the skin with even pressure.
    E. Stop when multiple fine bleeding points appear (punctate bleeding).
    F. Dermabrade down to the reticular dermis, leaving appendages to regenerate.

VII. Postoperative care
    A. Irrigate with normal saline.
    B. Use petroleum-based ointment coverage.
    C. Wash area several times per day with water and reapply ointment.
    D. Reepithelialization is usually complete in 7 days.
    E. Wait 10 days prior to using makeup.
    F. Avoid sun to minimize hyperpigmentation, which is usually more frequent than with peeling.

Laser Skin Resurfacing

Laser is becoming the treatment of choice for sun-damaged skin and fine rhytids. (See also Chapter 10, "Lasers in Plastic Surgery.") The char-free carbon dioxide laser enables precise surface tissue ablation, allowing skin resurfacing of wrinkles and removal of surface pigment abnormalities. Each laser pass removes 20 to 50 nm of skin.

I. Action
    A. The skin surface color is improved by mechanically removing damaged skin.
    B. Skin texture is improved via collagen shrinkage and remodeling.

II. Patient selection
    A. Careful patient selection should be performed to ensure predictable results.
    B. Fitzpatrick skin types I and II respond best with the fewest side effects.
    C. Patients with type III skin are at greater risk for pigmentation abnormalities.
    D. Patients with types IV, V, and VI skin are generally avoided.

III. Pretreatment
    A. All patients are treated with Retin-A 0.1% applied daily for 1 month prior to laser therapy.
    B. Type III patients are treated with Retin-A and hydroquinone for 1 month prior to laser resurfacing.

  C. Prophylactic antiviral and antibacterial agents are essential.
IV. Therapy
  A. Individual aesthetic units may be treated with local anesthesia.
  B. Full-face therapy can require general anesthesia.
V. Post-treatment care
  A. Wash the skin daily with a dilute acidic solution to decrease infection and avoid crust formation.
  B. After the skin reepithelializes, erythema occurs and usually persists for 3 to 6 months. Cosmetic camouflage may be used during this time.
  C. Sunscreen use should be encouraged.
VI. Complications
  A. Minor complications include milia and skin sensitivity.
  B. Major complications include infection, scarring, pigmentation alterations, and hyperpigmentation.

Botulinum Toxin

I. Introduction
  A. The toxin is produced by *Clostridium botulinum*, which is responsible for muscle paralysis from food poisoning.
  B. First used in the 1970s for the treatment of strabismus. Paralysis of specific extraocular muscles can improve ocular alignment in these patients.
II. Types of toxins: Seven different antigenic toxins are produced by different strains of *C. botulinum.*
  A. Type A: The most potent and the most commonly used type.
  B. Type B: Less potent; useful for patients who develop antibodies to type A.
III. Commercially available toxins
  A. Botox: Type A, made by Allergan, Inc., in Irvine, California. FDA approved for glabellar wrinkles in 2002.
  B. Dysport: Type A, made by Ipsen Limited in Maidenhead, Berkshire, United Kingdom.
  C. Myobloc/Neurobloc: Type B, made by Elan Pharmaceuticals in San Francisco, California.
IV. Mechanism of action
  A. Botulinum toxin acts at the presynaptic cholinergic neuromuscular end plate by inhibiting the release of vesicle-bound acetylcholine at presynaptic terminals.
  B. Toxins have different sites of action on soluble N-ethylmaleimide-sensitive factor attachment protein receptor (SNARE) proteins responsible for membrane docking and fusion of synaptic vesicles that release acetylcholine.
  C. Return of function is seen in 3 to 4 months, after new axonal sprouts replace nonfunctioning end plates.
V. Preparation of toxins
  A. Toxicity is measured in units. One unit (1 U) is equivalent to the amount of toxin that kills 50% of female Swiss-Webster mice after an intraperitoneal injection.
  B. Relative units: 1 U Botox = 3–5 U Dysport = 50–100 U Myobloc.
  C. The lethal dose of Botox for humans is 2,500 to 3,000 U for a 70-kg person.
VI. Clinical uses: Wrinkles or rhytids are produced by underlying hyperfunctioning muscles. With aging, ridges or wrinkles appear perpendicular to the causative muscle fibers. Chemical paresis created by botulinum toxin eliminates muscle contraction, thus decreasing dynamic wrinkles and furrows.
  A. Upper third of the face
    1. Glabellar furrows are formed by contractions of the procerus, corrugator supercilii, and medial fibers of the orbicularis oculi.
    2. Typically, five to seven sites are injected in the glabella/medial brow (2.5–4.0 U per injection), for a total of 20 to 25 units of Botox.

3. Chemical denervation can last for up to 6 months.
4. Transient ptosis is the most significant complication and can occur in up to 5% of patients.
5. A chemical brow lift can occur from unopposed action of the frontalis due to paralysis of the brow depressors.

B. Horizontal forehead lines
1. The frontalis muscle is responsible for horizontal forehead lines.
2. Typically, four to eight sites are injected in the forehead, 2 to 3 cm above the orbital rims.
3. Brow ptosis can occur if the frontalis is overinjected. Also, injecting lateral to the midpupillary line can cause drooping of the lateral eyebrow or eyelid, or both, and lead to a tired appearance.

C. Periocular "crow's feet"
1. Crow's feet are caused by contraction of the orbicularis oculi, risorius, and zygomaticus muscles.
2. The lateral orbicularis is injected in one to four sites with a total of 5 to 15 U Botox.
3. Avoid injecting too deeply to prevent paralysis of the extraocular muscles.

D. Middle third of the face
1. Vertical lip wrinkles are caused by contraction of the orbicularis oris muscle.
2. Injecting 1 to 2 U of Botox in each wrinkle can soften perioral rhytids.
3. Limit use to 2 U of Botox per side. Treat only two to three wrinkles at a time.

E. Marionette lines
1. Frown lines are improved by injecting the depressor anguli oris muscles.
2. Platysma injections can also help.
3. Overtreatment can cause difficulty with smiling. Injection in these areas is specifically not recommended for singers or musicians.

F. Mentalis: Prominent mentalis contraction can cause a pebbly or cobblestone chin that can benefit from Botox.

G. Nasolabial folds
1. Injection to paralyze the zygomaticus major has not given consistent results.
2. Injection into the levator superioris alaeque nasi may smooth the superomedial nasolabial fold.

VII. Adverse effects
A. There have been no reports of allergic reactions with facial aesthetic Botox procedures.
B. Transient bruising can be minimized by using a 30-gauge needle and applying postinjection pressure.

VIII. Contraindications
A. There have been no reports of teratogenicity with botulinum toxin.
B. Most physicians do not inject pregnant or lactating women.
C. A history of neuromuscular disease is a contraindication.
D. Known sensitivity to human albumin is a contraindication.
E. Aminoglycosides can potentiate the effects of Botox.
F. Areas of active infection should not be injected.

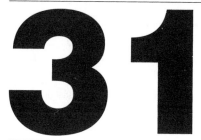

Body Contouring

Amy Alderman

Abdominoplasty

I. **Indications**
   A. Striae
   B. Excess abdominal skin
   C. Excess fatty tissue
   D. Musculoskeletal laxity

II. **Goals**
   A. **To achieve a flat abdomen** with normal-appearing umbilicus and inconspicuous scars
   B. **Skin resection and redraping,** subcutaneous tissue reduction, and correction of muscle diastasis
   C. **Potential impairments** to the goals: Intraperitoneal fat, perimenopausal changes, and relaxation of the musculoaponeurotic system

III. **Etiology**
   A. **Pregnancy:** "Biologic tissue expansion"
      1. Abdominal wall laxity and skin excess.
      2. Rectus abdominis diastasis.
      3. Striae gravidarum: Occurs in 90% of white women due to increased estrogen levels and tissue stress.
   B. **Weight loss or gain:** Damages skin elasticity, creating cellulite-type skin tone and/or leading to pannus formation
   C. **Aging**
      1. Increase in visceral fat.
      2. Decrease in skin elasticity.
   D. **Genetics:** Hereditary factors contribute to undesirable fat distribution.
      1. **Gynecoid distribution:** Excess fat in the lower abdomen, thighs, and hips.
      2. **Android distribution:** Excess fat in the flanks, abdomen, and chest.
   E. **Previous incisions**
      1. Hernias.
      2. Poorly draped skin.
      3. Unaesthetic scars.
   F. **Medications**
      1. Steroids (striae, lipodystrophy).
      2. Hormones (lipodystrophy).
      3. Antidepressants (lipodystrophy, fluctuations in weight).
   G. **Ultraviolet exposure:** Damages skin elasticity.

IV. **Anatomy**
   A. **Vascular anatomy** of the abdominal wall: Three zones described by Huger
      1. **Huger zone I:** Directly over the rectus abdominis: deep superior and inferior epigastric arteries.
      2. **Huger zone II:** Inferolaterally on the anterior abdominal wall: circumflex iliac system, superficial epigastric and superficial pudendal arteries.
      3. **Huger zone III:** Laterally over internal and external obliques: segmental lumbar and intercostal perforators.

    4. The abdominoplasty flap, in general, must rely on zone III for its blood supply; therefore, limit undermining/liposuction in this area.

B. Sensory innervation

    1. Anterior abdominal wall: Originates laterally from the sixth to twelfth thoracic nerves and the first lumbar nerve.

        a. Lateral to the anterior superior iliac spine (ASIS), the nerves are located between the internal oblique and the transversus abdominis muscles.

        b. Medial to the ASIS, the nerves run between the internal and external oblique muscles.

    2. Lateral femoral cutaneous nerve (L2-3): Sensation to the anterolateral thigh. Located 1 to 6 cm medial to the ASIS, this nerve can be injured during dissection and closure of an abdominoplasty, resulting in paresthesias or a painful neuroma.

    3. Ilioinguinal and iliohypogastric nerves: Can be injured with deep plication of the lower rectus abdominis.

C. Abdominal wall musculature

    1. Vertical layer (vertical pull).

        a. Paired rectus abdominis muscles.

            (1) Diastasis exists normally above and below the umbilicus to a varying degree.

            (2) Type III muscle: Deep superior and inferior epigastric pedicles.

            (3) Arcuate line of Douglas: Halfway between the umbilicus and the pubis. The anterior and posterior rectus fascia fuse, and both lie anterior to the muscle below this line.

        b. External oblique.

    2. Horizontal layer (horizonta pull).

        a. Internal oblique.

        b. Transversalis abdominis.

    3. Layers of the anterior abdominal wall lateral to the rectus abdominis: Skin, Camper's fascia, Scarpa's fascia, external oblique, internal oblique, transversalis fascia, peritoneum.

    4. Superficial fascial system (SFS) is composed of Scarpa's fascia; many recommend reapproximating this fascial layer in the closure for better postoperative results (provides a thigh lift and limits scar widening; see "Total Lower Body Lift").

D. Umbilicus

    1. Umbilical hernias frequently occur and can be repaired at the time of abdominoplasty.

    2. The umbilicus derives a dual blood supply from the deep layer and from the skin, which allows for either circumscribing the umbilicus on its stalk or transecting its base.

E. Aesthetic subunits

    1. Epigastrium.

    2. Periumbilical.

    3. Hypogastrium.

    4. Flanks.

    5. Mons pubis.

F. Gender differences

    1. Men

        a. Fat deposits preferentially in the flanks.

        b. Rectus diastasis in the *upper* abdomen.

        c. Thicker skin: Redundancy is rare and is usually associated with massive weight loss.

        d. Increased intraabdominal fat with aging.

    2. Women

        a. Narrow waistline.

        b. Rectus diastasis in the *lower* abdomen.

      c. Thinner skin: Skin redundancy and striae are more common and are increased by pregnancy.

V. Potential contraindications

  A. Supraumbilical scars (vascular compromise to the skin flap)

  B. Future pregnancy

  C. Chronic medical conditions (deep venous thrombosis, chronic obstructive pulmonary disease, diabetes mellitus)

  D. Combined procedures (may increase the risk of deep venous thrombosis or infection)

  E. Current nicotine or smoking history

VI. Surgical planning

  A. History: Assessment of relative contraindications

    1. Smoking: Increased risk of flap necrosis and wound-healing complications.

    2. Diabetes: Same as smoking.

    3. Chronic obstructive pulmonary disease (COPD): Increased risk of wound dehiscence with coughing; also increased postoperative pulmonary compromise.

    4. Use of steroids: Increased risk of wound dehiscence.

  B. Physical examination

    1. Evaluate height, weight, and body habitus: Morbidly obese patients are not candidates for abdominoplasty.

    2. Evaluate skin tone and elasticity.

    3. Measure subcutaneous fat with the "pinch test."

    4. Evaluate tightness of the musculoaponeurotic system and look for ventral hernia and rectus diastasis.

    5. Common preexisting abdominal scars.

      a. McBurney-type appendectomy incision: Little effect on surgical planning.

      b. Open cholecystectomy incision: Relative contraindication to a full abdominoplasty, due to interruption of blood supply through this area (Huger zone III).

      c. Midline abdominal incision: Disrupts cross-midline perfusion and can result in wound-healing complications.

      d. Lower abdominal scars to be excised with the pannus have no effect.

      e. Upper abdominal scars that will be transposed below the umbilicus are a relative contraindication for abdominoplasty and are an absolute contraindication to combined liposuction.

  C. Goals

    1. Skin resection and redraping.

    2. Subcutaneous tissue reduction.

    3. Correction of muscle diastasis and abdominal wall laxity.

VII. Surgical techniques

  A. Suction-assisted lipectomy (SAL) is indicated for patients with minimal skin excess, good skin elasticity, and adequate muscle tone (see "Liposuction").

  B. Endoscopically assisted abdominoplasty

    1. Indications.

      a. Minimal excess skin and/or skin with good elasticity that will retract after liposuction.

      b. Rectus abdominis diastasis.

    2. The endoscope allows for limited-access muscle plication; combine with liposuction as needed.

  C. Miniabdominoplasty

    1. Indicated for patients with lower abdominal contour deformity involving skin excess and musculofascial laxity.

    2. Liposuction as needed.

    3. A 6- to 15-cm long ellipse of midline lower abdominal skin is resected.

      a. Incision can often be limited to the pubic hairline.

      b. Height of resection is limited by the width of the incision and by tension on the umbilicus, which is not repositioned.

    4. Rectus abdominis plication is performed inferior to the umbilicus.

    5. Use closed suction drains.

    6. Postoperative compression garments and no heavy lifting are recommended for 6 weeks.

D. Modified abdominoplasty

    1. Indications.

        a. Excess supraumbilical skin.

        b. Insufficient skin laxity for resection up to umbilicus.

        c. Upper rectus diastasis, epigastric laxity.

        d. When wide undermining is contraindicated, such as preexisting abdominal scars.

    2. Incision is longer than in the miniabdominoplasty, but does not extend lateral to the ASIS.

    3. Undermining is performed above and below the umbilicus, with rectus plication from xiphoid to pubis.

    4. Consider transecting the umbilical stalk to allow redraping of excess abdominal wall skin.

    5. Postoperative care is similar to the miniabdominoplasty.

E. Full abdominoplasty

    1. Indicated for patients with significant skin excess and upper and lower rectus diastasis/abdominal wall laxity.

    2. Plan to remove all tissue inferior to the umbilicus.

    3. High-volume liposuction combined with elevating a large abdominal flap is associated with increased complication rates.

    4. Wide flap undermining.

        a. Incision extends laterally to the ASIS.

        b. Undermine to costal margins and xiphoid.

    5. Plicate rectus abdominis from xiphoid to pubis.

    6. Exteriorize umbilical stalk.

    7. Postoperative care: Suction drainage of wound, with or without abdominal binder, and no heavy lifting for 6 weeks.

F. High lateral tension abdominoplasty: Variation of the full abdominoplasty

    1. Undermining is limited to the paramedian area and discontinuous undermining (via liposuction) laterally, which keeps perforators intact over Huger zone III.

    2. High lateral skin resection.

    3. Superficial fascial system repair.

VIII. Complications

A. Seroma: 2% to 9%.

    1. Increased incidence when SAL is combined with flap elevation.

    2. Decreased incidence with wound drainage and tacking sutures.

    3. Occurrence can be delayed and persistent, often requiring percutaneous drainage.

B. Delayed wound healing: 5%.

C. Infection: 1% to 7%.

D. Toxic shock.

E. Hematomas: Should be drained promptly to avoid flap compromise or infection.

F. Abnormal-appearing umbilicus or necrosis.

G. Flap necrosis: Most commonly occurs in a major abdominoplasty with adjuvant liposuction.

H. Nerve damage: Entrapment of lateral femoral cutaneous, iliohypogastric, or ilioinguinal nerves.

I. Abnormal scars: 4%.

J. Pulmonary embolism: Less than 1%.

K. Deep venous thrombosis (DVT): Less than 1%.

L. Pulmonary fat embolism.

Total Lower Body Lift

I. Indications

A. Moderate to severe skin laxity of the buttocks, lateral and medial thighs, and lower trunk. Patients with lipodystrophy should initially be treated with liposuction prior to a lower body lift.

B. This procedure allows multiple areas with contour irregularities to be addressed in one stage, as opposed to previously performed multiple staged operations (buttock lift, medial thigh lift, flank excision, etc.).

II. Etiology: The etiology of soft tissue laxity of the lower trunk, thighs, and buttocks is similar to that listed for soft tissue laxity of the abdomen: solar damage, weight fluctuations, medications, pregnancy, and previous liposuction.

III. Goals: A total lower body lift should improve the contour irregularities from skin laxity in the lower trunk and thigh regions in a single stage without increased morbidity or complication rates.

IV. Patient selection

A. An assessment of the patient's general health should be performed, with particular attention to chronic illnesses such as diabetes, COPD, uncontrolled hypertension, coronary artery disease, or autoimmune disorders.

B. Smoking or nicotine history is important to obtain, because this is a contraindication to the procedure.

C. On examination, pinching the lateral hip area results in significant contour improvements in the lateral thighs.

D. The ideal candidate has a stable weight close to the ideal body weight with normal subcutaneous fat thickness but with excessive skin laxity of the lower trunk and thigh regions.

E. Patients with thick subcutaneous tissue are best approached with liposuction followed by a total body lift 3 to 6 months later.

V. Anatomy

A. The key to this operation is the superficial fascial system (SFS) as emphasized by Dr. Ted Lockwood. This is an extensive connective tissue framework in the subcutaneous tissue that connects skin and fat to the musculoskeletal system.

B. The function of the SFS is to encase the fat and subcutaneous tissue and provide support for this tissue layer. This layer is strong enough to anchor a resuspension of the thigh, which takes tension off the dermal/epidermal layer.

C. Using the SFS for support decreases the rate of wound dehiscence and scar widening, which often accompanies body contouring procedures that primarily rely on the skin for suspension.

VI. Surgical techniques

A. Markings

1. **Preoperative markings** should be performed in the standing position.

2. **The line of closure** should lie in the perineal-thigh crease, run vertically along the mons pubis, and then turn laterally 2 to 3 cm below the ASIS. Posteriorly, the incision gently curves down near the superior aspect of the gluteal crease.

B. Operative techniques

1. **Skin flaps** are elevated just above the muscle fascia, preserving the subcutaneous tissue and SFS in the elevated flap. Be careful to stay out of the lymphatics of the femoral triangle, and be aware of the location of the lateral femoral cutaneous nerve. Skin flaps are also raised in the gluteal region (but stay superficial to the gluteal vessels) and the greater trochanteric area (make sure to release any bands of adherence).

2. **Cannula undermining** is performed circumferentially in the thighs down to the level of the knees. This is performed without suction. The purpose is to loosen the SFS attachments without compromise to the lymphatics or vascular supply of the thigh.
3. **Excess skin** is resected. The SFS is repaired with permanent sutures; then the dermis and epidermal layers are closed. Suction drainage is required. The procedure is repeated on the opposite side.
4. Finally, the patient is placed in the supine position, frog-legged, and the perineal resections are performed. It is important to not disrupt the lymphatics in this medial thigh region. Perform a conservative resection to avoid distortion of the vulva. The SFS is used to suspend the medial closure to avoid vulvar lateral traction and widening.

VII. Complications: Wound infection, seromas, lymphoceles, lymphedema, prominent mons pubis or sacral fat, wound dehiscence

---

Liposuction

I. Anatomy

A. **Adipocytes** have two receptors for catecholamines, which regulate fat storage.
  1. **Beta-1 receptors**
     a. Located in areas of metabolically active fat such as upper body, face, and breast.
     b. Respond to catecholamines by releasing lipase, splitting triglycercides into glycerol and fatty acids.
  2. **Alpha-2 receptors**
     a. Located in diet-resistant areas such as the lateral thighs, buttocks, and abdomen.
     b. Antagonists of beta-1 receptors; block lipolysis.
B. **Adipocytes** are produced *in utero* and in early childhood and early adolescence and will not be replaced after liposuction. However, remaining adipocytes may hypertrophy.
C. **Retinacula cutis**
  1. Vertical fibrous septa connecting the dermis to fascia, which create a honeycomb network to support adipocytes. Responsible for dimples associated with obesity ("cellulite").
  2. Beta-1 receptors predominate.
D. **Reserve fat of Illouz**
  1. Deeper fat underneath the superficial fascia with horizontal fibrous septa.
  2. Alpha-2 receptors predominate.
E. **Anatomic considerations** with liposuction: The thighs have a definite deep subcutaneous fat layer that responds well to liposuction. Most vital structures lie deep to this plane, but be careful of the following.
  1. **Greater saphenous vein** medially (femoral artery also located medially but in a deeper location).
  2. **Supratrochanteric gluteal depression** laterally between the iliac crest and the saddle bag area (want to avoid with liposuction).

II. Patient evaluation

A. **Evaluate medical history** for eating disorders, weight fluctuations, thromboembolic disease, bleeding disorders, and chronic medical conditions such as COPD.
B. **Physical evaluation**
  1. The best candidates are thin overall, with isolated areas of lipodystrophy and with normal skin elasticity.
  2. Striae, cellulite, abdominal apron, and buttock ptosis respond poorly to liposuction and most often require dermolipectomy procedures.

3. Evaluate skin turgor and elasticity; skin that does not "snap back" quickly when pinched will respond poorly to liposuction.
4. Pinch test: Pinch at least 2 cm of fat to be a candidate for liposuction. Normal superficial fat in nonobese patients varies between 1.5 and 3.0 cm.
5. Liposuction of the medial thighs, especially in patients older than 35 years, is often disappointing. The skin in this area is thin and inelastic and often requires a lifting procedure.

III. Types of liposuction
A. Suction-assisted lipectomy, i.e., traditional liposuction (SAL)
1. **Indications:** Areas characterized by fatty deposits creating contour deformities. Excess fatty deposits are commonly found in the submental area, abdomen/flanks, thighs, medial knees, and calf/ankle.
2. **Mechanics:** Removal of fat cells through direct mechanical avulsion.
3. **Cannulas:** Blunt tips with lumens ranging from 1.5 to 6 mm. Smaller lumens are less prone to creating contour irregularities.
4. **Technique**
   a. Preoperative markings: Use both visual evaluation and manual pinch test to mark areas of lipodystrophy with the patient standing. These areas can become distorted when the patient is on the operating table. Depressions and valleys must be marked to minimize contour deformities.
   b. Wetting solution.
      (1) Fluid containing lidocaine and epinephrine is delivered to the subcutaneous tissue prior to suctioning, to provide anesthesia and hemostasis.
      (2) Use 50 mL of 1% lidocaine and 1 mL of 1:1000 epinephrine per liter of lactated Ringer's solution.
      (3) Tumescent technique: 1 cc of infiltrate per 1 cc of aspirate.
      (4) Superwet technique: 2 to 3 cc of infiltrate per 1 cc of aspirate.
      (5) The risk of lidocaine toxicity is minimal if lidocaine levels are kept to less than 34 mg/kg. Lidocaine is not necessary if the patient is under general anesthesia.
   c. Pretunnel: Create a pseudoplane deep to the superficial fascia to prevent skin dimpling by passing the cannula multiple times without suction.
   d. Superficial liposuction below the dermis is associated with significant contour deformities and should be avoided.
   e. Crisscross suctioning technique: Improved contouring performed via multiple access holes.
   f. Assess progress with repeated pinch tests. Do not overresect!
5. **Complications** (10% overall complication rate)
   a. Pulmonary fat embolus: Patients with a low serum albumin are predisposed to this complication. (Albumin is required to bind free fatty acids, which prevents a neutrophil-mediated response that causes injury to the lungs.)
   b. Hypovolemia: The most common etiology of liposuction fatalities. The risk is decreased with the use of superwet tumescent techniques.
      (1) Circulating blood volume continues to decrease 12 to 36 hours postoperatively, as fluid shifts into the resected areas.
      (2) For each 1 cc of aspirate, replace with 3 cc of intravenous fluid.
   c. Other complications: Lidocaine toxicity, contour irregularities, infection, seroma, hematoma, intraabdominal perforations, pigmentary changes, blood loss (1% drop in hematocrit for each 150 cc of fat removed).

B. Ultrasound-assisted liposuction (UAL)
1. **Indications:** May be more effective than SAL in fibrous areas (breast, back, etc.).
2. **Mechanics:** Cavitation created by ultrasonic energy liquifies adipocytes, facilitating the aspiration of fat.

3. Complications
  a. Same as with SAL.
  b. Skin burns due to "end hits" of the cannula, which delivers ultrasound to the dermis from below.

Pearls

1. Complications and blood loss significantly increase with liposuction aspirations of more than 1,500 cc.
2. Attempts to correct significant skin laxity without a full abdominoplasty will fail.
3. Discuss the issue of potential future breast reconstruction (inability to perform a rectus abdominis muscle [TRAM] flap procedure transverse after an abdominoplasty) with patients during the preoperative counseling.
4. Following SAL or UAL, patients remain candidates for TRAM flaps and full abdominoplasty.
5. Abdominoplasty performed in conjunction with another procedure such as a hysterectomy or tubal ligation has increased risk (infection and/or deep venous thrombosis).

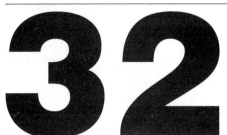

Breast Disease

Emily Hu

Anatomy and Development of the Breast

I. **Gland**
   A. **Boundaries**
      1. **Superior:** Second rib
      2. **Inferior:** Sixth rib
      3. **Medial:** Sternum edge
      4. **Lateral:** Midaxillary line
      5. **Deep**
         a. Superior and medial: Fascia of the pectoralis major muscle
         b. Inferior and lateral: Fascia of the serratus anterior muscle
      6. **Extension into the axilla:** The "tail of Spence"
   B. **Composition:** Skin, subcutaneous tissue, and breast tissue
      1. **10% to 15% is epithelial;** the remainder is stromal.
      2. **Breasts are composed of 15 to 20 radially arranged glandular lobes,** supported by fibrous connective tissue, interposed with adipose tissue.
         a. Lobes are subdivided into lobules, and then into tubuloalveolar glands.
         b. Each lobe concludes as a lactiferous duct.
         c. Lactiferous duct: 2 to 4 mm in diameter; dilates into a lactiferous sinus beneath the nipple.
   C. **Nipple-areolar complex**
      1. **Located at the fourth intercostal space** in nonpendulous breasts.
      2. **Composed of sebaceous glands** and apocrine sweat glands.
      3. **Montgomery glands:** At the areolar periphery, capable of secreting milk.
      4. **Tubercles of Morgagni:** Elevations at the gland openings.
      5. **Radial smooth muscle fibers** beneath the nipple contribute to nipple erection.
II. **Blood supply**
   A. **Internal mammary artery:** Perforating branches supply the medial and central portions of the breast.
   B. **Lateral thoracic artery:** Upper outer quadrant.
   C. **Anterolateral and anteromedial intercostal perforators.**
   D. **Venous drainage:** Follows the arterial supply.
III. **Innervation**
   A. **Medial:** Second through fifth anteromedial intercostal nerves.
   B. **Lateral:** Third through sixth anterolateral intercostal nerves.
   C. **Nipple-areolar complex:** Medial and lateral branches of the fourth intercostal nerve.
IV. **Lymphatic drainage**
   A. **Skin, nipple, and areola:** Superficial subareolar lymphatic plexus.
   B. **Breast:** Deep lymphatic plexus, which is connected to the superficial plexus. Seventy-five percent of the breast drains into the axillary basin; most of the

rest drains into the internal mammary nodes, and some to the inframammary lymph nodes.
  C. **Axillary space**
      1. **Borders:** Axillary vein superiorly, serratus anterior medially, latissimus dorsi laterally, pectoralis major anteriorly, and subscapularis posteriorly.
      2. **Important structures within the axilla:** Long thoracic nerve; thoracodorsal artery, vein, and nerve; and the intercostobrachial nerves.
      3. **Axillary nodes:** Embedded in fat; variable number.
          a. Level I: Inferior and lateral to the pectoralis minor muscle.
          b. Level II: Below the axillary vein and deep to the pectoralis minor muscle.
          c. Level III: Medial to the pectoralis minor muscle, against the chest wall.
          d. Rotter's nodes: Interpectoral nodes, between the pectoralis major and minor, along the lateral pectoral nerve.
  D. **Supraclavicular nodes:** Contiguous with the axillary apex.
  E. **Internal mammary nodes:** Within 3 cm of the sternal edge, in the first six intercostal spaces (the majority are found in the first three).
V. **Development**
  A. **Hormonal changes**
      1. **Primary modulator:** Hypothalamic-pituitary-gonadal axis.
      2. **In puberty, estrogen promotes ductal elongation and branching.**
      3. **Insulin-like growth factor (IGF)-1** is associated with growth stimulation; its pubertal peak is three times the adult concentration.
  B. **Somatic changes:** Tanner's clinical stages
      1. **Stage I:** Elevation of the papilla only; preadolescent.
      2. **Stage II:** Elevation of the breast and papilla; breast bud.
      3. **Stage III:** Further enlargement and elevation of the breast and areola, but no separation of contour.
      4. **Stage IV:** Projection of the areola and papilla to form a secondary mound above the breast.
      5. **Stage V:** Projection of the papilla only, with recession of the areola; mature.
  C. **Changes with menstrual cycle:** Secondary to cyclical increases in estrogen and progesterone.
      1. **Premenstrual:** Estrogen peak, breast sensitivity, fullness, and nodularity
      2. **Follicular phase (days 4–14):** Epithelial proliferation, increased mitoses
      3. **Luteal phase (days 5–28):** Predominantly progesterone; maximum proliferation; ductal dilatation and epithelial differentiation into secretory cells.
      4. **Menstruation:** Epithelial apoptosis, decline in secretions.

Clinical Evaluation of Breast Masses

I. **History**
  A. **Duration of lesion**
  B. **Pain, nipple discharge,** skin changes, weight loss and/or fatigue
  C. **Change in size with menstrual cycle**
  D. **Family history,** especially first-degree relatives with invasive cancer
  E. **Estrogen exposure:** Timing of menarche, pregnancy and menopause, and history of hormone replacement therapy (HRT)
II. **Physical examination**
  A. **Palpation of glandular tissue** is facilitated by having the sitting patient place her hands on her hips to contract the pectoralis muscles and by having the supine patient raise her arms and put her hands behind her head.
  B. **Axillary nodal basin** is assessed with the pectoralis muscles relaxed.
  C. **Masses and nodes** are characterized by their location, number, size, and firmness.

Table 32-1. Benign breast disease types

Category	Risk of Invasive Disease	Examples
Nonproliferative	No increased relative risk	Cysts, macro or micro Ductal ectasia Fat necrosis/lipoma Fibroadenoma Fibrocystic change Mastitis Metaplasia, squamous or apocrine Mild hyperplasia
Proliferative	Relative risk of 1.5 to 2 times	Papilloma Phylloides tumor Sclerosing adenosis Hyperplasia, moderate or severe
Proliferative with atypia	Relative risk of 4 to 5 times (9 times if there is a first-degree relative with breast cancer)	Atypical ductal hyperplasia Atypical lobular hyperplasia

Benign Breast Disease

I. **Types of benign breast disease** (Table 32-1)
   A. **Nonproliferative**
      1. **Most common;** 70% of palpable breast masses
      2. **No increased risk** of breast cancer
   B. **Proliferative:** Small increase in breast cancer risk, relative risk of 1.5 to 2.0 for developing invasive cancer
   C. **Proliferative with atypia**
      1. **Less common:** 3.6% of palpable breast masses, 7% to 10% of nonpalpable breast abnormalities
      2. **Relative risk of 4.0 to 5.0** for invasive cancer
      3. **Relative risk increases to 9.0 with a first-degree relative** with breast cancer

II. **Nonproliferative benign breast disease**
   A. **Cysts**
      1. **Etiology:** Lobular involution. Acini within the lobule distend to form microcysts; microcysts develop into macrocysts.
      2. **Presentation**
         a. Well-defined edges; mobile and firm.
         b. May fluctuate with the patient's menstrual cycle.
         c. Uncommon in postmenopausal women who are not on HRT.
         d. Peak incidence is from the mid-40s to the perimenopausal age group.
      3. **Definitive diagnosis**
         a. Ultrasound differentiates simple cysts versus complex cysts.
         b. Simple cyst: If asymptomatic, may be followed. If symptomatic, should be aspirated. If nonpalpable, no aspiration is needed.
         c. Complex cyst: Should be biopsied.
         d. Aspiration: May replace ultrasound as the initial step.
            (1) If the aspirate is nonbloody and the mass resolves, no further treatment is needed. If the mass persists, it should be biopsied.
            (2) If the aspirate is bloody, send it for cytology and obtain a surgical biopsy.

e. Surgical biopsy
  (1) Indications: Recurrent, bloody, persistent, and complex cysts.
  (2) Cyst wall tissue is required to determine the presence of malignancy.

B. Ductal ectasia
1. **Epidemiology:** Most common in multiparous women aged 40 to 50.
2. **Etiology:** Chronic intraductal and periductal inflammation causes dilation of mammary ducts and thickening of secretions.
3. **Presentation**
   a. A poorly defined, nontender, periareolar mass.
   b. Thick gray to black nipple discharge, nipple tenderness.
   c. Nipple retraction.
4. **Diagnosis and management**
   a. Biopsy.
   b. Once diagnosed, no further treatment is needed unless symptoms recur.

C. Fat necrosis and lipoma
1. **Etiology:** Trauma, breast surgery, infection, and radiation therapy; 50% are idiopathic.
2. **Presentation:** Poorly defined, painless, firm mass.
3. **Management.**
   a. Mammography.
   b. A biopsy is required to exclude malignancy.

D. Fibroadenoma
1. **Epidemiology.**
   a. Most common between the ages of 20 and 50.
   b. Accounts for 75% of breast biopsies in women younger than 20.
2. **Etiology:** Aberrant lobular development; proliferation of epithelial and fibrous tissues.
3. **Presentation.**
   a. Well-defined, palpable mass; averages 2 to 3 cm in diameter.
   b. Rubbery texture, mobile; also known as "breast mouse."
   c. Painless, slow-growing.
   d. Typically solitary (85%–90% of cases).
   e. Does not change significantly with the menstrual cycle.
   f. Often dramatically increases in size during pregnancy.
   g. Usually involutes after menopause.
   h. In postmenopausal women receiving just estrogen, masses may increase in size.
4. **Management.**
   a. Ultrasound shows a round, solid mass.
   b. Biopsy, excision.

E. Fibrocystic change or disease
1. **Heterogeneous group of processes,** physiologic and pathologic; thus not a particularly useful term.
2. **Epidemiology.**
   a. Most common of all the benign breast conditions.
   b. Most common during reproductive years, also during HRT after menopause.
3. **Presentation.**
   a. Cyclic, bilateral, and often diffuse pain, engorgement.
   b. Diffuse bilateral nodularity.
   c. Changes are most prominent just *before* menstruation.
   d. Secretory products in cysts can calcify.
4. **Management.**
   a. Fine-needle aspiration: Diagnostic and therapeutic.
   b. Open biopsy if:
     (1) Mammography is suggestive of malignancy.
     (2) A bloody fine-needle aspirate is obtained or the mass persists after aspiration.
     (3) Cyst recurs.

        c. Lifestyle changes: Beneficial to some patients.
           (1) Restriction of caffeine and methylxanthines.
           (2) Low-salt diet, vitamin E and/or a mild diuretic.
        d. Bilateral mastectomy: In severe cases with intractable pain.
     5. Prognosis: Fibrocystic changes alone do not confer an elevated risk of developing cancer.

F. Mastitis in lactating women
     1. Most common during the first 4 to 6 weeks postpartum.
     2. Etiology: *Staphylococcus aureus* is present in 50% of cases.
     3. Presentation.
        a. Fever (often >103°F), malaise, and general body aches.
        b. Unilateral erythema, tenderness and induration.
     4. Management.
        a. Antibiotics: Penicillinase-resistant cephalosporin.
        b. Continue breast-feeding to help drain the engorged breast.
        c. Consider abscess drainage if infection persists.
        d. Consider biopsy if it is refractory to treatment (to exclude malignancy).
     5. Distinguished from galactocele by the presence of fever.

G. Mastitis in nonlactating women
     1. Epidemiology.
        a. Usually occurs in premenopausal women.
        b. Associated with smoking.
     2. Etiology: Squamous epithelium extends abnormally into duct orifices, trapping keratin and causing dilation and eventual rupture of ducts.
     3. Presentation: Periareolar inflammation; purulent nipple discharge.
     4. Management
        a. Antibiotics: Aerobic and anaerobic coverage.
        b. Aspiration.
        c. Terminal duct excision if infections recur.
        d. Consider open drainage with biopsy if it is refractory to treatment.

III. Proliferative benign breast disease
A. Papilloma
     1. Etiology: Intraductal epithelial tumor.
     2. Presentation: Spontaneous bloody, serous, or cloudy nipple discharge; typically not palpable.
     3. Prognosis: Increased malignant potential after age 50 or with atypia.
     4. Management.
        a. Test discharge for occult blood; identify the quadrant of origin.
        b. Mammography: Masses, calcification, or dilated ducts.
        c. If mass present: Biopsy.
        d. If mass absent: Terminal duct excision.

B. Phylloides tumor
     1. Average age: 45 years.
     2. Etiology.
        a. Rapid growth of a fibroepithelial periductal tumor.
        b. Malignant degeneration to sarcoma is reported in 6% of cases.
     3. Presentation: Often a very large mass; spreads hematogenously, often to the lungs.
     4. Prognosis: The majority are benign, despite common use of the term "cystosarcoma phylloides." They may recur locally.
     5. Management.
        a. Not truly encapsulated; requires local excision with margins of more than 1 cm.
        b. No axillary node dissection is required.
        c. If very large and benign, a subcutaneous mastectomy is necessary.

IV. Proliferative benign breast disease with atypia
A. Atypical ductal hyperplasia
     1. Histologically similar to ductal carcinoma *in situ*.
     2. However, the lesion has a limited extent, and cells are not uniform.

B. Atypical lobular hyperplasia
1. Resembles lobular carcinoma *in situ*.
2. However, these do not fill more than 50% of an acinus within the lobule.
3. Extension into ducts: Increased risk of invasive carcinoma.

Premalignant (Noninvasive) Breast Disease

I. Lobular carcinoma *in situ* (LCIS)
A. Epidemiology
1. 15% of *in situ* breast disease
2. Predominantly occurs in premenopausal women (40–50 years old)
3. Decreased incidence after menopause
B. Etiology: Proliferation of uniform cells in one or more lobules
C. Presentation
1. **Almost never palpable**; thus, often an incidental finding
2. **No specific mammographic findings**
3. **High incidence of bilaterality** (50%–70%) and multicentricity
D. Prognosis: Not a malignant or true premalignant lesion, but rather a *marker* of risk for developing invasive cancer
1. **Relative risk** of breast cancer is 5% to 12% (1% per year).
2. **Risk is equal in both breasts.**
3. **Infiltrative ductal carcinoma** is still the most common after a diagnosis of LCIS.
E. Management
1. **Close monitoring** with or without tamoxifen.
2. **Bilateral total mastectomy** in select patients with high anxiety level and a first-degree relative with invasive disease (controversial).
II. Ductal carcinoma *in situ* (DCIS, or intraductal carcinoma)
A. Epidemiology: 85% of *in situ* breast disease
B. Etiology
1. **Cribriform proliferation** of cells into duct.
2. **Micropapillary growth** into lumen.
3. **Cells lack the ability to invade** the basement membrane, but can spread through the ductal system.
C. Presentation: Usually first noted on mammography as clustered microcalcifications
D. Prognosis
1. **Classified based on nuclear grade** (low, intermediate, and high) and necrosis.
2. **About 50% of local recurrences** after excision contain invasive carcinoma.
3. **Younger women** are at higher risk for recurrence.
E. Management
1. **Mammography** to evaluate the extent of involvement.
2. **Wide excision** with a breast-conserving approach is possible if the lesion size is suitable for an aesthetically acceptable result.
3. **Mastectomy** is performed if the lesion is too large for wide excision.
4. **Radiation therapy:** Most beneficial for large tumors (>15 mm), high-grade lesions, and excision margins of less than 10 mm.
5. **Tamoxifen.**
   a. Indicated for estrogen receptor–positive lesions.
   b. Reduces the risk of invasive carcinoma in DCIS patients.
   c. Beneficial with both positive and negative surgical margins.
III. Paget's disease of the nipple
A. **A form of DCIS** that spreads from nipple ducts into the surrounding skin of the nipple-areolar complex.
B. Findings: Fissured, ulcerated, and oozing nipple; local erythema.

C. **Palpable mass in 50% to 60% of cases;** associated with invasive carcinoma.

D. **Histologically,** malignant cells involving the epidermis are called *Paget cells.*

E. **Prognosis and treatment** depend on the extent of the underlying carcinoma.

Malignant (Invasive) Breast Disease

I. **Epidemiology**

   A. **Cells cross the basement membrane** and have the ability to distantly metastasize.

   B. **The most common cancer in American women.**

   C. **The second most common cause of death in American women** (heart disease is first).

   D. **Risk factors**

      1. **Age and ethnicity.**

         a. Greatest risk occurs after age 65.

         b. In the younger age group, breast cancer is more common in African American women than in white women.

         c. After age 40, white women are at higher risk.

      2. **Family history.**

         a. 20% to 30% of women with breast cancer have a contributory family history.

         b. Only 5% to 10% of these 20% to 30% have an inherited mutation in the breast cancer susceptibility gene.

         c. The majority of mutations occur in BRCA1 or BRCA2, with both maternal and paternal inheritance patterns.

         d. Mutations indicate a lifetime risk of breast cancer, with a high risk of contralateral breast disease and ovarian cancer; prostate cancer in the family; and an increased risk of male breast cancer.

      3. **Hormonal factors:** Risk is proportional to estrogen exposure.

         a. Premenopausal: Age at menarche (<12 years old), age of first pregnancy (age >35 years), or nulliparity (with an increased number of ovulatory cycles).

         b. Postmenopausal: Age at menopause.

         c. Obesity: Increased peripheral estrogen production.

         d. Estrogen replacement therapy: When used for longer than 5 years.

      4. **Environment and diet.**

         a. Ionizing radiation (medical or nuclear) of more than 90 rads.

         b. Increased alcohol intake (controversial).

      5. **Other risk factors.**

         a. Other neoplasms (contralateral breast, uterine, or ovarian cancer; major salivary gland carcinoma).

         b. Atypical hyperplasia.

         c. DCIS or LCIS.

II. **Definitive diagnosis**

   A. **Diagnostic mammography:** To evaluate a symptomatic patient

   B. **Fine-needle aspiration (FNA):** To obtain cells for histology

   C. **Image-guided core biopsy:** Preferred for calcific masses

   D. **Indications for surgical biopsy** after needle core biopsy: Atypical ductal hyperplasia, discontinuity between histologic diagnosis and mammographic appearance, nondiagnostic specimen

   E. **Needle localization with excision**

      1. **Advantages:** Complete pathologic characterization before local therapy is chosen; may suffice as the definitive treatment as a form of lumpectomy.

2. **Disadvantages:** Overresection of benign lesions, discomfort and cosmetic deformity; incomplete excision can occur, thus requiring reoperation.

3. **Specimen radiography:** Confirms that an intraoperative palpable mass corresponds to the mammographic lesion; confirms removal of calcifications.

III. Types of malignant breast lesions

A. Invasive ductal carcinoma

1. **Presentation:** Hard, irregular, and immobile.
2. **60% to 85% of cases of invasive breast cancer.**

B. Invasive lobular carcinoma: 10% of breast cancer cases

C. Histologic types

1. **Tubular:** Well differentiated; no myoepithelial cells; nodal metastases rare; best prognosis.
2. **Mucinous/colloid:** Cells have increased mucin content; prognosis is similar to tubular type.
3. **Medullary:** Large, pleomorphic nuclei; high mitotic rate; favorable prognosis.
4. **Cribriform:** Well differentiated.
5. **Adenocystic and secretory "juvenile":** Rare.

IV. Grading

A. Partially determines need for chemotherapy.

B. Nuclear: Well differentiated, intermediate or poorly differentiated.

C. Histologic: Cytologic differentiation, growth pattern, extent of tubules, mitotic rate.

V. Hormone receptors

A. Estrogen and progesterone receptors are nuclear hormone receptors.

B. Hormone receptors act like transcription regulators.

C. Receptor status determines candidacy for hormonal therapy.

VI. Staging

Table 32-2. TNM classification of breast cancer

Primary Tumor	
TX	Primary tumor cannot be assessed
T0	No evidence of a primary tumor
Tis	Carcinoma in situ or Paget's of nipple without tumor
T1	Greatest tumor diameter ≤2 cm
T2	Greatest tumor diameter 2 cm to ≤5cm
T3	Tumors >5 cm
T4	Tumor ≥5 cm, or extends to the chest wall (excluding any size, extending the pectoralis muscle), skin edema, skin ulceration or skin satellites, or inflammatory carcinoma
Regional Lymph Nodes	
NX	Nodes cannot be assessed
N0	No lymph node metastases
N1	Mobile metastases to ipsilateral axillary nodes
N2	Fixed metastases to ipsilateral axillary nodes
N3	Metastases to ipsilateral internal mammary nodes
Distant Metastases	
MX	Cannot be assessed
M0	None
M1	Distant metastases (including supraclavicular nodes)

Table 32-3. American Joint Committee on Cancer's staging of breast cancer

Stage 0	Tis N0 M0
Stage I	T1 N0 M0
Stage IIA	T0 N1 M0
	T1 N1 M0
	T2 N0 M0
Stage IIB	T2 N1 M0
	T3 N0 M0
Stage IIIA	T0 N2 M0
	T1 N2 M0
	T2 N2 M0
	T3 N1 M0
	T3 N2 M0
Stage IIIB	T4 Any N M0
	Any T N3 M0
Stage IV	Any T Any N M1

  A. Staging is generated from TNM classification (Tables 32-2 and 32-3).

  B. Tumor excision must have negative surgical margins in order to be staged.

  C. Staging provides the most accurate estimate of prognosis and end result.

VII. Treatment

 A. Local therapy

  1. Breast-conserving therapy (BCT): Removal of primary tumor with adequate (usually 1-cm) margins of normal tissue and subsequent radiation therapy (XRT).

   a. Contraindications.

    (1) Two or more tumors in different quadrants

    (2) Persistent positive margins after surgery

    (3) Pregnancy (first and second trimester; for third trimester, XRT can be given after delivery)

    (4) History of prior radiation

   b. In contrast to postoperative therapy, neoadjuvant therapy has not been shown to improve survival in BCT.

  2. Modified radical mastectomy (MRM): Removal of all breast tissue, fascia of the pectoralis major muscle, and level I and II axillary lymphatics. MRM is commonly used for the most invasive disease.

 B. Axillary node management

  1. Axillary node dissection

   a. Levels I and II: Standard; identifies metastases in 98% of patients.

   b. Level III: Reserved for patients with gross nodal metastases.

  2. Complications

   a. Major (rare): Injury to the axillary vein or motor nerves.

   b. Minor.

    (1) Intercostobrachial nerve paresthesia.

    (2) Pain and weakness: 20% to 30% of cases after 1 year.

    (3) Lymphedema: Risk related to extent of axillary dissection and postoperative radiation.

  3. Sentinel lymph node (SLN) biopsy

   a. The sentinel lymph node is the first lymph node receiving drainage from a primary tumor. It identifies axillary node involvement while minimizing morbidity from a full basin dissection.

   b. SLN biopsy involves injection of Lymphazurin blue dye, radioactive isotope-labeled colloid (i.e., technetium), or both. The sentinel node is detected via blue staining and/or "hot" counts with a Geiger counter.

      c. The SLN can be identified in 90% of patients and can predict the status of the remaining axillary nodes in more than 90% of those patients. The technique is highly operator dependent, with a steep learning curve.

      d. Contraindications.

        (1) Pregnant or lactating woman.

        (2) Multicentric carcinoma.

        (3) Palpable axillary adenopathy: A node filled with tumor will not take up mapping agent, giving a false negative result.

        (4) Use of preoperative chemotherapy.

        (5) Tumor size greater than 5 cm, or locally advanced disease.

C. Radiotherapy

  1. Reduces the risk of local recurrence and improves survival by eliminating local disease resistant to chemotherapy.

  2. Indicated for patients with four or more involved axillary nodes.

  3. Component of BCT (see "Local Therapy").

D. Adjuvant systemic therapy

  1. A large proportion of breast cancers are thought to have metastases at diagnosis. Chemotherapy is used to eliminate clinically occult metastases.

  2. Cytotoxic agents: Cytoxan, methotrexate, 5-fluorouracil, and paclitaxel.

  3. Endocrine agents: Selective estrogen receptor modulators (e.g., tamoxifen).

    a. Estrogen antagonist action: Competitive blockade of receptors in the breast.

    b. Estrogen agonist actions: Preserves bone density, lowers cholesterol levels, and increases the risk of endometrial carcinoma.

    c. Indicated for estrogen and/or progesterone receptor–positive tumors.

    d. Reduce the annual risk of recurrence by 47% and the annual risk of death by 26%.

Special Considerations

I. Gynecomastia

  A. Definition: Enlargement of the male breast

  B. Etiology

    1. Imbalance between estrogenic and androgenic effects, leading to hyperestrinism.

    2. External causes of hyperestrinism: Medications (e.g., spironolactone), cirrhosis, alcohol, marijuana, heroin, and anabolic steroids.

    3. May be a manifestation of Klinefelter's syndrome or of a functioning testicular neoplasm (Leydig cell or Sertoli cell).

  C. Presentation

    1. Unilateral or bilateral.

    2. Begins with subareolar enlargement.

  D. Management options

    1. Must rule out male breast cancer if asymmetric.

    2. A combination of liposuction and direct periareolar excision is the most common approach to resection.

II. Male breast cancer

  A. Risk factors

    1. Similar to those for women.

    2. Decreased testicular function (i.e., Klinefelter's syndrome).

    3. Gynecomastia is *not* a risk factor (except when associated with Klinefelter's syndrome).

  B. Epidemiology

    1. Mean age of 60 to 70 years.

    2. 1% of all breast cancer cases.

  C. Presentation

   1. **Mass beneath the nipple-areolar complex,** nipple ulceration.
   2. **Axillary node involvement is seen in about 50%** of cases at presentation.
D. **Diagnostic approach:** Same as with female breast cancer.
E. **Management**
   1. **Modified radical mastectomy.**
   2. **Partial pectoralis muscle excision:** If there is limited muscle involvement.
   3. **Radical mastectomy:** If there is extensive muscle involvement.
   4. **Hormonal therapy:** Most beneficial if the tumor is hormone receptor positive.
      a. Tamoxifen: No definitive studies yet.
      b. Orchiectomy: Reserved for patients refractory to other medical treatments.
F. **Prognosis:** When matched by stage, survival is similar to women with breast cancer, but it often presents at an advanced stage.

Pearls

---

1. Four nerves to locate and preserve during axillary dissection are the long thoracic nerve (of Bell), the thoracodorsal nerve, the medial pectoral nerve, and the lateral pectoral nerve.
2. The cutaneous nerve crossing the axilla transversely is the intercostobrachial nerve.
3. Skin retraction is often secondary to tumor involvement of the deep fibrous suspensory ligaments, called Cooper's ligaments.
4. The test of choice to evaluate a breast mass in women younger than 30 is ultrasound.
5. Mondor's disease is thrombophlebitis of the thoracoepigastric veins; palpable cords are often present.

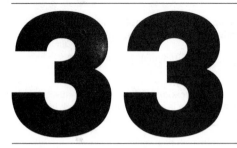

Reduction Mammoplasty, Augmentation Mammoplasty, and Mastopexy

Andrew H. Rosenthal

Breast Reduction (Reduction Mammoplasty)

I. Indications
  A. Physical and functional problems
    1. Back, neck, and shoulder pain
    2. Shoulder grooving
    3. Mastodynia
    4. Maceration and infections in the inframammary region
    5. Exercise restriction
    6. Problems with bra and clothing fit
  B. Psychological problems
    1. Embarrassment
    2. Feelings of physical unattractiveness
    3. Difficulty in social situations (e.g., swimwear, formal wear)
II. Preoperative considerations
  A. Workup
    1. A complete medical history should be obtained, including a family history of breast cancer, pregnancies, breast-feeding history, previous breast surgeries, and future childbearing plans.
    2. A complete physical examination should be performed, including a detailed breast exam.
    3. Preoperative mammograms should be taken if the patient is older than 35 (or younger, with a positive family history of breast cancer).
  B. Patient education for any breast reduction procedure should include counseling regarding the following.
    1. Significant scarring that may occur. "Having a breast reduction is trading large breasts for smaller breasts with scars."
    2. Asymmetries should be brought to the patient's attention prior to surgery.
    3. The inability to breast-feed is encountered in 20% to 30% of patients postoperatively.
    4. Changes in nipple sensibility: Breast reduction can lead to hypersensitivity or hyposensitivity, which is usually temporary but can be permanent.
    5. Nipple or flap loss and delayed healing: Smoking cessation may reduce the risk of tissue loss and delayed wound healing.
    6. Changes in breast shape or volume secondary to future pregnancies or changes in weight.
    7. The inability to completely predict the extent of improvement in symptoms.
III. Surgical approaches. The following is not a comprehensive list, but rather a collection of common approaches that deal with the issues set forth previously.
  A. General considerations: All approaches to surgical reduction of the breast must deal with the following four issues.
    1. Reduction and reshaping of the gland.
    2. Creation of a pedicle for the nipple-areolar complex.

3. Skin reduction and redraping.
4. Superior repositioning of the nipple-areolar complex.

B. **Inferior central pedicle techniques**
1. **The inferior pedicle** techniques are probably the most commonly used today.
2. **Wise pattern reduction**
   a. Gland reduction: Superior, medial, and lateral breast
   b. Nipple pedicle: Central, inferiorly centrally based
   c. Redraping: Easily accomplished as flaps are tailored
   d. Advantages
      (1) Fairly simple, safe, and popular
      (2) Applicable to large variety of breast shapes and sizes
      (3) Easy to resect large amount of extra skin
   e. Disadvantages
      (1) Tends to "bottom out" with time, leading to pseudoptosis
      (2) Produces more extensive scars than other techniques
3. **Markings** (Fig. 33-1)
   a. The sternal notch, inframammary folds, and midline are marked.
   b. The intended breast meridian is marked. A line is drawn from the mid-portion of the clavicle to the nipple. If this line is greater than 10 to 12 cm from the midline, then it should be relocated medially.
   c. The new nipple location is marked at the level of the inframammary fold (using the technique preferred by the surgeon). The distance from the sternal notch to nipple can be adjusted based on patient height, magnitude of the planned reduction, and surgeon preference.
   d. Eight-centimeter "vertical" limbs are drawn obliquely down from the intended new nipple center mark. The vertical limbs form an isosceles triangle. The base should be approximately 9 cm wide, depending on the degree of reduction desired.
   e. The bases of the vertical limbs are then connected medially and laterally to the inframammary fold via curvilinear markings.

C. **Vertical techniques**
1. **Lejour**
   a. Gland reduction: Lower central pole of breast, with reshaping by suturing gland into new position.
   b. Nipple pedicle: Superior.
   c. Redraping: Minimal; relies on wrinkling of the skin in vertical incision.
   d. Advantages.
      (1) Eliminates the incision in the inframammary fold (IMF).
      (2) Attractive breast shape without areolar enlargement.
      (3) Not likely to bottom out.
   e. Disadvantages.
      (1) There is a steep learning curve.
      (2) Immediately postoperatively, the breast shape and wrinkling are unattractive. It can take 3 to 4 months for the breast to settle into the final, desired shape.
2. **Asplund and Davies**
   a. Gland reduction: Lower pole of breast, reshaping by (minimal) suture.
   b. Nipple pedicle: Medial (from internal mammary artery perforators).
   c. Redraping: Minimal; relies on wrinkling of the skin in the vertical incision.
   d. Advantages.
      (1) Eliminates the incision in the IMF.
      (2) The medial pedicle prevents excessive periareolar tension and assists in nipple repositioning.
      (3) Attractive breast shape.
      (4) Not likely to bottom out.

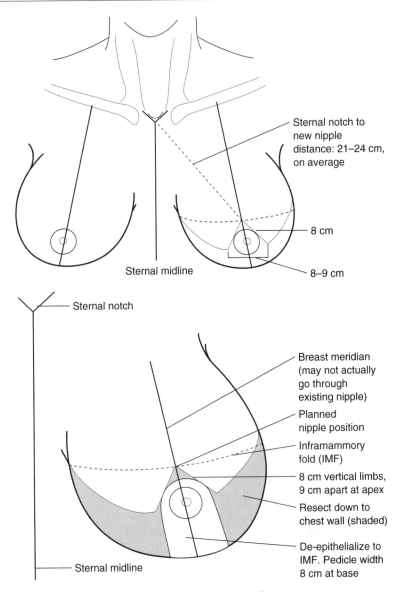

Sternal notch to new nipple distance: 21–24 cm, on average

8 cm

8–9 cm

Sternal midline

Sternal notch

Breast meridian (may not actually go through existing nipple)

Planned nipple position

Inframammory fold (IMF)

8 cm vertical limbs, 9 cm apart at apex

Resect down to chest wall (shaded)

De-epithelialize to IMF. Pedicle width 8 cm at base

Sternal midline

Fig. 33-1. Inferior pedicle design for reduction mammoplasty.

     e. Disadvantages
       (1) Has a steep learning curve.
       (2) Wrinkling immediately postoperatively is unattractive, like the Lejour technique.
  D. SPAIR technique (**s**hort scar, **p**eriareolar, **i**nferior pedicle **r**eduction)
    1. Developed by Dr. Dennis Hammond
    2. Gland reduction: Mostly periareolar, but can be tailored
    3. Nipple pedicle: Inferior

      4. Redraping: Relies on wrinkling of the skin around the nipple.

      5. Advantages.

        a. Eliminates incision in IMF.

        b. Attractive breast shape without areolar enlargement.

        c. Not likely to bottom out.

      6. Disadvantages.

        a. Shape and position rely on extensive glandular suturing.

        b. Requires more extensive intraoperative decision making.

        c. Learning curve is steep.

E. Free nipple techniques

      1. Indicated for very large reductions (or for breasts with an IMF-to-nipple distance of >17 cm) where the nipple will likely not survive on a pedicle.

      2. Nipple is removed and replaced as a full-thickness skin graft.

      3. Advantages.

        a. Simple to perform.

        b. Fast.

        c. May therefore allow patients not in perfect health to undergo breast reduction.

      4. Disadvantages.

        a. No possibility of nursing.

        b. Loss of sensation to nipple-areolar complex.

        c. Possible loss of nipple graft.

F. Suction-assisted lipectomy

      1. Liposuction can be used alone to reduce the breast or as an adjunct to other procedures.

      2. Advantages.

        a. Minimal external scarring.

        b. Symmetry easily achieved.

        c. Maximal preservation of breast neurovascular anatomy.

      3. Disadvantages.

        a. Inability to change nipple position or reduce skin laxity.

        b. Traditional liposuction may be difficult due to density of breast in some patients.

        c. Inability to examine specimen pathology.

IV. Potential problems and complications

    A. Changes in nipple sensitivity

    B. Unacceptable scarring

    C. Asymmetry

    D. Unappealing shape

    E. Nipple loss

    F. Fat necrosis

    G. Hematoma

    H. Infection

    I. Dissatisfaction with breast size

    J. Inability to breast-feed

Breast Augmentation

Breast augmentation is one of the most common aesthetic procedures in plastic surgery. The surgeon must have a clear understanding of the patient's desires as well as motivations. The patient must have realistic expectations as well as a clear understanding of the risks, benefits, and postoperative restrictions and limitations of breast implants.

I. Preoperative considerations

    A. A comprehensive history, including a family and personal history of breast disease, should be obtained.

B. **A complete physical examination,** including the breasts and axillary nodal basins, should be performed.

C. **A social history,** including exploration of the motives for breast augmentation, family situation, and recent life changes, should be determined.

D. **The patient's goals and expectations** should be discussed. The patient should describe what is displeasing about her breasts.

E. **The impact of implants on cancer monitoring** (see "Mammographic Interference") should be discussed.

F. The patient must be made aware that many implants need to be removed or exchanged.

G. **Mammograms should be obtained** (controversial for patients younger than 35).

H. **Preoperative photographs** should be taken, and any preoperative asymmetry should be discussed, since it may be accentuated postoperatively.

II. **Operative considerations**

A. **Anesthesia** may be provided by a general anesthetic or by intravenous sedation and intercostal nerve blocks.

B. **Implant size** should be roughly determined in preoperative discussions.

C. **Implant shell types**

1. **Textured silicone elastomer shells**

a. Had fewer capsular contractures when associated with gel implants, but not of proven benefit with saline implants.

b. More visible wrinkling.

c. Implant "fixed" to capsule.

2. **Smooth silicone elastomer shell**

a. Higher capsular contracture rate versus textured gel, but no difference versus textured saline.

b. Allows the implant to move more naturally.

D. **Implant fill type**

1. **Saline filled**

a. The most common type currently used in the United States.

b. Leaks lead to complete deflation.

c. All air should be removed to prevent "sloshing."

d. Overfilling leads to less wrinkling, but also makes the implant more firm.

2. **Silicone gel filled**

a. Not currently approved for use in the United States.

b. More natural consistency.

c. Leaks can go undetected for long periods of time.

d. Silicone gel can cause granulomas in the surrounding tissues.

3. **"Composite" implants** (inner gel and outer saline) are still under investigation.

E. **Implant shape**

1. **Anatomic:** Used for all textured and some smooth implants to decrease upper pole projection.

2. **Round:** Smooth round implants assume a teardrop shape in a standing patient.

F. **Pocket position**

1. **Submuscular placement:** Provides better protection for the implant from being seen and felt, and may reduce capsular contracture rates (not proven in saline implants). Can be either partially (upper pole under pectoralis major) or totally (under pectoralis major and serratus) submuscular. Most important, submuscular placement obscures less of the gland on mammography.

2. **Subglandular placement:** Obscures more of the gland on mammography. It may be considered as an alternative for very active, muscular women because the pectoralis can squeeze the implant, producing an unnatural appearance.

G. **Incision location (surgical exposure)**

1. **Inframammary:** Simple, with good control of implant position, but the scar may be prominent.

2. **Periareolar:** The scar is fairly inconspicuous, but exposure is limited, resulting in more trauma to the gland.
3. **Axillary:** The scar is inconspicuous, but the exposure is difficult, especially in the lower portion of the pocket. The use of the endoscope improves visualization, but IMF irregularities and asymmetries plague this approach.
4. **Transumbilical breast augmentation (TUBA):** A "blind" procedure.

III. **Potential complications**
   A. **Hematoma:** 1% to 3%.
   B. **Seroma:** Typically self-limiting.
   C. **Changes in nipple sensibility** (hypersensitivity or hyposensitivity).
   D. **Arm sensibility changes** from injury to intercostobrachial nerve (with the transaxillary approach).
   E. **Infection:** 2%. *Staphylococcus aureus* and *S. epidermidis* are the most commonly offending organisms. The implant is typically not salvageable.
   F. **Pneumothorax:** Very rare.
   G. **Asymmetry**
   H. **Wrinkling**
   I. **Capsular contracture**
      1. Contraction of the bursalike cavity around the implant creates a tight cavity, which squeezes the implant.
      2. **The Baker classification** describes the degree of capsular contracture.
         a. I: Soft
         b. II: Palpable firmness, but not visible
         c. III: Palpable and visible firmness
         d. IV: Painful, firm contracture
      3. **Grade III and IV contractures** can be treated only by incising and/or excising the capsule surgically.
      4. **Closed capsular release** is not recommended.
      5. **The use of leukotriene inhibitors** has been reported to possibly reduce capsular contractures.
   J. **Implant rupture**
      1. The failure rate is generally quoted as 1% per year for the first 10 years; it is unknown thereafter.
      2. **Ultrasound** is the best screening tool for a suspected implant rupture.
      3. **Magnetic resonance imaging (MRI)** is the most sensitive imaging modality.
   K. **Tissue thinning/implant extrusion**
   L. **Pathologic cutaneous scarring**

IV. **Mammographic interference**
   A. Breast implants interfere with mammographic cancer surveillance.
   B. **Subglandular implants:** Can obscure 50% to 80% of the breast parenchyma. This amount can be reduced to around 40% with special (Eklund) displacement views, in which the implant is manually displaced during imaging.
   C. **Subpectoral implants:** Obscure approximately 30% of the breast parenchyma. This can be reduced to 10% with Eklund views.
   D. Breast tissue is never completely visualized, even for breasts without implants.
   E. Capsular contracture worsens the quality of mammographic monitoring.

V. **The implant controversy:** In the 1980s, a number of silicone breast implant patients alleged that a variety of diseases, mostly connective tissue disorders, were directly related to silicone exposure. The Food and Drug Administration called for a moratorium on the use of silicone breast implants until further study could be performed. These implants may be used today only under very strictly controlled study guidelines. No studies to date have been able to prove that silicone exposure contributes to this spectrum of diseases or any other systemic disease. However, because of the limitations of statistics, it is impossible to conclusively prove that silicone exposure *does not* cause disease.

Mastopexy

I. **Pathophysiology of ptosis**
   A. **Normal breast anatomy**
      1. The gland spans from the second to the sixth rib.
      2. The nipple-areolar complex is situated superior to the IMF and is centralized over the breast mound.
      3. The sternal notch-to-nipple distance is 17 to 21 cm.
      4. The IMF-to-nipple distance is 7 to 8 cm.
   B. **Ptotic breast anatomic changes**
      1. The nipple moves inferiorly.
      2. The breast parenchyma hangs over the IMF.
      3. The sternal notch-to-nipple distance is increased.
      4. Connective tissues stretch with loss of elasticity.
      5. Etiologies include gravity, hormonal changes, weight loss, and glandular atrophy.
II. **Patient evaluation:** As in all breast surgery, evaluation should include a complete history and physical with efforts to look for breast pathology with mammogram where appropriate (see above).
   A. **Assessment of breast ptosis**
      1. **Size, shape, and density** of the breast tissue should be noted.
      2. **The degree of ptosis** should be recorded.
         a. Grade 1 (minor ptosis): The nipple lies *above* the IMF.
         b. Grade 2 (moderate ptosis): The nipple lies *at* the IMF.
         c. Grade 3 (major ptosis): The nipple lies *below* the IMF.
      3. **Patient weight and body habitus** should be noted.
      4. **Asymmetries** should be noted and discussed preoperatively.
   B. **Ideal candidates** for mastopexy include patients with the following.
      1. **Adequate breast parenchyma.** Those with inadequate breast parenchyma should consider augmentation with delayed mastopexy.
      2. **Ptosis of the nipple-areolar complex.**
      3. **Willingness to accept scarring.**
III. **Operations**
   A. **Operative treatment** is almost identical to breast reduction without gland resection. The general operative sequence consists of the following.
      1. Reshaping and/or repositioning of the gland
      2. Skin reduction and redraping
      3. Superior repositioning of the nipple-areolar complex
   B. **Types of mastopexy procedures**
      1. **Periareolar mastopexy (Benelli)**
         a. Attractive consideration due to inconspicuous scarring.
         b. Can lead to widening of the nipple-areolar complex unless a permanent purse-string suture is used around the areola.
      2. **Wise pattern ("inverted T")**
         a. Very predictable.
         b. Extensive scarring compared with other procedures.
      3. **Vertical pattern**
         a. Allows more tailoring than with the periareolar incision alone.
         b. Fewer scars than with the Wise pattern.
      4. **Implant placement**
         a. Breast implant placement can "fill out" the existing skin envelope and accomplish or assist with the goals of mastopexy.

   b. However, breast implant benefit is often moderate, and it is difficult to completely augment women out of ptosis. It is often recommended to perform the augmentation and mastopexy in a staged fashion to reduce the risk of tissue loss.

C. Degree of ptosis determines the type of mastopexy procedure.

   1. Grade I (minor ptosis)

   a. If skin quality is good:

   (1) Augmentation only, or

   (2) Circumareolar mastopexy

   b. If skin quality is fair (lacks tone):

   (1) Circumareolar mastopexy, or

   (2) Augmentation and delayed mastopexy (two stages)

   2. Grade II (moderate ptosis)

   a. If skin quality is good to fair:

   (1) Vertical scar mastopexy

   (2) Can add augmentation if glandular hypoplasia is present

   b. If skin quality is fair to poor:

   (1) Vertical scar mastopexy with short vertical component

   (2) Can add augmentation if glandular hypoplasia is present

   3. Grade III (major ptosis): Inverted-T Wise pattern mastopexy is usually the best choice.

IV. Potential problems and complications

   A. Changes in nipple sensitivity

   B. Hematoma

   C. Unacceptable scarring

   D. Asymmetry

   E. Unappealing shape

   F. Infection

   G. Implant-related problems

   H. Recurrent ptosis

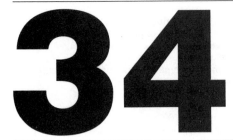

**Breast
Reconstruction**

Catherine Curtin

Basics

I. Goals
   A. "First do no harm": Reconstruction should not interfere with oncologic treatment (i.e., should not significantly delay chemotherapy or radiation therapy).
   B. Reconstructive procedures should not add unacceptable risks of delay of diagnosis of recurrent disease or of operative morbidity or mortality.
   C. Provide careful preoperative counseling to educate patients about the many options currently available.
   D. Establish patient preferences, and determine level of social support and physical condition, in order to determine the best treatment option.
   E. Produce an optimal aesthetic result, depending on the patient's preferences. For some patients, merely creating a breast mound that looks acceptable in clothing is sufficient, whereas others would prefer supple soft tissue with a complete nipple reconstruction.
II. Timing of reconstruction
   A. Factors to consider
      1. Patient preferences
      2. Oncologic factors, including stage of disease and the need for adjuvant therapy
      3. Recommendations of a multidisciplinary team that includes general surgeons, medical oncologists, and radiation oncologists
   B. Immediate reconstruction (mastectomy and reconstruction performed on the same day)
      1. Ideal for patients with early disease (stage I or II)
      2. Advantages
         a. Decreased psychological trauma.
         b. Less expensive.
         c. Does not increase the rate of local recurrence.
         d. Compared with delayed reconstruction, immediate reconstruction generally produces a better aesthetic result because the skin envelope and the inframammary fold are maintained.
      3. Disadvantages
         a. Potential delay of adjuvant therapy if postoperative complications occur.
         b. The reconstructive plan may be adversely affected by the oncologic procedure (e.g., mastectomy flaps are too thin, vascular pedicle is damaged or in spasm).
      4. Contraindications
         a. Advanced disease (stage III or greater, relative contraindication).
         b. Postoperative radiation (relative contraindication).
         c. Medical comorbidities (severe obesity, cardiopulmonary disease).
   C. Delayed reconstruction
      1. Advantages
         a. Fewer complications compared with immediate reconstruction.

  b. Final pathology results are available, and thus a more informed decision regarding reconstruction in the context of the entire treatment regimen can be made.

 2. Disadvantages

  a. Prolongs overall treatment.

  b. Sometimes technically more challenging.

  c. Thoracodorsal pedicle may be unusable (for free flap inflow) if it is enveloped in scar tissue.

Reconstructive Techniques

I. Direct implant placement without tissue expansion

 A. Simplest

 B. Dependent upon sufficient skin after mastectomy to cover implant

 C. Rarely feasible without prior expansion

 D. Generally discouraged

II. Tissue expansion followed by permanent implant placement

 A. Advantages

  1. No flap donor site.

  2. Less invasive surgery; less operative time; easier postoperative recovery.

 B. Disadvantages

  1. Saline implants feel unnatural.

  2. Implants lack natural ptosis.

  3. Reconstruction with tissue expanders takes several months and multiple clinic visits, and requires at least one additional operation for implant exchange.

  4. Complications include infection, capsular contracture, deflation, extrusion, and visible wrinkling of the implant.

 C. Patients appropriate for implant reconstruction

  1. Patients who are not suitable for autologous reconstruction.

  2. Patients who do not want additional donor scars.

  3. Patients who prefer a speedier recovery.

  4. Ideal for small-breasted women.

 D. Contraindications

  1. Completed or planned radiation therapy to the breast (relative contraindication).

  2. Thin skin flap coverage.

 E. Most common technique for reconstruction with an implant.

 F. Allows for the development of adequate soft tissue coverage for the implant.

 G. The expander size is chosen by preoperatively measuring the chest wall base dimensions of the breast.

 H. Must have viable mastectomy flaps (if the mastectomy flaps are compromised, it is best to delay placement of the expander).

 I. The expander is placed in a submuscular pocket.

  1. The pocket dimensions should match the expander (do not let expander roll up at edges).

  2. Do not alter (undermine) the inframammary fold.

  3. The pocket is developed beneath the pectoralis major, and sometimes additionally beneath the serratus and rectus abdominus to achieve total coverage.

 J. Expansion may begin 2 to 3 weeks postoperatively if the wounds are healed.

 K. Inflate expander weekly or more often, with the volume instilled depending on patient comfort and overlying skin quality and changes with expansion (e.g., tightness, erythema).

 L. Overexpand by 25% to 50% to improve skin drape over the implant, to allow for differences in profile of implant versus expander, and to allow for skin recoil postexpansion.

    M. After expansion is completed, allow an additional 2 to 4 months for tissue equilibrium to occur prior to operative implant exchange.

III. Pedicled autologous reconstruction

A. Advantages

1. Natural-feeling breast mound.
2. Able to achieve more natural ptosis.
3. Reconstruction of the breast can often be achieved in a single stage.

B. Disadvantages

1. Donor site morbidity.
2. More complex operation; longer operative time.

C. Latissimus dorsi flap (muscle or myocutaneous).

1. **Blood supply** (type V muscle).
   a. Thoracodorsal artery (dominant).
   b. May also be sustained from retrograde flow from the serratus branch if the thoracodorsal vessels are damaged proximally from the mastectomy

2. **Advantages**
   a. Reliable workhorse flap.
   b. Excellent soft tissue for coverage of implant, if needed.
   c. Can provide a single-stage implant reconstruction.

3. **Disadvantages**
   a. Significant donor site scar, especially if a skin paddle is harvested.
   b. Seroma formation is problematic in the donor site in about half of patients.
   c. Often there is insufficient tissue for total autologous reconstruction, and therefore the patient requires an implant and/or tissue expander.

4. **Indications**
   a. Reconstruction after transverse rectus abdominus muscle (TRAM) flap or implant failures.
   b. Partial defects.
   c. Obese patients.
   d. TRAM vascular supply not available.
   e. Patient preference.

D. Pedicled TRAM

1. **Anatomy**
   a. Type III muscle: Superior epigastric (used for pedicled flap) and deep inferior epigastric (used for free flap) arteries.
   b. The cutaneous portion of the flap is divided into four zones (order of reliability: zones 1, 3, 2, 4) (Fig. 34-1).
   c. Periumbilical perforators supply the skin and subcutaneous tissues of the flap.

2. **Advantages**
   a. Excellent aesthetic results in most cases.
   b. Usually enough tissue for total autologous reconstruction.
   c. Tolerates radiation well.

3. **Disadvantages**
   a. Significant amount of surgery, requiring several days of hospitalization and fairly intensive pain management.
   b. Fullness medially or inferiorly from the pedicle (this can be minimized with adequate tunnel dissection).
   c. Complications.
      (1) Hematoma
      (2) Seroma
      (3) Partial or total flap loss
      (4) Hernias and abdominal wall laxity
      (5) Fat necrosis, which can confound cancer monitoring
      (6) Necrosis of the umbilicus

4. **Patient selection**
   a. Patients must have adequate abdominal tissue for creation of a breast mound.

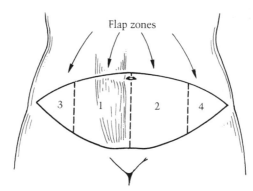

Fig. 34-1. Vascular zones of the TRAM flap. Zones 1 and 3 are on the side ipsilateral to the pedicle and zones 2 and 4 are on the contralateral, less vascularized side. (From Maxwell P. and Hammond D Breast reconstruction following mastectomy and surgical management of the patient with high-risk breast disease. In *Grabb and Smith's Plastic Surgery*, 5th ed. Aston SJ, Beasley RW, Thorne CH, eds. Philadelphia, Lippincott-Raven, 1997. With permission.)

  b. Evaluate the abdomen for old scars that may have previously divided the pedicle.
  c. A TRAM flap is contraindicated in patients who have had previous abdominoplasty.
  d. A TRAM flap should be avoided in significantly overweight patients, due to the unreliability of the skin and subcutaneous flap.
  e. Patients must be medically appropriate.
  f. Relative contraindications include smokers and patients with vascular disease.
 E. Bipedicled TRAM: Utilizes a flap based on both rectus muscles to reconstruct one breast.
  1. Used if large amount of tissue is required for reconstruction.
  2. Improves blood supply.
  3. Indicated in patients with a higher risk for partial loss of flap (smoker, obese).
  4. A mesh closure of the abdominal wall is needed to prevent abdominal laxity.
 F. Delay procedure for pedicled TRAM
  1. The inflow to the perforating vessels of the flap is most direct from the inferior pedicle. When a superior pedicle (i.e., pedicled TRAM) is used, the flow must traverse the choke vessels between the superior and inferior epigastric arteries before reaching the perforators to the flap. In order to improve blood flow to the flap through these vessels, many surgeons advocate utilizing a delay procedure.
  2. The inferior epigastric pedicle or pedicles are divided several weeks before the planned breast reconstruction.
  3. Dilates choke vessels.
  4. Increases the robustness of the superior epigastric pedicle.
  5. Used for patients with risk factors for tissue necrosis of flap (e.g., smokers, patients with excess lower abdominal subcutaneous tissues) and for those in whom a large amount of lower abdominal tissue is required for the reconstruction.
 G. Supercharging procedure for TRAM: In a pedicled TRAM, the inferior epigastric vessels can be anastomosed microsurgically to the thoracodorsal or internal mammary vessels to improve arterial inflow and/or venous outflow.
IV. Microvascular reconstruction
 A. Free TRAM

1. **Blood supply:** Deep inferior epigastric artery (the dominant blood supply to the skin paddle) and its venae comitantes are anastomosed to the thoracodorsal or internal mammary vessels.

2. **Advantages**
   a. Can be used for patients in whom the superior epigastric artery has been previously divided.
   b. More robust blood supply to the flap perforating vessels.
   c. Some surgeons argue that there is a lower rate of flap loss and fat necrosis versus the pedicled flap, but results are highly operator dependent.

3. **Disadvantages**
   a. Increased operating time and cost.
   b. Contraindicated in patients with lower abdominal incisions in which the pedicle vessels might have been divided or are encased in scar tissue (including inguinal hernia repair).
   c. Requires microsurgical expertise.
   d. Potential for total flap loss.

B. **Deep inferior epigastric artery perforator (DIEP) flap**
   1. The cutaneous flap is raised like a free TRAM, but with the blood supply to the flap based on only one or two perforators from the deep inferior epigastric artery, sparing harvest of the rectus muscle.

   2. **Advantages**
      a. No muscle harvested, although some portion is divided from its innervation.
      b. Less incidence of abdominal wall weakness, laxity, and hernia formation.
      c. Less pain.

   3. **Disadvantages**
      a. Technically challenging.
      b. If the perforator is damaged, the entire flap can be lost.
      c. Less robust blood supply, leading to increased risk of fat necrosis.

C. **Other free flap options**
   1. **Superior/inferior gluteal flaps**
      a. Advantage: Majority of patients have tissue available for transfer.
      b. Disadvantages.
         (1) A technically challenging flap to raise.
         (2) Donor site pain if the sciatic nerve is not sufficiently padded.
         (3) Potentially disfiguring donor site.
   2. **Thigh flap:** Often unacceptable donor site.
   3. **Rubens flap**
      a. Based on the deep circumflex iliac pedicle.
      b. Indicated in patients who have had previous abdominoplasty.

V. **Treatment of the contralateral breast**
   A. To achieve symmetry, the contralateral breast must be evaluated.
   B. Alteration of the contralateral breast to optimize symmetry may include augmentation, reduction, or mastopexy.
   C. Federal law assures insurance coverage of alteration of the contralateral breast in cases of breast cancer reconstruction.

VI. **Nipple and areolar reconstruction**
   A. Nipple and areolar reconstruction is a separate procedure performed once the reconstructed breast has achieved a stable form (usually at least 6 to 8 weeks postreconstruction).
   B. **Nipple position** is marked preoperatively with the patient upright, symmetric to the contralateral side.
   C. The technique chosen is dependent upon surgeon preference and the size of the opposite papule.
   D. A variety of local flaps have been developed to improve projection, including the **skate flap.**
      1. Two wings are elevated laterally at the level of the deep dermis.
      2. The wings are then wrapped around themselves.

3. Projection will reliably decrease postoperatively, so overcorrect by roughly one-half.

E. **A composite graft** from the opposite nipple can be used if the contralateral nipple is large or ptotic.

F. **Reconstruction of the areola** is most often achieved with a full-thickness skin graft, although some prefer to use tattooing alone. Donor sites include the following.

   1. The TRAM abdominal incision
   2. Medial thigh
   3. Breast mastectomy scar

G. **Color match** can be achieved through medical tattooing.

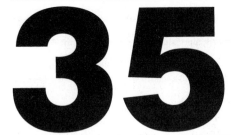

Hand and Wrist Anatomy and Examination

Steven C. Haase

I. **Before you begin**
   A. **Remember the ABCs of trauma** for all injured patients—do not assume that there is an isolated hand/wrist injury.
   B. Take a focused history.
      1. Age, handedness, vocation and avocations, smoking status.
      2. Time of last meal and drink, allergies, current medications, medical problems.
      3. Exact mechanism of injury (crush/avulsion, sharp/dull, dirty/clean).
   C. Order appropriate x-rays.
   D. **Examine the joint(s) proximal and distal to the injury** to detect associated injuries in the limb.
   E. Administer tetanus booster and antibiotics if needed (open injuries).
II. **Common abbreviations**
   A. **Digits**
      1. IF: Index finger
      2. MF: Middle finger
      3. RF: Ring finger
      4. LF: Little finger (or SF, small finger)
   B. **Joints**
      1. IPJ: Interphalangeal joint
      2. DIPJ: Distal interphalangeal joint
      3. PIPJ: Proximal interphalangeal joint
      4. MPJ: Metacarpophalangeal joint
   C. **Muscles**
      1. FCR/FCU: Flexor carpi radialis/ulnaris
      2. FPL/FPB: Flexor pollicis longus/brevis
      3. FDS: Flexor digitorum superficialis
      4. FDP: Flexor digitorum profundus
      5. ECRL/ECRB: Extensor carpi radialis longus/brevis
      6. ECU: Extensor carpi ulnaris
      7. EDC: Extensor digitorum communis
      8. EIP: Extensor indicis proprius
      9. EDM: Extensor digiti minimi (or EDQ, extensor digit quinti)
      10. EPL/EPB: Extensor pollicis longus/brevis
      11. PL: Palmaris longus
      12. PT: Pronator teres
      13. PQ: Pronator quadratus
      14. AdP: Adductor pollicis
      15. APL/APB: Abductor pollicis longus/brevis
III. **Vasculature**
   A. **Arterial supply**
      1. The radial artery supplies the deep palmar arch.
      2. The ulnar artery supplies the superficial palmar arch.
      3. The radial artery is usually dominant, but ulnar dominance and codominance can exist.
   B. **Venous drainage**
      1. Dorsal (subcutaneous) venous network and palmar venous arch.

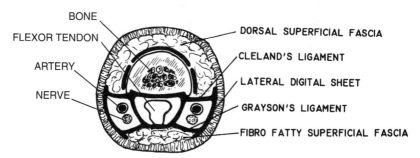

Fig. 35-1. Cross-section of the digit. (From Sherman R and Isenberg S Principles of soft-tissue reconstruction of the lower extremity. In *Plastic, Maxillofacial, and Reconstructive Surgery*, 3rd edition. Georgiade G, Riefkohl R, Levin S. Philadelphia, Williams & Wilkins, 1997. With permission.)

> **2.** Drain into the cephalic vein (originates near the "anatomic snuffbox") and the basilic vein (originates on the dorsoulnar aspect on hand).

  C. Allen's test: Compress the radial and ulnar arteries at the wrist, and have the patient make a tight fist (to exsanguinate) and then relax; release one or the other artery to check blood supply to the hand and patency of the palmar arch via that artery.

  D. A digital Allen's test can also be performed.

  E. Arterial location relative to accompanying nerves.
>   **1.** In the palm: Arteries are volar to the nerves.
>   **2.** In the digits: Arteries are dorsal to the nerves (Fig. 35-1).

  F. Capillary refill should be 2 to 3 seconds; best place to check is the nail bed or eponychial fold.

IV. Nerves

  A. Radial nerve anatomy
>   **1.** Passes between heads of the supinator and enters the forearm between the brachioradialis and the ECRL/ECRB.
>   **2.** Branches
>   **a.** Posterior interosseous nerve: Innervates the EDC, EDM, APL, EPB, EPL, EIP, and ECU; sensory branch to the wrist capsule (deep within fourth dorsal compartment of the wrist); makes a good donor for digital nerve grafts.
>   **b.** Superficial radial nerve: Sensory to the dorsum of the thumb, first web space, IF, MF, and radial RF up to the level of the PIP joints (Fig. 35-2).

  B. Median nerve anatomy
>   **1.** Enters the forearm with the brachial artery, emerging between the heads of the pronator teres; innervates the pronator teres, FCR, palmaris longus, and FDS.
>   **2.** Branches.
>   **a.** Anterior interosseous nerve innervates FPL, radial two FDP (IF and MF), and pronator quadratus; sensory to wrist capsule.
>   **b.** Remainder of median nerve enters the carpal tunnel.
>   **(1)** Motor branch: Innervates the two lumbricals, **o**pponens pollicis (OP), **A**PB, and **F**PB (LOAF).
>   **(2)** Sensory: Palmar cutaneous branch, digital nerves (thumb, IF, MF, and radial RF) (Fig. 35-2).

  C. Ulnar nerve anatomy
>   **1.** Enters forearm behind the medial epicondyle; innervates the FCU and ulnar two FDP (RF and LF).
>   **2.** Travels under the FCU to the wrist, forming the following branches.
>   **a.** Deep palmar branch: Innervates abductor digiti minimi, flexor digiti minimi brevis, opponens digiti minimi, all interosseous muscles, medial lumbricals (two) and AdP.

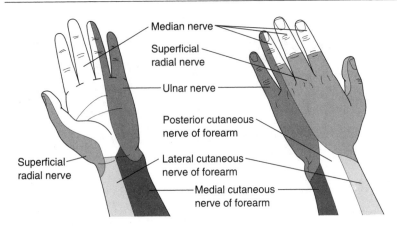

Fig. 35-2. Cutaneous sensory innervation of the hand, volar and dorsal surfaces.

        b. Superficial branch: Innervates palmaris brevis; sensory palmar digital
        nerves to LF and ulnar RF (Fig. 35-2).

        c. Dorsal branch: Sensory to the dorsum of the LF and ulnar RF (Fig. 35-2).

     3. Martin Gruber anastomosis: An anatomic variant in which the median
     nerve crosses over to contribute to the ulnar nerve. The two most com-
     mon variations are as follows.

        a. Median nerve in proximal forearm contributes to the ulnar nerve in the
        distal forearm.

        b. Anterior interosseus nerve contributes to ulnar nerve.

     4. Riche-Cannieu anastomosis: A more distal variant in which ulnar fibers
     contribute to median nerve branches in the palm.

  D. "Quick and simple" nerve exam

     1. Median nerve: Sensation at tip of IF (light touch and two-point discrimina-
     tion); ability to make "OK" sign (demonstrates FPL, FDP, and OP).

     2. Ulnar nerve: Sensation at tip of LF; ability to abduct/fingers "wave hello"
     and cross fingers (interossei working).

     3. Radial nerve: Sensation at dorsal first web space; ability to give "thumbs
     up" (EPL working).

V. Tendons and muscles

  A. Flexors

     1. Flexor tendon zones (Fig. 35-3)

        a. Zone 1: Middle of middle phalanx to fingertip (distal to insertion of
        FDS, includes only FDP).

        b. Zone 2: Distal palmar crease to middle of middle phalanx (both FDS
        and FDP tendons, with FDP volar, proceeding distally).

        c. Zone 3: Transverse carpal ligament to distal palmar crease.

        d. Zone 4: Under transverse carpal ligament (in carpal tunnel).

        e. Zone 5: Proximal border of transverse carpal ligament to musculo-
        tendinous junction.

     2. Flexor muscle mass originates largely at the medial epicondyle.

     3. The carpal tunnel contains the median nerve and nine tendons: FDP
     (four), FDS (four), and FPL (Fig. 35-4).

        a. FDS is superficial to the FDP in the carpal tunnel.

        b. FDS (MF and RF) is superficial to FDS (IF and LF)—the "hard way" to
        cross your fingers.

     4. Flexor digitorum superficialis

        a. Splits into radial and ulnar slips prior to inserting into the proximal as-
        pect of the respective middle phalanges.

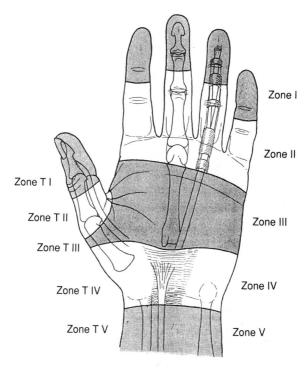

Fig. 35-3. Flexor tendon zones. (From Zidel P. Tendon healing and flexor tendon surgery. In *Grabb and Smith's Plastic Surgery*, 5th ed. Aston SJ, Beasley RW, Thorne CH, eds. Philadelphia, Lippincott-Raven, 1997. With permission.)

    b. FDP passes between the two slips of FDS, through a space called "Camper's chiasm."

    c. To test: Lay hand flat on exam table, palm up. With other fingers held in extension (blocks FDP), test active flexion (and to resistance) at each PIPJ.

5. Flexor digitorum profundus

    a. Inserts into proximal volar aspect of respective distal phalanges.

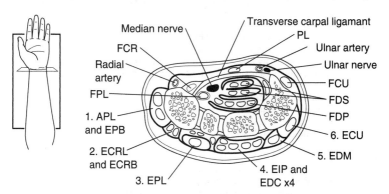

Fig. 35-4. Cross-section through the wrist, including extensor tendon compartments 1 to 6.

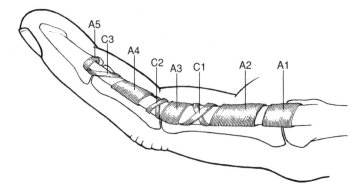

Fig. 35-5. Flexor sheath pulley system. A1–A5: annular pulleys; C1–C3: cruciate pulleys. A2 and A4 should be preserved to prevent bowstringing. (From Hoffman L. Mackenzie D., and Schwartz M. Common inflammatory disorders of the upper limb. In *Grabb and Smith's Plastic Surgery*, 5th ed. Aston SJ, Beasley RW, Thorne CH, eds. Philadelphia, Lippincott-Raven Publishers, 1997. With permission.)

    b. To test: With PIPJ held in extension (examiner's pressure on middle phalanx), test active DIPJ flexion (and to resistance).

6. **Flexor pollicis longus**
    a. Inserts into distal phalanx of thumb.
    b. To test: Look for active flexion of IPJ ("OK" sign).

7. **Pulleys:** Prevent bowstringing and increase the mechanical effectiveness of pull across the joints (Fig. 35-5).
    a. Five annular pulleys (A1–A5).
        (1) A2 and A4 are the most critical to finger function; located on the proximal and middle phalanx, respectively.
        (2) A1, A3, and A5 are at the MPJ, PIPJ, and DIPJ, respectively.
    b. Three cruciate pulleys (C1–C3) interdigitate between A2, A3, A4, and A5.
    c. The thumb has three pulleys: A1, A2, and oblique, which are located over the MPJ, IPJ, and proximal phalanx, respectively. The oblique pulley is the most mechanically important.

B. **Extensors**
  1. **Zones:** The extensor tendons have nine zones. The odd-numbered zones (1–7) lie over joints, with the even-numbered zones in between (see Chapter 37, "Tendon Injuries and Tendonitis").
  2. The extensor muscle mass (also known as the "mobile wad"): Originates largely at the lateral epicondyle.
  3. **Junctura tendinae:** Interconnect tendons on the back of the hand and may mask an extensor rupture, as pull from a proximal tendon from another finger can be transmitted via a junctura to the distal extensor tendon of the injured finger.
  4. **Wrist compartments** (radial to ulnar) (Fig. 35-4)
    a. Compartment 1: APL, EPB
    b. Compartment 2: ECRL, ECRB
    c. Compartment 3: EPL
    d. Compartment 4: EDC, EIP
    e. Compartment 5: EDM
    f. Compartment 6: ECU
  5. **EIP, EDM**
    a. These tendons lie *ulnar* to their accompanying EDC tendons.
    b. To test: Independent extension of the IF and LF with other fingers flexed.

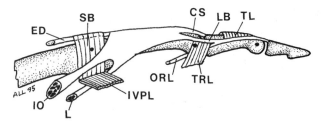

Fig. 35-6. Extensor tendon anatomy. (From Lluch A. Repair of the extensor tendon system. In *Grabb and Smith's Plastic Surgery*, 5th ed. Aston SJ, Beasley RW, Thorne CH, eds. Philadelphia, Lippincott-Raven Publishers, 1997. With permission.)

      6. EPL: To test, check ability to raise thumb off table with hand prone.

      7. Extensor mechanism (Fig. 35-6).

        a. Extensor digitorum communis (plus EIP in the index finger and EDM in the small finger) expands over the MPJ to form the extensor hood.

        b. The lumbrical and interosseus tendons join the hood laterally, providing MPJ flexion.

        c. The extensor hood divides into three components over the proximal phalanx. The central slip of the extensor hood inserts on the base of the middle phalanx, while the two lateral bands continue distally, then fuse prior to inserting on the base of the distal phalanx (the terminal tendon).

C. Intrinsic muscles

    1. ADP: Test for key pinch (thumb to side of IF) by having patient hold a piece of paper here and resist the paper being pulled away; if FPL takes over (DIPJ flexes), this is a positive "Froment sign" and implies that AdP function is absent or diminished (compare simultaneously to the opposite side).

    2. Interosseus muscles: Test for abduction/adduction of fingers (including to resistance).

    3. Intrinsic tightness test.

      a. With the wrist in neutral position, hyperextend the MPJ to relax the extrinsics.

      b. Measure passive flexion of PIPJ ("intrinsic tightness").

        (1) Mild: 60 to 80 degrees.

        (2) Moderate: 20 to 59 degrees.

        (3) Severe: Less than 20 degrees.

    4. Extrinsic tightness test

      a. With the wrist in neutral position, flex the MPJ, to relax the intrinsics.

      b. Check for resistance to PIPJ flexion, which will indicate extrinsic tightness.

VI. Bones and joints

  A. Wrist

    1. Radius and ulna articulate with each other and with the carpus.

    2. Conceptually, the radius rotates around the fixed ulna at the wrist.

    3. Normal alignment is reviewed in Chapter 36, "Fractures and Dislocations of the Hand and Wrist."

  B. Carpus

    1. Eight bones (scaphoid, lunate, triquetrum, pisiform, trapezium, trapezoid, capitate, hamate). Mnemonic: "**S**cared **L**overs **T**ry **P**ositions **T**hat **T**hey **C**annot **H**andle."

    2. The pisiform is actually a sesamoid bone, imbedded in the FCU tendon.

    3. Normal alignment: The capitate is collinear with the lunate and the third metacarpal.

4. Gilula's lines consist of arcs formed by the outlines of the carpal bones seen on anteroposterior radiographs of the wrist. The proximal row (scaphoid, lunate, and triquetrum) forms the proximal arcs, and the proximal edge of the distal row (trapezoid, trapezium, capitate, and hamate) forms the distal arc. The arcs should be smooth and continuous; otherwise, a fracture or dislocation may be present.

C. Fingers

1. Five metacarpals, 14 phalanges (three per finger, two per thumb)
2. Joint mechanics (see Chapter 36, "Fractures and Dislocations of the Hand and Wrist")

D. Normal ranges of motion (approximate)

1. Finger MPJ: 0 to 45 degrees hyperextension, 90 degrees flexion
2. Finger PIPJ: 0 degrees extension, 100 degrees flexion
3. Finger DIPJ: 0 degrees extension, 70 to 80 degrees flexion
4. Thumb MPJ: 10 degrees hyperextension, 55 degrees flexion
5. Thumb IPJ: 15 degrees hyperextension, 80 degrees flexion
6. Wrist: 70 degrees extension, 75 degrees flexion, 20 degrees radial deviation, 35 degrees ulnar deviation
7. Forearm: 70 degrees pronation, 85 degrees supination

VII. Tourniquet use

A. Never put on a finger tourniquet without establishing a prominent, obvious reminder to remove it (e.g., hemostat, sterile glove).

B. Blood pressure cuffs make good arm tourniquets in the emergency room.

C. Tourniquet pressure should be about 125 to 150 mm Hg above systolic pressure (usually set around 230–250 mm Hg).

D. Limit tourniquet time to 2 hours to prevent permanent damage.

1. Nerves are the most vulnerable structures to pressure and hypoxia.
2. Blood flow should be returned to the ischemic part for 5 minutes for every 30 minutes of ischemia (i.e., deflate tourniquet for 20 minutes every 2 hours).

VIII. Nerve blocks (see Chapter 8, "Local Anesthetics")

A. Median nerve

1. Place needle at the distal wrist crease between the PL and FCR; enter at 45-degree angle to the forearm. Usually a "pop" is felt as the deep fascia is penetrated.
2. If there is no "pop," insert until paresthesias or bone is encountered, at which time the needle is withdrawn slightly and 3 to 5 cc of local anesthetic is injected.

B. Ulnar nerve

1. Place needle just proximal to the ulnar styloid; enter behind the FCU tendon with the needle directed from ulnar to radial in the coronal plane.
2. Once the needle is just past the FCU, inject the anesthetic (3–5 cc).

C. Radial nerve

1. Must block a wide area: Start proximal to the radial styloid and inject the subcutaneous tissue.
2. Extend the field block in both directions (volar and dorsal) around the distal forearm.

D. Digital block

1. **Dorsal approach** (some think is less painful): Subcutaneous wheal over the extensor tendon to block the dorsal nerves. Two injections just proximal to the web, one on either side of the digit—advance the needle until the tip approaches the palmar skin surface and then withdraw while injecting slowly.
2. **Volar approach:** A subcutaneous wheal is placed directly over the flexor tendon and then laterally near the digital neurovascular bundles.
3. **Sheath approach:** Insert the needle volarly, just distal to the distal palmar crease, down into the flexor tendons. With slight pressure on the syringe plunger, withdraw the needle slowly until there is a loss of resistance (indicating injection into the potential space of the flexor sheath).

Inject a couple of cc's of local. Sometimes, a fluid wave can be felt distally in the finger over the sheath. This technique reliably results in digital anesthesia with one injection, but is not very effective in cases of sheath violation, such as distal amputation.

IX. Incisions on the hand

    A. When planning incisions, avoid crossing flexion creases at a right angle.

        1. Midaxial incisions: With the finger fully flexed, mark the radial and ulnar extent of the flexion crease at each finger joint.

        2. Bruner incisions: Flexor surface incisions that zigzag from midaxial line to midaxial line.

    B. On the extensor surface, longitudinal, curvilinear, "gentle-S," and transverse incisions are all usually acceptable.

Pearls

1. Do not forget that hand trauma patients are also *trauma* patients.

2. When unsure of anatomy, physiology, or pathology, compare the injured hand with the contralateral (uninjured) one—most people are symmetric.

3. Always document a neurovascular examination *before* injecting local anesthetic.

4. Always test a tendon or muscle against *resistance*—you may detect a partial injury that is otherwise compensated.

5. Always incorporate a "reminder" with finger tourniquets, such as a hemostat.

Fractures and Dislocations of the Hand and Wrist

John C. Austin

General Principles

I. **Classification of fractures:** Universal descriptive system
   A. **Open versus closed**
   B. **Orientation** (transverse, oblique, spiral, or comminuted)
   C. **Location** (base, shaft, neck, head, or condyle)
   D. **Displaced versus nondisplaced**
   E. **Level of comminution**
   F. **Degree of rotation, angulation, or shortening**
II. **Salter-Harris classification of pediatric fractures**
   A. **Type I:** Fracture through physis only
   B. **Type II:** Involves physis and metaphysis
   C. **Type III:** Involves physis and epiphysis
   D. **Type IV:** Fracture extends from metaphysis through physis, into epiphysis
   E. **Type V:** Crush injury to physis
III. **Stability:** Key to the management of fractures and dislocations
   A. **Stable fractures:** Once reduced, are able to resist deforming forces
   B. **Unstable fractures:** Significant tendency to redisplace once reduced
IV. **Treatment:** Best results are achieved by the following.
   A. **Anatomic reduction**
   B. **Appropriate immobilization**
      1. Length of time needed is determined by fracture location and severity.
      2. General guidelines
         a. 2 to 4 weeks for phalangeal and metacarpal fractures
         b. 4 to 6 weeks for distal radius fractures
         c. 8 to 12 weeks or more for scaphoid fractures
   C. **Early mobilization with occupational therapy**
      1. Fingers are generally mobilized early, since they can develop contractures faster.
      2. The wrist generally recovers mobility better than the fingers.
V. **Assessment of healing**
   A. **Serial x-rays** (fracture callus, new bone formation)
   B. **Physical examination** (loss of tenderness to direct palpation at the fracture site)

Fractures

I. **Phalangeal fractures**
   A. Phalangeal and metacarpal fractures are common (about 10% of all fractures).
   B. **Evaluation**
      1. Swelling, pain, decreased range of motion (ROM), deformity, and associated injuries.

2. **Distal phalanx fractures.**
   a. Evaluate for nail bed injury.
   b. Evaluate for mallet finger (flexion deformity of distal interphalangeal joint due to disruption of the extensor mechanism).
3. **Deformity is based on key deforming forces.**
   a. Middle phalanx fractures.
      (1) Proximal to flexor digitorum superficialis (FDS) insertion: Apex dorsal tendency.
      (2) Distal to FDS insertion: Apex volar tendency.
   b. Proximal phalanx fractures: Apex volar tendency, due to the following.
      (1) Flexion of proximal fragment (interosseous muscles).
      (2) Extension of distal fragment (extensor mechanism via central slip).
4. **Radiographs:** Anteroposterior (AP), lateral, and oblique x-rays in varying amounts of flexion to isolate affected digit(s).

C. **Treatment:** Guided by reducibility and stability
1. **Reducible and stable:** Usually treated closed with buddy taping, splinting, or casting.
2. **Reducible and unstable:** Require percutaneous pinning or open reduction and internal fixation (ORIF) to maintain reduction.
3. **Irreducible:** Require ORIF.
4. **Fixation choices**
   a. K-wires (percutaneous or buried).
   b. Plates and screws (e.g., modular hand system).
   c. Lag screws.
   d. Interosseous wires.

D. **Complications**
1. **Tendon adhesions** (to fracture site).
   a. Early ROM minimizes scarring.
   b. Tenolysis has variable success.
2. **Malunion.**
   a. Rotational deformity can be treated with derotational osteotomy.
   b. Angular deformity can be treated with closing wedge osteotomy.
3. **Symptomatic hardware.**
   a. Prominent plates or screws can lead to pain and tenosynovitis.
   b. Treatment: Hardware removal after fracture has healed.
4. **Pin-tract infections.**

II. **Metacarpal fractures**
A. **Evaluation:** Similar to that for phalangeal fractures
B. **Metacarpal head fractures**
1. Undisplaced fractures: Treated with immobilization alone.
2. Displaced oblique fractures: ORIF with K-wires or small screws.
C. **Metacarpal neck fractures** (e.g., Boxer's fracture, little finger metacarpal)
1. Result of a direct blow to metacarpal head; common in little and ring fingers.
2. Metacarpal head is usually depressed (apex dorsal); closed reduction should be attempted. Acceptable residual deformity postreduction:
   a. Index finger (IF) or middle finger (MF): Less than 10 degrees.
   b. Ring finger (RF): Less than 30 degrees.
   c. Little finger (LF): Less than 40 degrees.
   d. More angular deformity is allowed at little and ring metacarpals due to increased carpometacarpal joint motion relative to index and middle fingers.
   e. The allowable residual deformity should be individualized for each patient. Untreated residual angulation can result in the patient feeling the metacarpal head in the palm with gripping, and result in a loss of strength with power grip.
3. No rotational deformity is acceptable for any of the metacarpals.
D. **Metacarpal shaft fractures**
1. **Transverse fractures:** Can often be treated with closed reduction and splint or cast.

2. Spiral and long oblique fractures.
  a. More unstable; prone to shortening and malrotation.
  b. ORIF indicated if:
   (1) Concern regarding shortening/rotation and desire to get moving earlier to prevent stiffness associated with splinting.
   (2) Greater than 3 mm shortening.
   (3) Angulation greater than 10 degrees (index/middle metacarpals).
   (4) Angulation greater than 20 degrees (ring/little metacarpals).
   (5) Multiple fractures.
3. Fractures with excessive comminution, open fractures with severe soft tissue injury, and fractures with segmental bone loss may require external fixation.

E. Metacarpal base fractures
 1. When central digits are involved (IF, MF, RF), usually immobilization alone is sufficient.
 2. Base of thumb metacarpal is less protected.
  a. Bennett's fracture-dislocation.
   (1) Oblique intraarticular fracture of the base of the thumb metacarpal.
   (2) Small volar ulnar fragment remains attached to anterior oblique ligament ("volar beak ligament").
   (3) Larger (distal) fragment is displaced proximally and abducted by pull of abductor pollicis longus (APL).
   (4) Usually repaired with closed reduction and percutaneous pinning.
  b. Rolando's fracture
   (1) Comminuted intraarticular fracture of the base of the thumb metacarpal.
   (2) Comminution results in T- or Y-shaped fracture lines.
   (3) Usually requires ORIF (i.e., plate and screws).
 3. Base of little finger metacarpal.
  a. "Baby Bennett's" or reverse Bennett's fracture.
  b. Analogous to Bennett's fracture, but deforming force on main metacarpal fragment is the extensor carpi ulnaris (ECU).

III. Scaphoid fractures
A. Introduction.
 1. Most common carpal bone fracture.
 2. Common in young men.
 3. Scaphoid waist fractures are most frequent.
B. Anatomy
 1. Principal blood supply enters the distal pole of the scaphoid.
 2. Proximal pole receives blood supply via intraosseous branches from distal pole, leading to slower healing and higher rates of nonunion in proximal pole fractures.
C. Physical examination suggestive of scaphoid pathology
 1. "Anatomic snuffbox" tenderness (between extensor pollicis longus [EPL] and extensor pollicis brevis [EPB] tendons).
 2. Watson's scaphoid shift test (palmar pressure at proximal pole while radially deviating the wrist; the scaphoid flexes volarly with radial deviation of wrist) is positive (scaphoid flexion is able to be counteracted with examiner's pressure) in cases of ligamentous injury and/or fracture.
D. Radiographs
 1. Standard wrist x-ray series with scaphoid view (posteroanterior wrist in ulnar deviation).
 2. Undisplaced scaphoid fractures may take up to 2 weeks to become visible on radiographs (fracture resorption improves visualization).
E. Treatment
 1. Splint or cast all suspected cases (mechanism, tenderness) of scaphoid fractures for 1 to 2 weeks, with follow-up exam and x-rays, because many scaphoid fractures are unrecognized on initial x-rays.

    2. Undisplaced waist and distal pole fractures: Usually stable; treat with short-arm thumb spica cast for 6 to 12 weeks.

    3. Undisplaced proximal pole fractures: Heal more slowly (12–24 weeks); treat with long-arm thumb spica cast for first 6 weeks, followed by short-arm thumb spica cast. Consider ORIF.

    4. Displaced fractures (>1 mm displacement or any angulation): Unstable and require ORIF via dorsal or volar approach. Herbert or Acutrak screws (headless, variable, or multipitch screws) are used to compress the fracture; immediate ROM is possible with rigid fixation.

F. Complications

   1. Nonunion

    a. Defined as failure to heal after 6 months.

    b. Incidence increases for proximal pole fractures and displaced fractures (up to 90%, versus 5%–10% for waist fractures).

    c. Risk factors: Delay in diagnosis, inadequate immobilization and associated ligamentous instability. If left untreated, post-traumatic arthritis and carpal collapse often follow.

    d. Evaluation: Thin-cut computed tomographic (CT) scan to determine exact anatomy.

    e. Treatment: ORIF with bone grafting if articular surfaces are intact and reduction is possible; salvage procedures (proximal row carpectomy, intercarpal arthrodesis) are indicated in advanced cases (carpal collapse, arthritis, etc.).

   2. Malunion

    a. Occurs when angulated fracture heals without anatomic reduction.

    b. Usually heals with apex dorsal angulation (humpback deformity); this leads to dorsal intercalated segmental instability (DISI), as evidenced by an increased scapholunate angle.

    c. End result: Post-traumatic arthritis, loss of motion, and decreased grip strength.

   3. Post-traumatic arthritis

    a. Associated with scaphoid nonunion and malunion.

    b. Scapholunate advanced collapse (SLAC), a pattern of post-traumatic arthritis, can result from scaphoid nonunion and malunion.

   4. Avascular necrosis

    a. Risk is 90% in proximal pole fractures; risk is 30% to 50% in waist fractures.

    b. Evaluation: X-rays reveal sclerosis in the proximal fragment; magnetic resonance imaging (MRI) is the most sensitive and specific test and is indicated when x-rays are equivocal.

    c. Treatment: ORIF with bone grafting in select cases; vascularized bone graft from distal radius has been successful; salvage procedures include proximal pole excision, proximal row carpectomy, and various subtotal and total wrist fusions.

IV. Distal radius fractures

  A. General information

    1. Most common fracture of the upper extremity.

    2. Very heterogeneous group of injuries; wide variety of patients.

    3. Management remains controversial and challenging; consistently good clinical outcomes are difficult to obtain.

    4. Residual articular incongruity results in post-traumatic arthritis in most patients.

    5. Maximum functional recovery may take 6 to 12 months or longer.

  B. Anatomy

    1. Distal radius has three concave articular surfaces: scaphoid fossa, lunate fossa, and sigmoid notch.

    2. Distal radioulnar joint (DRUJ): Sigmoid notch articulates with ulnar head.

    3. Triangular fibrocartilage complex (TFCC): Soft tissue structure between the ulna and the carpus; may be injured in distal radius fractures.

       4. Radius normally carries about 80% of axial load across the wrist; increased radial shortening or dorsal tilt with fractures can lead to greater loads shifted to the ulna.

C. History

1. Mechanism.
   a. Most common: Compressive loading on dorsiflexed wrist ("fell on an outstretched hand")
   b. Others: Excessive force placed on flexed wrist, shearing mechanism, or direct blow
2. Osteoporosis is a significant predisposing factor.
3. Degree of comminution is proportional to the energy transferred to the bone.

D. Physical examination

1. Wrist tenderness, swelling, deformity.
2. More severe swelling with high-energy injuries.
3. "Silver fork deformity": Dorsal displacement of distal radius (classic Colles' pattern).
4. Skin integrity (abrasions from fall versus open fractures).
5. Neurovascular status.
   a. Median nerve compromise is relatively common.
   b. Reassess after fracture reduction.

E. Radiographs and imaging

1. Posteroanterior (PA) and lateral x-rays: Oblique views are often helpful.
2. Scaphoid series (PA wrist with wrist in ulnar deviation and fist clenched): Helps evaluate associated scaphoid fracture and/or scapholunate ligament injury.
3. Radiographic measurements: Assess severity of fracture and evaluate reduction (Fig. 36-1).
   a. Radial inclination: Average is 23 degrees (PA view).
   b. Radial length: Average is 12 mm (PA view).
   c. Volar tilt: Average is 11 degrees (lateral view).
   d. Also assess Gilula's arcs/lines, scapholunate interval, associated ulna fractures (especially ulnar styloid), and DRUJ.
4. Subtle or complex fractures may require other imaging modalities.
   a. CT: Best for evaluating complex or comminuted fractures (e.g., articular depression fractures).
   b. MRI: Best for evaluating soft tissue injuries.

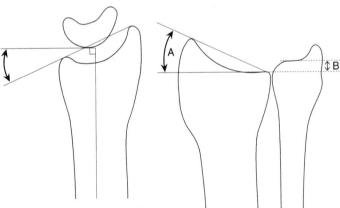

A Volar tilt (lateral radiograph)
    Normal = 12°
    Acceptable ≥ 0°

B Radial inclination (A) and ulnar variance (B) (PA radiograph)

Fig. 36-1. Distal radius, normal angles of inclination. **A:** Lateral view and **B:** PA view.

F. Fracture description or classification
   1. Numerous classification systems exist (Frykman, Melone, AO/ASIF, Rayhack).
   2. None is universally accepted; each has its shortcomings.
   3. The descriptive system is most practical (see "General Principles").
G. Eponyms and named fractures
   1. Historically used, but many fracture patterns do not fit into one specific pattern.
   2. **Colles' fracture:** Extraarticular fracture with dorsal comminution, dorsal displacement of distal fragment, and radial shortening.
   3. **Smith's (reverse Colles') fracture:** Volar displacement of distal fragment.
   4. **Barton's fracture:** Intraarticular fracture (wrist fracture-dislocation); can be volar or dorsal, usually unstable.
   5. **Chauffeur's fracture:** Intraarticular fracture of radial styloid.
   6. **Die-punch fracture:** Intraarticular depression fracture of lunate fossa.
H. Associated injuries
   1. **Median nerve compression or neurapraxia.**
      a. Usually improves after reduction.
      b. If not improved after 48 hours, exploration and carpal tunnel release are indicated.
   2. **Compartment syndrome:** Fewer than 1% of distal radius fractures (see Chapter 45, "Hand Infections, Compartment Syndrome, and High-Energy Injuries").
   3. **TFCC injury:** Associated with fractures at the base of the ulnar styloid.
   4. **Ligament injury:** Carpal ligament injury is common (e.g., scapholunate ligament).
I. Treatment principles
   1. **Goal: Anatomic reduction**
      a. Maximizes function and minimizes the risk of post-traumatic arthritis.
      b. The younger and more active the patient, the more critical it is to achieve anatomic reduction.
   2. **Stability**
      a. Stable, reduced fractures: Usually treat nonoperatively.
      b. Unstable and/or irreducible fractures: Usually treat operatively.
         (1) Articular depression greater than 2 mm.
         (2) Radial shortening greater than 5 mm.
         (3) Dorsal tilt greater than 20 degrees.
         (4) Excessive comminution.
   3. **Timing**
      a. In most cases, initial reduction and splinting can be performed in the emergency room.
      b. Operative intervention, if required, can be scheduled within 7 to 10 days.
   4. **Immobilization**
      a. Initial splint is usually sugar-tong type, to allow for some swelling and to prevent pronation/supination.
      b. May change to a removable splint or short- or long-arm cast, depending on individual patient and fracture pattern.
      c. If uninjured, fingers should be free and patient should work on finger ROM as early as 1 to 2 weeks after injury.
      d. Do not immobilize the shoulder, because of the risk of rotator cuff tendonitis and adhesive capsulitis.
      e. Undisplaced fractures: Usually immobilize for 4 weeks.
      f. Displaced fractures (reduced): Usually immobilize for 6 weeks.
         (1) Less in children.
         (2) Less when stable ORIF performed.
         (3) More for complex fractures.
J. Treatment algorithm
   1. **Open fractures**
      a. Washout in the operating room is generally required.

   b. Thoroughly debride all contamination and nonviable tissues.

   c. Controversy exists regarding immediate versus delayed fracture fixation.

   d. Consider external fixation.

  2. Closed fractures

   a. Undisplaced fractures: Immobilization alone is usually sufficient.

   b. Displaced fractures: Attempt closed reduction (see below).

    (1) Adequate reduction.

     (a) Stable.

      (i) Immobilization may be sufficient.

      (ii) Weekly x-rays to check reduction.

     (b) Unstable: Operative fixation required.

    (2) Inadequate reduction: Operative fixation required.

K. Closed reduction

 1. Relies on ligamentotaxis to restore anatomic alignment

 2. Procedure

  a. Hang hand from finger traps with shoulder abducted 90 degrees and elbow flexed 90 degrees.

  b. Anesthesia: Conscious sedation and/or hematoma block (plain lidocaine injected into fracture hematoma site).

  c. Longitudinal traction is provided by weights (usually 10–20 pounds) hung from stockinette just proximal to elbow.

  d. Fracture reduction maneuvers.

   (1) Re-creation of injury pattern (e.g., wrist hyperextension for Colles' fractures) under continuous longitudinal traction.

   (2) Followed by reduction move (e.g., palmar translating force for Colles' fractures) distal to fracture site.

  e. C-arm guidance may be used to assess adequacy of reduction.

  f. Apply sugar-tong splint and obtain postreduction x-rays.

 3. Guidelines for adequate closed reduction

  a. Articular incongruity less than 2 mm.

  b. Radial shortening less than 5 mm.

  c. Dorsal tilt less than 10 degrees.

L. Operative reduction and fixation

 1. Closed reduction with percutaneous pinning (CRPP)

  a. Generally for unstable and/or irreducible extraarticular fractures.

  b. Kapandji technique (intrafocal pinning).

   (1) Heavy K-wire is directed through the fracture line dorsally or radially.

   (2) Use K-wire as lever arm to reduce fracture.

   (3) Drive K-wire into opposite cortex for stabilization.

 2. Open reduction and internal fixation

  a. Many types of implants are available: K-wires, screws, intraosseous wiring, plates and screws, and manufacturer-specific fracture fixation systems.

  b. Limited approaches are preferred for simple, intraarticular fracture patterns such as radial styloid fractures and articular margin fractures.

  c. Complex articular fractures require more complete exposure and/or multiple approaches.

  d. Surgical approaches

   (1) Volar: Between flexor carpi radialis (FCR) and radial artery; indicated for volarly displaced distal radius fractures; allows for concomitant carpal tunnel release.

   (2) Dorsal: Through third dorsal extensor compartment; indicated for complex intraarticular fractures.

   (3) Dorsal radial: Used for displaced radial styloid fractures.

 3. External fixation

  a. Indicated for unstable fractures with excessive comminution.

  b. Maintains length of the distal radius while healing occurs.

  c. Avoid overdistraction: Can lead to finger stiffness and fracture nonunion or delayed union.

  d. Avoid leaving wrist in flexion: Can lead to median nerve compression.

  e. Place pins with open technique to avoid eccentric pin placement and injury to radial sensory nerve.

 4. Arthroscopy

  a. Can be used to confirm reduction (i.e., check articular surface).

  b. Can be used to diagnose and treat ligamentous tears, TFCC tears.

 5. Bone grafting

  a. Indicated when articular depression, bone loss, and extensive comminution are present.

  b. Example: Die-punch fracture—the articular fragment is elevated, and bone graft is placed proximally in the created metaphyseal defect.

  c. Bone graft source is often allograft or bone substitute materials (nonunion is rare in distal radius fractures).

 6. Combinations of the previously listed options: Complex fracture patterns frequently require combinations of the above (such as ORIF, external fixation, and bone grafting).

M. Complications

 1. Malunion: Relatively common (e.g., dorsal tilt and loss of radial length can lead to ulnocarpal impaction, DRUJ incongruity, pain, weakness, and decreased ROM).

 2. Nonunion: Rare except in cases of overdistraction during external fixation.

 3. Tendon rupture: Usually EPL (a late complication).

 4. Post-traumatic arthritis.

 5. Complex regional pain syndromes (CRPS).

Dislocations and Ligamentous Injuries

I. Phalangeal dislocations

A. Distal interphalangeal (DIP) joint dislocations

 1. Anatomy and mechanism

  a. Usually dorsal dislocation; due to hyperextension injury of the DIP joint.

  b. About 60% are associated with a volar laceration.

  c. Often involve disruption of both collateral ligaments and the volar plate.

 2. Treatment

  a. Simple (reducible)

   (1) Closed reduction under metacarpal block: Extend distal phalanx, then push dorsally over condyles of middle phalanx.

   (2) Check x-rays to confirm joint congruity and rule out associated fracture; splint for 2 weeks.

  b. Complex (irreducible)

   (1) Open reduction is required.

   (2) Possible causes include interposition of the profundus tendon (implies disruption of at least one collateral ligament), volar plate, or displaced articular fracture fragment.

 3. Complications: Recurrent instability, post-traumatic arthritis

B. Proximal interphalangeal (PIP) joint dislocations

 1. Anatomy and mechanism

  a. PIP joint is a hinged joint with articular congruity between the two condyles of the proximal phalanx and two concave surfaces of the middle phalanx.

  b. Strong volar plate and collateral ligaments provide additional stability.

 2. Dorsal dislocation

  a. More common than volar dislocation.

  b. Obvious deformity with dorsal location of middle phalanx.

    c. Radiographs may reveal an avulsion fracture from the volar surface of the middle phalanx (distal volar plate insertion site).

    d. Treatment.

        (1) Closed reduction under metacarpal block with longitudinal traction.

        (2) Stable reductions are treated with extension block splinting or buddy taping for 3 weeks and early ROM.

        (3) Unstable reductions are treated with extension block splinting in 20 degrees of flexion for about 3 weeks.

    e. Rotational deformity of the finger may suggest displacement of the middle phalanx between the central slip and lateral band.

3. Volar dislocation

    a. Lack of active extension of middle phalanx against gentle resistance indicates central slip rupture.

    b. Radiographs may reveal avulsion fracture from dorsum of middle phalanx (central slip insertion).

    c. Treatment

        (1) Closed reduction with longitudinal traction and flexion at PIP joint.

        (2) After reduction, must assess PIP joint extension.

            (a) If central slip intact: Immobilization with buddy taping and early ROM.

            (b) If central slip disrupted: Treat as per central slip rupture (see Chapter 37, "Tendon Injuries and Tendonitis").

    d. Complications: Progressive boutonnière deformity, PIP joint stiffness.

4. PIP joint fracture-dislocations

    a. Can be quite disabling.

    b. Radiographs are essential. Injuries range from a small articular fragment to pieces involving more than 50% of joint surface.

    c. Treatment.

        (1) Stable PIP joint with less than 30% articular surface involved: Dorsal extension block splinting.

        (2) Unstable PIP joint and/or more than 30% of articular surface involved: ORIF.

        (3) Comminuted fractures: Volar plate arthroplasty (volar fragment excision and advancement of volar plate distally on middle phalanx).

    d. Complications: Persistent instability; joint stiffness.

C. Metacarpophalangeal (MP) joint dislocations

    1. Less common than PIP joint dislocations

    2. Dorsal dislocations are more common; usually involve the index or little fingers.

    3. Evaluation.

        a. Simple (reducible): Notable deformity with marked MP joint hyperextension.

        b. Complex (irreducible).

            (1) Deformity not as obvious; MP joint only slightly hyperextended.

            (2) Cannot be reduced, due to interposition of the volar plate ("buttonhole effect"; look for puckering of volar skin and/or presence of a sesamoid bone in widened MP joint) or trapping of metacarpal head between lumbrical (radially) and flexor tendon (ulnarly).

    4. Treatment.

        a. Simple dislocations.

            (1) Closed reduction via gentle hyperextension at MP joint followed by relocating proximal phalanx onto metacarpal head.

            (2) After reduction, splinting with MP joints in 50 degrees of flexion for 7 to 10 days followed by buddy taping. ORIF is recommended if associated joint subluxation and/or intraarticular fracture involving more than 20% of joint surface is present.

      b. Complex dislocations: Usually require open reduction (via dorsal or volar approach).

II. Thumb dislocations

A. Thumb MP joint dislocation

1. Multiaxial diarthrodial joint: Allows for flexion, extension, limited adduction, abduction, and circumduction.
2. Stability is critical for grip and pinch.
3. **Dorsal dislocation.**
   a. Simple: Closed reduction and thumb spica splint immobilization.
   b. Complex: Irreducible; usually due to volar plate or FPL interposition; requires operative reduction and soft tissue repair followed by splinting.
4. **Volar dislocation:** Rare.

B. Thumb ulnar collateral ligament (UCL) injuries

1. Injury produced by forceful radial deviation of thumb.
   a. Acute rupture: "Skier's thumb".
   b. Chronic attenuation: "Gamekeeper's thumb".
2. Physical examination and treatment.
   a. Tenderness over ulnar collateral ligament; ligamentous laxity should always be compared with the contralateral (healthy) thumb.
   b. Partial tear: Opens less than 45 degrees with radial stress; requires thumb spica splinting with thumb MP joint held in slight flexion for 4 to 6 weeks.
   c. Complete tear: Opens more than 45 degrees with radial stress.
      (1) Can be associated with a (palpable) Stener lesion (interposition of adductor pollicis aponeurosis between torn end of UCL and its insertion at the base of proximal phalanx).
      (2) Requires operative repair with suture anchor or pullout button.

C. Thumb radial collateral ligament (RCL) injuries

1. Rare and less debilitating than ulnar collateral ligament injuries.
2. Treated nonoperatively with splint or cast.

III. Carpal dislocations and ligamentous injuries

A. Anatomy

1. **There are seven carpal bones** (excluding pisiform, a sesamoid bone within FCU tendon).
2. **Row theory** (traditional wrist model) divides carpal bones into two rows.
   a. Proximal row: Scaphoid, lunate, triquetrum.
   b. Distal row: Trapezium, trapezoid, capitate, hamate.
3. **Wrist ligaments.**
   a. Intrinsic ligaments.
      (1) Connect carpal bones within a carpal row.
      (2) Most important are scapholunate (SL) and lunotriquetral (LT) ligaments.
   b. Extrinsic ligaments
      (1) Connect bones between carpal rows (spans midcarpal joint).
      (2) Volar extrinsic ligaments are stronger than dorsal extrinsic ligaments.
4. **Kinematics.**
   a. Wrist motion is complex and occurs primarily at radiocarpal and midcarpal interface.
   b. Proximal carpal row flexes with radial deviation of wrist and extends with ulnar deviation. This function is impaired with SL and LT ligament disruptions.

B. Injury types

1. No single classification system effectively describes all of the various patterns of injury.
2. **Perilunate injury.**
   a. Occurs in stages as ligaments sequentially fail around the lunate.
      (1) Stage I: Scapholunate ligament tear.
      (2) Stage II: Capitolunate ligament tear.

(3) Stage III: Lunotriquetral ligament tear (dorsal perilunate dislocation).

(4) Stage IV: Dorsal radiolunate ligament tear (volar lunate dislocation).

   b. Note that **dorsal** perilunate dislocation (stage III) is caused by the same injury pattern as **volar** lunate dislocation (stage IV).

3. Greater and lesser arc injuries.

   a. Perilunate carpal disruptions can be purely ligamentous or can have associated carpal fractures.

   b. Greater arc injury (involves carpal fracture).

      (1) Combines carpal bone fracture with perilunate dislocation.

      (2) Fractures occur because injury pattern involves an arc of greater radius around lunate that passes through surrounding osseous structures.

      (3) Transscaphoid perilunate fracture-dislocation

         (a) Combines scaphoid fracture with perilunate dislocation.

         (b) Most common type of greater arc injury.

         (c) Immediate treatment: Closed reduction and splinting to minimize damage to neurovascular structures.

         (d) Definitive treatment.

            (i) Volar approach: Allows for scaphoid fracture ORIF with screw or K-wires; repairs volar ligament injury.

            (ii) Dorsal approach: Assists with anatomic reduction of carpal bones (restores lunate in its fossa in distal radius and capitate in fossa in distal lunate articulation).

      (4) Transradial styloid perilunate fracture-dislocation.

         (a) Combined radial styloid fracture with perilunate dislocation.

         (b) Immediate treatment: Closed reduction and splinting as in above injuries, with adequate reduction of radial styloid fragment.

         (c) Definitive treatment.

            (i) ORIF of radial styloid fracture.

            (ii) Reduction, soft tissue repair, and K-wire fixation of perilunate injury are then performed as in isolated perilunate dislocations.

   c. Lesser arc injury (purely ligamentous injury).

      (1) No fractures because pattern of injury is via an arc of smaller radius through ligaments immediately adjacent to lunate.

      (2) Most common injury patterns are dorsal perilunate (lunate remains in its fossa in distal radius with dorsal dislocation of capitate and rest of carpus) and volar lunate (lunate displaced from fossa of distal radius) dislocations.

      (3) Perilunate dislocation (dorsal perilunate and volar lunate dislocations).

         (a) Immediate treatment.

            (i) Closed reduction and splinting to minimize damage to neurovascular structures.

            (ii) Open reduction is often required in volar lunate dislocations.

         (b) Definitive treatment.

            (i) ORIF via combined dorsal (between third and fourth compartments) and volar (via carpal canal) approaches.

            (ii) Repair volar ligament injury.

            (iii) K-wires secure scaphoid, lunate, and capitate in their respective anatomic positions.

            (iv) Pins remain in place for 8 to 12 weeks.

4. Axial (longitudinal) carpal instability.

   a. Rare, high-energy injuries associated with significant soft tissue disruption.

   b. Direction of disruption is in longitudinal plane that is perpendicular to plane of perilunate injury.

c. Radial axial injuries: Involve separation of first and second metacarpals and trapezium/trapezoid from remaining ulnar part of hand and carpus.

d. Ulnar axial injuries: Involve separation between third and fourth metacarpals and capitate/hamate.

e. Treatment: ORIF via dorsal approach.

C. Instability patterns

1. Carpal instability dissociative (CID): Includes intrinsic ligament disruptions that occur within a carpal row.

   a. Dorsal intercalated segmental instability (DISI; rotatory subluxation of the scaphoid).

   (1) Scaphoid and lunate dissociated due to scapholunate ligament disruption or scaphoid fracture.

   (2) Lunate rotated dorsally via the LT ligament as the counterbalancing force of the SL ligament is lost.

   (3) Physical examination: Watson test.

   (a) Identifies SL ligament disruption.

   (b) Palpable clunk present with thumb pressure applied dorsally over volar scaphoid tubercle during radial and ulnar wrist deviation.

   (4) Radiographs.

   (a) Lateral wrist x-ray.

   (i) Increased dorsal tilt of lunate (radiolunate angle >15 degrees).

   (ii) Increased scapholunate angle (>60 degrees).

   (b) PA x-ray.

   (i) Widened scapholunate interval (>3 mm) or scaphoid fracture.

   (ii) Cortical ring sign ("double density" appearance of shortened scaphoid) occurs due to abnormal scaphoid rotation.

   (5) Early diagnosis and treatment of SL ligament rupture can prevent DISI deformity and associated carpal arthritis (SLAC wrist).

   (6) Treatment of acute SL injuries.

   (a) ORIF with direct SL ligament repair.

   (b) Dorsal approach between third and fourth dorsal compartments.

   (c) K-wires passed from scaphoid to lunate and capitate.

   (d) Suture anchors: Allow for anatomic repair of ligament to bone when possible.

   (e) Blatt capsulodesis: Repair augmented with dorsal capsule if SL ligament attenuated.

   (f) Pins removed after 8 to 12 weeks.

   (7) Treatment of chronic SL injuries (>6–8 weeks old).

   (a) No associated arthritis: Treat as acute injury with Blatt capsulodesis.

   (b) Associated arthritis present or irreducible dislocation: Treat with limited arthrodesis (scaphotrapezial-trapezoid fusion; scapholunate fusion; scaphocapitate fusion).

   (8) Scapholunate advanced collapse (SLAC wrist).

   (a) Systematic progression of intercarpal degenerative arthritis following chronic SL ligament rupture or scaphoid fracture nonunion with collapse.

   (b) Four stages.

   (i) Stage I: Stylocarpal arthritis.

   (ii) Stage II: Scaphoid fossa involvement.

   (iii) Stage III: Capitolunate arthritis.

   (iv) Stage IV: Diffuse carpal arthritis.

   (c) Treatment.

   (i) Scaphoid excision with four-corner fusion.

(ii) Other options: Proximal row carpectomy, complete wrist fusion, and wrist arthroplasty.

b. **Volar intercalated segmental instability (VISI).**
   (1) Much less common and not understood as well as DISI.
   (2) Thought to be due to disruption of both LT ligament and dorsal radiocarpal ligaments.
   (3) Lunate is rotated volarly via forces applied through SL ligament alone (because the LT ligament is disrupted).
   (4) Physical examination: Shuck test.
      (a) Identifies LT ligament disruption.
      (b) Triquetrum and lunate shifted volarly and dorsally to elicit instability or discomfort.
   (5) Radiographs: Lateral wrist x-ray reveals decreased SL angle (<30 degrees) and increased radiolunate angle (>15 degrees).
   (6) Treatment.
      (a) Isolated LT ligament tears: Nonoperative management with nonsteroidal anti-inflammatory agents and splinting.
      (b) LT tears associated with VISI deformity.
         (i) Management controversial
         (ii) Options include soft tissue reconstruction with dorsal capsule or tendon autograft or arthrodesis (such as four-corner fusion).

2. **Carpal instability nondissociative (CIND).**
   a. Extrinsic ligament disruption between carpal rows.
   b. Midcarpal instability.
      (1) Frequently insidious onset.
      (2) Common in patients with increased ligamentous laxity.
      (3) Sudden painful clunk often present when shift occurs between the two carpal rows.
      (4) Diagnosis.
         (a) Physical examination (palpable clunk).
         (b) Stress radiographs.
         (c) Fluoroscopic examination under anesthesia.
      (5) Treatment.
         (a) Soft tissue reconstruction (if no associated arthritis).
         (b) Midcarpal arthrodesis (in chronic cases with associated arthritis).

3. **Carpal instability complex (CIC).**
   a. Combines CID and CIND (both intrinsic and extrinsic ligament disruption patterns are present).
   b. Perilunate dislocations.

4. **Static versus dynamic instability.**
   a. Static instability patterns.
      (1) Fixed.
      (2) Clearly seen on routine radiographs.
   b. Dynamic instability patterns.
      (1) Transient.
      (2) Not present on routine radiographs.
      (3) Require stress x-rays or fluoroscopy for diagnosis.
      (4) Example: Clenched-fist PA view to identify dynamic SL ligament instability.

D. **Acute versus chronic injury.**
   1. **Acute injury.**
      a. Readily identifiable injury with associated pain and swelling.
      b. Complete neurovascular evaluation important.
   2. **Chronic injury.**
      a. Injury patterns more subtle than acute injuries both clinically and radiographically.
      b. Additional studies often needed.

(1) Wrist arthrography, fluoroscopy, and MRI have been used historically.
(2) Wrist arthroscopy.
　　(a) Becoming more popular as the most complete and direct means of carpal ligament evaluation.
　　(b) Also provides for examination of carpal bones (osteochondral defects, arthritis assessment) and synovium (hypertrophy, inflammation).

Pearls

1. Use the universal descriptive system for all fractures.
2. The choice of fixation must maximize rigidity while minimizing exposure (periosteal stripping).
3. Sometimes a more invasive approach to fixation allows earlier mobilization and a better result overall.
4. In the adult patient, interphalangeal joint stiffness should be avoided at all costs—get the fingers moving as soon as possible!
5. Recovery from a wrist fracture can take 6 to 12 months or longer; prepare patients for the long haul.

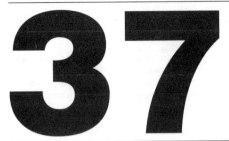

Tendon Injuries and Tendonitis

Michelle S. Caird

Tendon Blood Supply and Healing

I. **Anatomy and general considerations**
   A. **Definition:** Strong, dense connective tissues that attach muscle to bone.
   B. **Tendon makeup:** Type 1 collagen → longitudinal bundles → fibrils → fascicles → tendons.
   C. **Paratenon-covered tendons and synovial tendons** have different blood supply and methods of healing.
   D. **Three phases of healing**
      1. **Inflammatory (first week):** Cell proliferation and cleanup.
      2. **Proliferative (weeks 2–4):** Fibroblasts and capillary buds migrate in and produce random collagen.
      3. **Remodeling (months 2–6):** Longitudinal organization of collagen fibers in line with stress.

II. **Tendons with paratenon**
   A. **In general, tendons that move in straight lines** (no sharp turns) have paratenon (e.g., extensor carpi radialis longus [ECRL] and extensor carpi radialis brevis [ECRB]).
   B. **Paratenon** is composed of loose connective tissue, continuous with the tendon surface.
   C. **Blood supply emanates** from vessels in the perimysium, at the bony insertion, and at **many points** along the course of the tendon, forming a longitudinal anastomotic capillary system.
   D. **Healing from paratenon:** Fibroblasts and capillary buds migrate into the injured area.

III. **Tendons with synovial sheath**
   A. **In general, tendons that take sharp turns around joints (e.g., flexor tendons)** have synovial sheaths.
   B. **The tendon sheath** surrounds the tendon and produces synovial fluid for low-friction gliding.
   C. **Blood supply emanates** from vessels in the perimysium, at the bony insertion, and through mesotendon conduits (vincula) at discrete points along the tendon.
   D. **Areas of relative avascularity** exist along the tendon, which receive nutrition by synovial diffusion.
   E. **Healing (controversial)**
      1. **Extrinsic:** Fibroblasts migrate from the sheath into the injured site (also form adhesions).
      2. **Intrinsic:** Tendon cells can migrate across closely approximated ends and heal with nutrients from synovial fluid.

Timing of Repair

I. **Acute and subacute repair**

    A. If the condition of the soft tissues allows, primary tendon repair should be performed on an urgent basis (within several days).

    B. After 1 week: Increased risk of adhesions with primary repair.

    C. After 3 weeks: Muscle contraction interferes with primary repair.

II. Delayed reconstruction

    A. Flexor tendon injuries

        1. One-stage reconstruction with a tendon graft is used *only* if the flexor sheath is intact and full passive motion is present.

        2. Two-stage reconstruction is preferred if the above conditions are not met and after soft tissues are quiet (3–4 weeks after injury).

            a. First stage: Temporary silicone implant (Hunter rod) to create a bed for the graft.

            b. Second stage: Wait at least 2 to 3 months, then exchange the rod for a tendon graft (palmaris longus, extensor digitorum longus, or plantaris).

    B. Extensor tendon injuries

        1. Frequently need staged reconstruction after degloving injuries to the hand.

        2. Two-stage reconstruction

            a. First stage: Obtain adequate skin coverage with or without placement of silicone implants.

            b. Second stage: Wait about 3 months, and then perform tendon graft.

III. Tenolysis

    A. Indicated if discrepancy exists between active and passive range of motion (ROM).

    B. Timing

        1. After maximized therapy for full passive motion of all joints.

        2. After soft tissues achieve equilibrium and tendon is healed.

    C. In flexors, preserve A2 and A4 pulleys to prevent bowstringing.

Tendon Suture Techniques

I. General considerations

    A. Atraumatic handling of tendon ends, synthetic braided nonabsorbable suture, and end-to-end repair.

    B. Sheath repair is controversial. The theory is that closure improves synovial nutrition for healing, but this has not been proven.

    C. Tensile strength–time relationship

        1. Weakest 7 to 10 days after repair.

            a. Postoperative day 10 is the most common time for rupture after primary repair.

            b. Treat with prompt exploration and repair.

        2. Most strength has returned 4 to 6 weeks after repair.

        3. Maximum strength 6 months after repair.

II. Core suture (Fig. 37-1)

    A. Strength of repair is proportional to the number of core strands crossing the repair.

    B. There are a number of ways to suture a tendon, but all have common features.

        1. Small grasping stitches avoid pullout.

        2. Knots buried in the repair site assist in smooth gliding.

    C. Most common: Modified Kessler stitch.

III. Epitendinous suture

    A. Consists of a running stitch along the edges of the tendon repair after the core sutures are placed.

    B. Leads to decreased gap formation, which is the first step toward failure.

    C. Smoothes edge for gliding.

    D. Decreases adhesion formation.

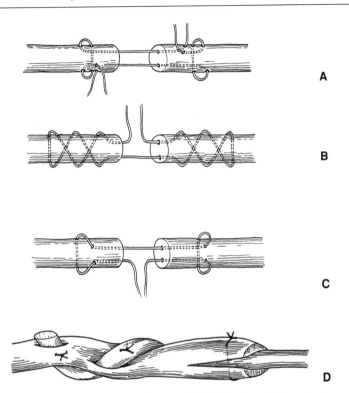

Fig. 37-1. Flexor tendon suturing techniques. **A:** Kessler suture. **B:** Bunnell suture. **C:** Modified Kessler suture. **D:** Pulvertaft weave suture results in a very strong juncture, but is not suitable for use within the flexor tendon sheath due to its bulk. (From Zidel P. Tendon healing and flexor tendon surgery. In *Grabb and Smith's Plastic Surgery*, 5th ed. Aston SJ, Beasley RW, Thorne CH, (eds). Philadelphia, Lippincott-Raven, 1997. With permission.)

Therapy Protocols

I. **General considerations**
   A. **Early controlled motion** prevents adhesions and improves healing and strength of tendon repairs.
   B. **Requires a cooperative patient** and close interaction with physician and hand therapist.
II. **Splinting**
   A. **Flexor tendons:** In general, wrist and metacarpophalangeal (MP) joints flexed; interphalangeal (IP) joints extended. Allows passive flexion of IP joints, if wrist flexed.
   B. **Extensor tendons:** Extension splinting of involved joints.
   C. **Small children or noncompliant patients** may need above elbow splint of cast to prevent removal.
III. **Therapy**
   A. **Tendon therapy** is a whole practice unto itself.
   B. **Flexor tendon therapy.**
      1. **Combine dynamic splints** with particular protocols.

2. **Active extension** with rubber band flexion (Kleinert and modifications), controlled passive motion (Durand and similar), and controlled active motion protocols all have their advocates.

C. **Extensor tendon therapy:** A variety of early controlled motion protocols are available, depending on the injury.

Extensor Tendon Injuries

I. **Management by zones**

  A. **General considerations.**

  1. **The dorsum of the hand and forearm** are divided into nine zones, which guide management and predict outcome.

  2. **Odd zones are over each joint;** even zones are in between.

  3. **Multiple attachments limit retraction** of extensors and allow emergency room (ER) repair of many injuries.

  B. **Zone I:** Over the distal interphalangeal (DIP) joint; commonly called mallet finger and classified into four types.

  1. **Type I:** Rupture at insertion. Treat with extension splinting of DIP joint for 6 weeks (Stack splint).

  2. **Type II:** Laceration. Treat with repair and extension splinting. Repair can be performed as a single layer with the skin, using nonabsorbable (nylon) sutures.

  3. **Type III:** Abrasion with tendon loss and overlying soft tissue injury. Treat with coverage and graft or joint fusion.

  4. **Type IV:** Avulsion fracture (bony mallet). Treat with extension splinting if fragment reduces or with internal fixation if joint is subluxed.

  C. **Zone II:** Over the middle phalanx. Assess active and passive extension.

  1. **If active extension is intact** and tendon ends do not move, use simple splinting.

  2. **If full, active extension is not intact** or ends separate, repair.

  D. **Zone III:** Over the proximal interphalangeal (PIP) joint: central slip injury.

  1. **Laceration:** Treat with repair and extension splinting (of PIP only; leave DIP joint free to flex, as this action draws lateral bands and central slip distally, taking pressure off the central slip repair).

  2. **Avulsion:** Commonly from jammed finger. Treat with extension splinting (of PIP only).

  3. **If injury is missed, lateral bands** can sublux volarly and result in a boutonnière deformity.

  E. **Zone IV (and zone II of the thumb):** Over the proximal phalanx. Treat like a zone II injury.

  F. **Zone V (and zone III of the thumb):** Over the MP joint, at extensor tendon or sagittal bands.

  1. **Simple laceration:** Explore and repair tendon or sagittal band.

  2. **Beware of the "fight bite" or human bite wound** with injury in this location (suspect even if not the history given).

    a. Acute: Explore, repair tendon, give antibiotics, and leave skin open.

    b. Old/chronic: May require delayed treatment of tendon, until infection is controlled and soft tissue equilibrium is reached.

    c. The lacerations of the skin, tendon, and joint may not line up directly in the position in which the wound is explored (compared with the position in which the injury occurred): Be wary of deeper penetration.

    d. Suspect and rule out joint involvement.

  G. **Zone VI (and zone IV of the thumb):** Over the metacarpals. If tendon ends are easily retrievable, repair in ER (separate layer to skin repair, using nonabsorbable braided suture—horizontal mattress is acceptable); otherwise, repair in operating room.

H. **Zone VII:** Beneath the extensor retinaculum. Repair tendon with or without partial retinacular excision to prevent adhesions.

I. **Zone VIII:** Over the distal forearm. Treat as zone VI. May require tendon transfers if function lost.

J. **Zone IX:** Muscles of proximal forearm. Difficult to repair: Use large bites of large braided nonabsorbable sutures. May require transfers if function lost.

II. **Outcomes and complications**
   A. **With early treatment, most do fairly well.**
   B. **Worse outcome is associated with the following.**
      1. Distal injuries (zones I–IV).
      2. Infection.
      3. Associated bony and soft tissue injuries.
   C. **Adhesions and extrinsic tightness:** Treat with therapy, followed by tenolysis versus tendon release.
   D. **Missed injuries or late presenting injuries**
      1. **Fight bite:** Septic arthritis and/or cellulites. Needs aggressive irrigation and debridement. Can result in amputation.
      2. **Central slip injuries:** Can result in boutonnière deformity.
      3. **Sagittal band injury:** Subluxation of extensor tendon ulnarly (most common) or radially (rare).

Flexor Tendon Injuries

I. **Pulley system**
   A. **General considerations**
      1. **Pulleys are thickenings along flexor sheaths,** lined with synovium.
      2. **They improve biomechanics of flexor tendons** by preventing bowstringing of tendons during flexion.
   B. **Finger: Annular (five) and cruciate (three) pulleys** (see Fig. 35-5)
      1. **Annular pulleys**
         a. A1 at MP joint, A2 over proximal phalanx, A3 at PIP joint, A4 over middle phalanx, A5 at DIP joint.
         b. A2 and A4 are the most important biomechanically to prevent bowstringing.
      2. **Cruciate pulleys** are between the annular pulleys; they are thinner and less biomechanically important than annular pulleys.
   C. **Thumb:** Annular (two) and oblique (one) pulleys
      1. **Annular pulleys:** A1 at MP joint and A2 at IP joint.
      2. **Oblique pulley:** Extension of adductor pollicis attachment. Lies between A1 and A2. Most important pulley to prevent bowstringing in thumb.

II. **Management by zones** (see Fig. 35-3)
   A. **General considerations**
      1. **Hand and wrist** are divided into five zones, which guide management and help predict outcome.
      2. **The small number of attachments allows for proximal retraction** of lacerated tendons and therefore usually requires exploration and repair in the OR.
      3. **Associated neurovascular injury is common,** so a detailed examination is paramount prior to local anesthetic infiltration.
   B. **Zone I:** Middle of middle phalanx to fingertip (distal to insertion of flexor digitorum superficialis [FDS]; includes only flexor digitorum profundus [FDP]).
      1. **Laceration**
         a. Treat with direct repair.
         b. Avoid advancement, which can result in the **quadrigia effect:** incomplete flexion of FDPs of uninjured fingers when the shortened FDP reaches maximum flexion too early.

2. **Profundus avulsion (jersey finger):** Classification and treatment are based on the level of retraction of the tendon end.
   a. Type I: Into palm. Vincula are disrupted. Requires early treatment.
   b. Type II: Retracts to level of PIP joint because the long vinculum remains intact. Treatment can be performed up to a few months out.
   c. Type III: Retracts to A4 pulley (middle of middle phalanx) because a bony avulsion fragment gets stuck on the pulley. Avulsion fragment should be fixed back into position.
C. **Zone II:** Distal palmar crease to middle of middle phalanx (both FDS and FDP tendons, with FDP volar, proceeding distally).
   1. **Both tendons should be repaired.**
   2. **Tendon lacerations** may not match level of skin laceration or each other, depending on the joint positions at the time of injury.
   3. **Formerly known as "no man's land"** due to high risk of adhesions and poor rehabilitation outcomes.
D. **Zone III:** Transverse carpal ligament to distal palmar crease.
   1. **No sheath here;** outcome is generally better.
   2. **Associated injury to the common digital nerves** and superficial palmar arch is common.
E. **Zone IV:** Under transverse carpal ligament (in carpal tunnel).
   1. **Treat with operative repair** with or without lengthening of transverse carpal ligament.
   2. **Examine median nerve closely for injury.**
F. **Zone V:** Proximal border of transverse carpal ligament to musculotendinous junction. Generally has the best outcomes.
III. **Partial injuries**
A. **Full ROM is present,** but patient has weakness or pain with resisted flexion.
B. **Should be explored.**
   1. **Repair if laceration is greater than 60%,** due to risk of late rupture.
   2. **If less than 60%,** laceration should be left alone because the repair may impede blood supply or create adhesions, or both.
C. **If partial injuries are missed, or fail to present,** late rupture, adhesions, or triggering can result.

Trigger Finger and Thumb

I. **Definition and epidemiology**
A. **Stenosing tenosynovitis of flexor tendons.**
B. **A nodule forms in the flexor tendon,** creating a size mismatch between the tendon and the annular pulley.
C. **A1 pulley**
   1. **The most common site.**
   2. **Proximal edge** is located at the distal palmar crease in the little and ring fingers, between the proximal and distal creases in the middle finger, and at the proximal crease in the index finger and thumb.
D. **Middle-aged women** are the most commonly affected group.
E. **Increased incidence is seen with diabetes, rheumatoid arthritis, gout, and amyloidosis.**
II. **Complaints and examination findings**
A. **Catching, sticking, or occasional locking of fingers in flexed position.**
B. **Pain in distal palm,** or commonly referred to as the PIP joint.
C. **Pain and sticking are often worse on awakening.**
D. **More common in the thumb, long, and ring fingers.**
E. **Slight tenderness volarly over the tendon at the A1 pulley.** Nodule is palpable on tendon with movement. Popping or clicking on flexion/extension, as nodule moves through pulley.
III. **Treatment**

A. Injection
  1. **Most successful for recently acquired cases of triggering.**
  2. **Inject steroid plus local anesthetic** (50% Kenalog-40, 50% plain 1% lidocaine) into tendon sheath at the level of the A1 pulley (locate as above).
  3. **Use a small needle.** Insert down to bone; back out slowly, with pressure on plunger, stopping when solution flows easily into tendon sheath. A fluid wave can be felt down the finger in most cases.
  4. **Remind diabetics** that steroids will affect their blood sugar levels.
B. Splinting
  1. **Low success rate.**
  2. **Extension splint of affected digits** (especially at nighttime if there are morning symptoms).
  3. **Alone or with steroid injections.**
C. Surgery
  1. **Indications.**
    a. Long-standing triggering
    b. Persistent triggering that fails injection and splinting
  2. **Procedure:** Small transverse or Bruner-type incision at proximal edge of pulley (see above). Division of A1 pulley under direct vision.
  3. **Watch and protect the digital neurovascular bundles,** especially at the thumb where the radial bundle courses directly over the A1 pulley.
  4. **Release the entire pulley and have (awake) patient actively test in OR.**

Tenosynovitis

I. De Quervain's tenosynovitis
  A. **Definition: Stenosing tenosynovitis** of the tendons in the first dorsal compartment of the wrist (abductor pollicis longus [APL] and extensor pollicis brevis [EPB]).
  B. **Most common in middle-aged women.**
  C. **Symptoms and signs.**
    1. **Radial-sided wrist pain** with thumb use.
    2. **Positive Finkelstein's test:** Pain with thumb tuck and ulnar deviation of wrist.
    3. **Tenderness over first dorsal compartment.**
    4. **No pain with axial grind test,** which is positive in first carpometacarpal joint arthritis.
  D. Treatment
    1. **Injection with steroid** plus lidocaine into first dorsal compartment.
      a. Inject at distal end of compartment.
      b. Often fails due to multiple slips of APL, each in their own subcompartment.
    2. **Forearm-based thumb spica splinting.**
    3. **Surgery:** Release the first dorsal compartment and perform tenosynovectomy.
      a. Release of all subcompartments must be confirmed: As above, APL can have multiple slips, and fool the surgeon into thinking both APL and EPB have been released.
      b. Superficial radial nerve should be avoided during dissection to prevent paresthesia or painful neuroma formation.
II. Intersection syndrome
  A. **Definition: Inflammation and pain at the site where the first dorsal compartment tendons** (APL and EPB) cross the second dorsal compartment tendons (ECRL and ECRB).
  B. **Associated with repetitive wrist motion.**
  C. **Pain and crepitation with wrist motion at the intersection site.**
  D. **Treatment.**

1. Forearm-based wrist splinting.
2. Activity modification and rest.
3. Injection with steroid and lidocaine.
4. Surgery uncommon.

III. **Other common forms of tendonitis**
   A. **Flexor carpi radialis/ulnaris (FCR/FCU) tendonitis.**
      1. Associated with forceful repeated wrist flexion (overuse).
      2. Inflammation and tenderness along **FCR/FCU** and pain with resisted wrist flexion and radial/ulnar deviation.
      3. **Treatment:** Nonsteroidal antiinflammatory drugs (NSAIDs), splinting, activity modification, occasionally injection; surgery is uncommon.
   B. **Extensor carpi ulnaris (ECU), extensor pollicis longus (EPL), and extensor indicis proprius (EIP) tendonitis also occur.**
      1. Associated with overuse.
      2. **Treatment:** NSAIDs, splinting, activity modification, occasionally injection.
      3. Surgery for EPL tendonitis to prevent rupture.
   C. **Rheumatoid arthritis–related** tendon attrition and rupture: See Chapter 40, "Rheumatoid Arthritis, Osteoarthritis, and Dupuytren's Contracture."

Amputation, Replantation, and Fingertip and Nail Bed Injuries

Keith G. Wolter

Amputation

I. Emergency department assessment
    A. What is the level of the injury?
    B. What is the mechanism and type of injury (sharp, dull, compression, avulsion, crush)?
    C. What are the patient's occupation, mental health, and level of cooperativeness?
    D. Which is the dominant hand?
    E. Is the patient a smoker? How much?
    F. What are the patient's perceptions of injury as it relates to body image? (May have a cultural component.)
    G. What are the patient's expectations? (May be unrealistic.)
    H. What is the patient's age? (Children heal more quickly and adapt more easily to changes in form and function.)
    I. What other injuries exist?
    J. Is replantation possible? Is it a worthwhile option? (See "Replantation.")

II. Amputation goals
    A. Preserve function
    B. Create a durable amputation site
    C. Preserve sensation; prevent neuromas
    D. Minimize disfigurement of adjacent joints
    E. Allow early return to work and activity

III. Distal finger amputations
    A. Assess injury
        1. Dorsal versus volar
        2. Angle of injury
        3. Involvement of nail and/or nail bed (see "Fingertip and Nail Bed Injuries")
        4. Exposure of bone
    B. If no exposed bone
        1. Secondary intention healing.
            a. Gives the best results in most cases.
            b. Treat with dressing changes and antibiotic ointment to keep moist and clean.
            c. Cold intolerance is common, but no worse than with other treatment options.
        2. Primary closure is an option only if tissue loss is minimal; otherwise, tight closures can limit function and cause pain.
        3. Skin grafts
            a. Recovery of sensation is not as good as with secondary intention healing.
            b. If used, the best alternative is a full-thickness skin graft. The best donor site options include the following:
                (1) Original skin (if salvageable). This skin should be aggressively trimmed of all fat and even some dermis.

        (2) Skin from ulnar/hypothenar aspect of hand.

        (3) Volar wrist skin.

        (4) Antecubital skin.

    c. Split-thickness skin grafts should only be used on noncritical areas (i.e., ulnar side of index, middle, and ring fingers).

C. If bone is exposed

    1. Completion amputation: Bone shortening and primary closure.

      a. Allows quick return to work.

      b. Best option for a patient unlikely or unwilling to do dressing changes.

    2. Bone shortening and healing by secondary intention.

      a. Patients are often skeptical about outcome initially.

      b. If patient is able to tolerate dressing changes, then this is a good option.

    3. Fingertip flaps (see "Fingertip and Nail Bed Injuries").

      a. Many surgical options have been described; however, these procedures will not necessarily result in better outcomes or quicker recovery.

      b. Individual patient presentation and the surgeon's preference and expertise play large roles in determining the treatment method to use.

IV. Proximal finger amputations

  A. Amputations through joints (distal interphalangeal or proximal interphalangeal joints)

    1. The bone end must be debrided. Use a rongeur to smoothly contour the distal end by removing the condylar prominences and irregular bone spikes.

    2. Digital nerves must be transected proximally to prevent painful neuroma formation.

    3. The extensor and flexor tendons should be debrided, but take care not to suture the ends of them together, as this will limit the excursion of both.

      a. If the flexor digitorum profundus (FDP) tendon is shortened and tethered, then the **quadrigia effect** can occur. The FDP tendons share a common muscle belly. If one tendon is shortened, than the others cannot be fully contracted, leading to the inability to make a fist.

      b. Another potential problem in amputations at the distal interphalangeal (DIP) level is the **lumbrical-plus deformity**. If the FDP is severed from its insertion and migrates proximally, it pulls on the lumbrical; attempts to flex the digit cause proximal interphalangeal (PIP) extension (from FDP pull on lumbrical tendon, pulling on extensor mechanism). Sectioning of the lumbrical tendon is the treatment.

  B. Middle and proximal phalanx amputations

    1. A fish-mouth closure of the skin is used, with the incision oriented transversely across the end of the stump.

    2. Tendons, when preserved, are secured to their insertion on the phalanx.

    3. If an amputation occurs too proximally along the middle phalanx to allow resecuring of the tendon to the bone, or if the tendon is missing, then use of the next joint will be limited. Length preservation remains preferable, even if the joint is nonfunctional. In this case, the joint should be fused.

    4. Amputations near the metacarpophalangeal (MP) joint often result in problems with small object manipulation, especially in ring and middle finger amputations.

      a. Consideration should be given to eventually converting to a ray amputation to maximize function.

      b. Alternatively, prosthetic finger replacement is possible.

V. Metacarpal and carpal amputations

  A. Ray amputations

    1. Injuries at or near the level of the MP joint usually benefit from removal of most of the bone and closure of the space between remaining digits.

      a. Leaving a "gap" in the fingers can allow small objects to slip through.

      b. An amputation of the index finger at the MP level leaves a stump that can interfere with thumb use and creates a bulky web space.

       c. The overall appearance of the hand is better if the stump is removed and any gap closed, although the palm is made narrower in the process.

    2. Ray amputations are carried out electively at a later time, after the wound has healed.

    3. Central ray (middle or ring finger) amputations leave defects that must be closed between the remaining metacarpals.

B. Carpal amputations

    1. Initially, the treatment is tissue preservation.

    2. Functional recovery is poor. Some patients may opt for more proximal amputation, followed by fitting with a hand prosthesis.

    3. Alternatively, the tissue at the hand base can be preserved and used to anchor a nonfunctional cosmetic appliance.

VI. Amputations at and proximal to the wrist

A. Wrist disarticulation.

    1. Once felt to be inferior to a long below-elbow amputation; now performed increasingly, in part because of improvement in prostheses.

    2. Preserving the radioulnar joint allows for a full range of pronation and supination.

    3. A fish-mouth skin closure, with a longer skin flap on the palmar side, is used.

B. Below-elbow amputation: The goal is length preservation. More length preservation of the radius and ulna means greater pronation and supination; ideally, 65% to 80% of length should be preserved for maximal function.

C. Elbow and above-elbow amputations.

    1. Humeral condyle preservation, when possible, allows for translation of rotation to the eventual prosthesis. Therefore, an elbow disarticulation is a very adequate level of amputation.

    2. In above-elbow amputations, length preservation is key. Amputations proximally, at or above the axillary fold, have no real advantage versus shoulder disarticulations.

Replantation

I. Evaluation for replantation

A. "Life before limb": Patients may have other serious injuries, which must be addressed prior to any attempt at replantation.

B. Assess injury, as outlined earlier in "Amputation" section.

C. Additional history is needed before considering replantation.

    1. Overall patient health and comorbidities.

    2. Previous injuries to this extremity.

    3. Willingness of patient to comply with rehabilitation and to tolerate lengthy time off work (average time until return to work is 7 months), as well as future operations.

D. Obtain x-rays of both the hand and the amputated part. Give the patient a tetanus update and/or antibiotics if indicated, check the hematocrit, and perform fluid resuscitation.

E. Assess the amputated part and stump site.

    1. Sharp amputations do better than avulsion or crush amputations.

    2. Length of ischemia time of the amputated part is critical.

        a. Digits can tolerate up to 12 hours of warm ischemia time or 24 hours (or more) of cold ischemia time.

        b. More proximal amputations, which include muscle, tolerate less ischemia: 6 hours of warm ischemia or 12 hours of cold ischemia is considered the limit of viability for wrist or more proximal replantations.

II. Indications for replantation

A. Indications to attempt replantation.

    1. Thumb amputations.

    2. Multiple-finger amputations.

3. Amputation in child.
4. Amputation at the palm, wrist, or forearm level.
5. Single-digit injury distal to flexor digitorum superficialis (FDS) insertion (does well functionally).

B. Absolute contraindications to replantation.
1. Life-threatening injuries.
2. Prolonged ischemia time of part.
3. Part in multiple pieces (i.e., transected at more than one level).

C. Relative contraindications.
1. Severe crush/avulsion amputations.
2. Injuries at multiple levels.
3. Severe preexisting illness.
   a. Diabetes mellitus.
   b. Heart disease and/or atherosclerosis.
   c. Recent stroke and/or myocardial infarction.
   d. Psychiatric disorders.
4. Gross contamination of site.
5. Prior surgery or trauma to amputated part.
6. Smoking history.

D. A number of controversies persist.
1. Amputation proximal to the elbow: Technically possible, but functional outcomes are quite poor. The success is greater in children.
2. Amputation of single finger proximal to the FDS insertion: Some surgeons feel that poor functional outcome negatively affects the use of the remaining digits and leads to a less functional situation than amputation.

III. Preoperative care
A. Care of amputated parts: The part should be gently cleaned, wrapped in saline-moistened gauze, and placed in a sealed plastic bag. The bag is stored at 4°C for transport.
1. Saline-ice bath will maintain the proper temperature.
2. Do *not* place the finger directly on ice; freezing the part is worse than warm ischemia.

B. Consent.
1. Obtaining surgical consent for replant *attempts* is not trivial.
   a. The patient and/or family will likely have unrealistic expectations prior to counseling.
   b. The extensive recovery time, the need for rehabilitation, and the likely amount of optimal function should be explained in detail prior to replantation attempts.
   c. The possibility of long hospitalizations, multiple operations, heparinization, and blood transfusions must be recognized.
   d. The significant chance of failure must also be addressed.
2. Consent must provide for a number of contingencies.
   a. Vein graft.
   b. Nerve graft.
   c. Skin graft.
   d. Flap for coverage.
   e. Revision amputation.

IV. Operative techniques
A. Amputated part
1. Begin work preparing the amputated part on the "back table" prior to patient arrival to the OR.
2. Carefully expose the vessels and nerves, and tag their ends with fine Prolene suture.
   a. For fingers, use midaxial longitudinal incisions.
   b. A corkscrew appearance to the arteries suggests traumatic stretch from an avulsion. These will need debridement.
   c. Bruising of the neurovascular bundle also suggests avulsion or traction injury.

3. Preservation of "spare parts" may optimize outcome.
   a. Heterotopic replants transfer tissue from one site to another (e.g., thumb restoration with another amputated digit when the thumb is unsalvageable).
   b. Use of components from one amputated part for another part's replant is economical (e.g., digital nerves from another amputated, but unreplantable, finger).
4. When the amputation is more proximal, the part will contain muscle, which will swell after reperfusion. Therefore, any fascial compartments in the part must be released.

B. **Operative overview**
1. **The recommended replant sequence is as follows.**
   a. Prepare the stump; debride the wound.
   b. Identify arteries, veins, nerves, and tendons; place tagging sutures.
   c. Stabilize the bone(s).
   d. Repair extensor tendons and muscles, then flexor tendons and muscles.
   e. Coapt nerves.*
   f. Anastomose arteries.*
   g. Anastomose veins.*
   h. Cover wound with soft tissue and/or skin.
2. The sequence for the repairs marked by asterisks is altered depending on circumstances and surgeon preference.
   a. In patients with short ischemia times, some authors feel nerve repair can and should precede vascular repair.
   b. In amputations involving a part with significant muscle, the risk of prolonged ischemia and subsequent reperfusion injury is high. Therefore, arteries should be repaired first, then nerves, and finally veins. This sequence provides inflow to the amputated part and the "flushing out" of toxic metabolites while the nerves are being fixed, before the veins are anastomosed.

C. **Stump preparation:** Avulsion injuries involving tendons sometimes require fasciotomy or carpal tunnel release, or both, because swelling proximal to the level of the amputation will occur.

D. **Bone fixation**
1. Bone should be debrided. Shortening is beneficial in that it decreases tension on anastomoses and skin repairs.
2. Fixation can be achieved via various methods.
   a. Kirschner wires: Simple; very useful for fingers. Placed retrograde in amputated part first.
   b. Interosseous wires: Used to augment K-wire repairs.
   c. Plate fixation: Not typically necessary for phalanges; useful for amputation at or proximal to the metacarpals.
   d. External fixation: May be useful for forearm replants.

E. **Tendon and muscle repair**
1. Clean the tendon edges, but do not shorten excessively.
2. Extensor tendons are repaired first, with two or three horizontal mattress sutures using 4–0 braided polyester.
3. Next, repair flexor tendons with a core suture technique, such as a modified Kessler or Tajima repair (see Chapter 37, "Tendon Injuries and Tendonitis").

F. **Vessel anastomoses**
1. **Arterial repair**
   a. The artery must be trimmed back to healthy intima.
   b. Vein grafts of the appropriate size may be found in the volar forearm, in the dorsal foot, or in "spare" amputated parts.
   c. Papaverine and/or lidocaine is used to minimize vasospasm.
   d. Repair of two arteries to a digit yields a higher successful replantation rate than repair of a single artery, but one good anastomosis is adequate.

    2. Venous repair
- **a.** Two vein repairs per artery are preferred.
- **b.** Tension on venous repair must be minimal to prevent congestion.

G. Nerve coaptation
1. Trim the nerves back to undamaged areas.
2. Realign fascicles when possible to maximize the return of sensibility.

H. Coverage
1. Skin is closed loosely over repaired vessels. A tight closure will restrict venous outflow.
2. Split-thickness skin grafts are used as needed.
3. For more proximal replants, local or free muscle flaps are used to cover the operative site and protect the anastomoses.
4. A well-padded splint, with absolutely no circumferential pressure, should be made to protect the replant. It should extend above the elbow to prevent any rotational movement. A poorly made dressing can foil the whole case.

V. Postoperative care

A. Acute care
1. **Aggressive hydration** to keep vessels patent (usually a total fluid intake of one and a half maintenance).
2. **Avoid *any* vasoconstrictors** for the first several days after the operation, including caffeine and nicotine.
3. **Analgesia** is important to minimize catecholamine release. The patient should be resting comfortably.
4. **Medical therapies** used to diminish complication rates.
   - **a.** Systemic heparinization should be used in cases of wide vessel damage, such as in crush amputations. Initiate therapy intraoperatively for the best result.
   - **b.** Dextran 40 infusion is used by many replant surgeons for its plasma expansion and antiplatelet effects. A dosage of 500 cc is administered per day in adults (or 25 cc/hr). A test dose of 5 cc is usually administered in the operating room. Although statistical proof of efficacy is lacking, side effects (anaphylaxis, acute renal failure, pulmonary edema) are rare.
   - **c.** Aspirin 325 mg a day is given for 3 weeks to retard platelet aggregation.
   - **d.** Other agents are advocated by some authors, including chlorpromazine (Thorazine), dipyridamole (Persantine), and calcium channel blockers.
5. Objective monitoring of the replant can be done in a number of ways.
   - **a.** Temperature probes: Probably the most reliable.
   - **b.** Laser Doppler flowmetry.
   - **c.** Pulse oximetry.
6. Frequent evaluation by the surgeon and staff for color and capillary refill (subjective monitoring) is essential and represents the best monitoring method.

B. Failing replant
1. **In the acute setting,** the problem is usually vascular, either inflow or outflow.
   - **a.** Arterial insufficiency: Cool, pale replant; no capillary refill; pin prick produces little or no bleeding.
   - **b.** Venous insufficiency: Congested replant; increased tissue turgor; pin prick yields copious bleeding with dark blood.
2. **Initial treatment options** include nonoperative measures.
   - **a.** Elevate hand and arm.
   - **b.** Loosen dressing; if needed, relax or release sutures.
   - **c.** Add medical therapies (heparin, Thorazine, etc.).
   - **d.** Use better pain control (e.g., axillary block).
   - **e.** Use medicinal leeches.

        (1) Can reduce venous congestion.

        (2) Secrete hirudin, a potent anticoagulant that remains localized.

        (3) Treatment lasts for up to 6 days.

        (4) Patients should be placed on a third-generation cephalosporin to protect from *Aeromonas hydrophila* infection.

     f. Use of thrombolytics in replants is controversial.

   3. Reexploration is the definitive treatment for vascular problems.

     a. Functional outcomes are poorer in patients requiring reoperation.

     b. Outcomes are best when reoperation is performed within 6 hours of loss of perfusion.

VI. Outcomes

A. With good patient selection, replant failure rate is low, on the order of 20%. However, that number may be deceiving, because *viable* replants are not always *valuable* replants.

B. Late complications diminish the value of a replantation.

   1. Decreased range of motion in joints.

     a. Due to tendon adhesions and joint contracture.

     b. Many patients undergo one or more secondary procedures to address these problems and improve replant function, especially in more proximal amputations.

   2. Decreased sensation is a function of injury mechanism, repair technique, and level of injury.

   3. Loss of motor function is a problem in more proximal amputations, where the slow axonal regeneration limits muscle reinnervation.

   4. Chronic pain, including chronic regional pain syndrome (CRPS).

   5. Cold intolerance is a very common postreplant complaint. It typically improves over 2 years, but some intolerance is often permanent.

C. Functional outcome depends on multiple factors.

   1. Sharp amputations always have better recovery of sensation and function than crush or avulsion amputations.

   2. Children have better outcomes.

   3. Thumb replants do best. Even if mobility is poor, the replant has value as a sensate post.

   4. Zone I finger replants regain an average of 82 degrees of motion at the PIP joint.

   5. Zone II finger replants regain an average of 35 degrees of motion at the PIP joint.

   6. The average two-point discrimination in a finger replant is 11 mm.

Fingertip and Nail Bed Injuries

I. Overview

A. Everything distal to the DIP crease is considered the fingertip (Fig. 38-1).

B. The fingertip is the most sensitive part of the hand.

C. The glabrous skin on the fingertip is specialized for **pinch** and **grasp** functions.

D. The nail protects the distal phalanx and provides counterforce to the tip pulp.

E. Fingertips are essential for normal hand appearance.

F. Fingertips are commonly injured.

   1. Fingertip and nail injuries account for 45% of all hand injuries seen in the emergency room.

   2. The middle fingertip is most commonly injured, followed by the ring fingertip.

   3. Thumb tip injury is least common.

G. Fingertip injuries can have a great impact.

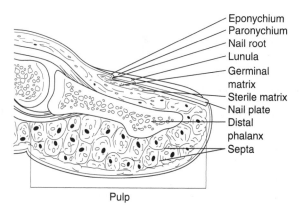

Fig. 38-1. Anatomy of the fingertip.

     1. May appear minor, but can have serious implications because of the effect on so many activities.

     2. Typically result in lost work (sometimes the end of a career).

   H. Immediate repair is preferable for the best outcome. Repair can often be performed in the emergency room.

II. Preparation and examination

   A. A digital nerve block is usually sufficient.

   B. In sterile fashion, prep the hand to the forearm, and secure on an arm board or table.

   C. Place a tourniquet on the finger, using a Penrose drain and hemostat or similar method to ensure tourniquet removal. Do *not* roll a cut glove finger onto the digit, because this band may be forgotten and can result in digit loss. A simple sterile glove secured by a hemostat works very well.

   D. Surgical loupes are helpful.

   E. Irrigate the fingertip first, then debride any clearly nonviable tissue.

   F. Have a low threshold for moving to the operating room when necessary.

III. Fingernail injuries

   A. Nail bed hematomas

     1. If less than 25% of surface of the nail in size, drain by lancing the nail with cautery or a heated paperclip end.

     2. If greater than 25%, remove the nail to repair the nail bed.

   B. Nail bed lacerations

     1. Use a Freer elevator or tenotomy scissors to separate the nail from the eponychium and underlying matrix.

     2. Set the nail aside in sterile saline.

     3. Repair the nailbed with 6–0 or 7–0 absorbable suture material. Use precise, interrupted stitches under loupe magnification.

     4. Maintain the eponychial fold with a stent. One can use the trimmed nail if available, or other material such as the foil from a suture pack. This is usually considered helpful to prevent the formation of painful split nails.

   C. Avulsed nail bed

     1. If attached to nail, replace as an onlay graft.

     2. If the nail bed is missing, use a split-thickness nail bed graft from another nail to fill the defect (usually electively).

   D. Amputations through the lunula/germinal matrix: If unable to repair or replant, remove the remaining germinal matrix before closure. Otherwise, the remaining matrix will form an irritating, painful nail remnant.

IV. Flaps for fingertip repair

A. As discussed earlier, healing by secondary intention often gives as good or better outcomes than flap repairs. A variety of techniques can be used to repair fingertip injuries. The angle of injury or amputation, as well as individual surgeon experience, determines when and where to use a given technique.

B. Advancement flaps

1. Lateral V-Y advancement flaps (Kutler flaps)

a. Most useful for transverse amputations.

b. Bilateral triangles are advanced and sutured to distal nail bed.

c. Can advance up to 5 mm if skin alone, and up to 14 mm if a neurovascular flap is elevated down to the level of the periosteum.

d. Disadvantages.

  (1) Vascular supply is sometimes unreliable.

  (2) Scar is at the tip; may be painful or insensate.

2. Volar V-Y advancement flap (Atasoy-Kleinert flap)

a. Most useful for dorsal oblique amputations.

b. Triangular flap, with base no wider than nail bed.

c. Skin incisions are through the dermis; deep aspect is dissected off of phalanx.

d. Advancement of up to 10 mm.

e. Good survival; disadvantages include possible hypersensitivity or hook nail.

3. Volar neurovascular advancement flap (Moberg flap)

a. Best sensation preservation.

b. Longitudinal incisions are made on both sides, dorsal to the neurovascular structures. Nerves and arteries are contained in the flap.

c. Advanced to cover tip defect.

d. Requires some joint flexion during healing; therefore, there is a high risk of flexion contracture.

e. Used for the thumb tip, when padding and sensation are critical and some flexion contracture can be tolerated. The Moberg flap should generally not be used for fingers.

C. Regional flaps

1. Cross-finger flap

a. Dorsal skin from one digit is transferred to the injured area of an adjacent digit; can be used for volar or dorsal amputations.

b. Pedicled flap with delayed division, usually in 2 to 3 weeks.

c. Donor site requires a skin graft.

2. Thenar flap

a. The injured digit is flexed and tucked into the thenar area, and the palmar skin is used to cover the tip.

b. Advantage: No defect on fingers adjacent to injury.

c. Disadvantage: PIP flexion contracture of recipient finger. Therefore mostly used in children.

3. Neurovascular island transfer flap (Littler flap)

a. Used for insensate fingers following trauma to recreate sensibility in the tip.

b. Usually reserved for thumb, index finger, or ulnar little finger.

c. Must balance recipient sensation restoration with donor site loss.

d. Flap pedicle is composed of digital vessels and nerve.

e. Typically raised from the ulnar aspect of the ring or middle finger; raised at the level of the flexor sheath.

f. Donor site is closed either with graft or primarily.

Nerve Injuries, Compression Syndromes, and Tendon Transfers

39

Keith G. Wolter

Nerve Injury

I. **Peripheral nerve anatomy**
  A. **Neurons:** The basic unit of nervous tissue.
   1. **Motor neurons**
      a. Large, multipolar cell body, with multiple dendrites and a long axon.
      b. The cell body is located in the ventral horn of the spinal cord; the axon leaves the spinal cord via the ventral root.
      c. Terminate on the motor end plate of the innervated muscle.
   2. **Sensory neurons**
      a. The cell body is found in the dorsal root ganglion.
      b. Unipolar, with a single axonal process running from the periphery (either an encapsulated receptor in the skin or a terminal branch in tissue), through the dorsal root ganglion, and into the spinal cord.
      c. Terminate in the dorsal horn of the spinal cord, or may ascend to the brainstem.
   3. **Sympathetic neurons**
      a. Control vasomotor and pilomotor function.
      b. Axons are unmyelinated.
  B. **Glial cells:** Produce myelin to insulate axons and increase conduction speed.
   1. **Schwann cells** are the primary glial cell of the peripheral nervous system.
      a. Schwann cells produce a sheath of myelin that wraps multiple times concentrically around the axon.
      b. Each Schwann cell covers a segment of axon 1 mm in length.
      c. Spaces between Schwann cells are the nodes of Ranvier.
   2. Peripheral nerve fibers can be myelinated or unmyelinated.
  C. **Connective tissue:** Makes up 25% to 75% of the cross-section of nerves; it has three layers.
   1. **Endoneurium**
      a. Within the fascicle, individual axons are surrounded by endoneurium.
      b. Unmyelinated nerve fibers have a diameter ranging from 0.2 to 3.0 μm.
      c. Myelinated fibers have diameters ranging from 2 to 25 μm.
   2. **Perineurium**
      a. Surrounds individual fascicles within nerves.
      b. Each fascicle represents a group of nerve fibers.
      c. Fascicular diameter ranges from 0.04 to 3.0 mm.
   3. **Epineurium**
      a. **External epineurium** surrounds the whole nerve as an outer sheath.
      b. **Internal epineurium** is composed of loose connective tissue and serves to cushion the fascicles from trauma.
      c. Contains a longitudinal plexus of blood vessels.
      d. Usually the site for suturing during nerve reconstruction.
  D. **Nerve topography**
   1. Peripheral nerves can be:

      a. Monofascicular (e.g., terminal skin branch): One fascicle, either pure motor or sensory.

      b. Oligofascicular (e.g., common digital nerve): Either purely motor or sensory, or mixed function.

      c. Polyfascicular (e.g., radial nerve): Major nerves contain fibers for a variety of functions.

   2. The organization of the fascicles in the major (polyfascicular) upper extremity nerves has been mapped, with detailed study of the pattern of motor and sensory axons along the length of the nerve. These maps are critical during fascicular nerve repair procedures.

II. Chronology of nerve injury: Degeneration followed by regeneration.

A. Nerve degeneration

   1. Cell bodies of injured axons swell, and alter their metabolism to produce proteins needed to rebuild the axons.

   2. Wallerian degeneration occurs along the axon at and distal to the level of injury. The distal axon degrades, and Schwann cells withdraw. Macrophages clear debris from the axonal tract. Wallerian degeneration can also extend up to 2 cm proximal to the injury site.

   3. Synapses distal to the nerve injury degrade.

B. Nerve regeneration

   1. Injured peripheral nerves can regenerate, provided continuity with the distal portion of the nerve tract is maintained or is reestablished surgically.

   2. Nerve growth factors, secreted by target cells (postsynaptic neurons or muscle cells) and by Schwann cells, are required for axonal regrowth.

   3. Macrophages secrete interleukins that induce Schwann cell proliferation.

   4. Schwann cells along the distal axonal tract express laminins and adhesion molecules, which help guide the regenerating axon.

   5. Axonal sprouts from the proximal cut end must enter the distal tract to regrow. If disruption of the nerve is severe and/or scarring is great, the budding axons cannot cross the gap, and regeneration does not occur.

   6. Prior to any regeneration, degradation and clearing of debris takes approximately 15 to 30 days.

   7. Once growth is initiated, axons extend by approximately 1 mm a day.

III. Nerve injury classification

A. Seddon nerve injury classification system: Described by Sir Herbert Seddon.

   1. Neuropraxia: Local transient block of conduction along a nerve. The anatomy of the nerve is preserved, and no Wallerian degeneration occurs. Recovery is usually rapid, but may take several months. Selective demyelination of fibers may occur.

   2. Axonotmesis: Axonal damage within the nerve. Anatomic continuity is preserved. Wallerian degeneration occurs. Recovery rate is 1 mm per day along the nerve, once healing begins. Fibrillations are present on electromotor testing. Recovery is typically complete eventually (without surgery).

   3. Neurotmesis: Nerve is transected. Continuity of the nerve is lost, and Wallerian degeneration occurs. Some recovery may occur, but it is never complete; surgical repair is needed for the best outcome.

B. Sunderland nerve injury classification system (with Mackinnon modification)

   1. First-degree injury: Nerve is demyelinated, resulting in a local conduction block. Treatment is nonoperative, and recovery is complete within approximately 12 weeks.

   2. Second-degree injury: Some nerve fibers are disrupted, but the endoneurial sheaths remain intact. Wallerian degeneration occurs with second-degree and higher injuries. Tinel's sign indicates an advancing growth cone. Treatment is nonoperative. Complete recovery is expected.

3. **Third-degree injury:** Some endoneurial sheaths are disrupted with scarring, while the perineurium remains intact. Incomplete recovery; some nerve fibers do not reinnervate their target. Treatment is usually nonoperative.
4. **Fourth-degree injury:** Loss of continuity of the perineurium. Scar blocks all fiber growth; little or no nerve recovery. Treatment is operative.
5. **Fifth-degree injury:** The nerve is completely transected. The epineurium is disrupted. No recovery is expected without operative management.
6. **Sixth-degree injury:** Added to Sunderland's classification scheme by Susan Mackinnon.

Nerve Compression Syndromes

I. **General principles**
   A. **Pathophysiology**
      1. **Ischemia:** Pressure on the nerve leads to loss of blood flow (Table 39-1).
      2. **Fibrosis:** Ischemia leads to nerve fibrosis, which worsens in progressive stages (Table 39-2).
      3. **Traction:** Entrapment can limit nerve excursion. With limb motion, this can lead to additional traction-induced conduction block.
      4. **Double-crush phenomenon:** A given locus of compression impairs axonal transport along the nerve, lowering the threshold for a second locus to become symptomatic (e.g., thoracic outlet plus carpal tunnel syndrome).
      5. **Systemic conditions:** Can depress peripheral nerve function, which in turn lowers the threshold for symptoms (diabetes, alcoholism, hypothyroidism, and exposure to industrial solvents).
   B. **Diagnostic testing**
      1. **Sensory testing:** Use threshold tests to evaluate compression neuropathies.
         a. **Semmes-Weinstein test:** Monofilament test for slow-adapting touch fibers.
         b. **Vibration test:** Best test for quick-adapting touch receptors.
      2. **Tinel's sign:** The skin is percussed over the course of the nerve. Tingling over the nerve distribution indicates a partial lesion of the nerve. After nerve repair, this may be a positive finding, indicating nerve regeneration.
      3. **Phalen's test:** The wrist is palmar flexed to 90 degrees (can be accomplished by having the patient press the backs of his or her hands together) and held in this position for 60 seconds. Patients with carpal tunnel syndrome will exhibit hypesthesia/paresthesia in the median nerve distribution of the affected hand(s).
      4. **Electrodiagnostic testing:** The gold standard; provides objective data to support or disprove a compression neuropathy.

Table 39-1. Effects of increasing pressure on peripheral nerves

Pressure (mm Hg)	Effect on Nerve
20–30	Reduced epineurial blood flow
30	Impaired axonal transport
30–40	Paresthesias
50 (for 2 hr)	Epineurial edema; axonal transport block
>60	Complete intraneural ischemia

Table 39-2. Management and outcome of fibrosis of peripheral nerves

Stage	Treatment	Expected Outcome
Early	Splinting, steroids	Full recovery
Intermediate	Operative release	Full recovery
Advanced	Operative release	Permanent nerve loss

   a. Electrodiagnostics are limited by operator experience and reliability.
   b. Typically, nerve conduction studies and electromyography (EMG) are performed at the same time to assess both nerves and muscles.
   c. In compression mononeuropathies, there is a drop in amplitude of nerve action potentials, decreased nerve conduction velocity, and prolonged latency.
   d. Results are more useful if compared with old tests on the same individual and/or on contralateral nerves; population norms may be used, but individual patient values can vary widely.
   e. Nerve conduction and EMG can help establish a diagnosis, but in isolation do not establish one. Patients must have symptoms first to have a diagnosis made.
  5. Radiologic studies: Plain films and/or magnetic resonance imaging (MRI) as needed, to rule out the following.
   a. Fractures and post-traumatic deformities (e.g., hamate fracture).
   b. Congenital deformities (e.g., cervical rib).
   c. Neoplasms and masses (e.g., Pancoast's tumor).
II. Median nerve
 A. Carpal tunnel syndrome (CTS) is the most common mononeuropathy.
  1. Epidemiology
   a. Mean age of diagnosis is 50 years.
   b. Intrinsic risk factors: Female gender, pregnancy, diabetes, and rheumatoid arthritis.
   c. Controversial risk factors: Repetitive or forceful tasks, mechanical stress; occupational posture; vibration and/or temperature.
   d. *Not* a risk factor: Anatomically small carpal tunnel.
  2. Anatomy
   a. Carpal tunnel boundaries.
    (1) Dorsal and lateral: The carpal bones.
    (2) Volar: The flexor retinaculum, consisting of the deep forearm fascia, transverse carpal ligament (TCL), and the distal fascia between the thenar and hypothenar muscles.
   b. The carpal tunnel contains the median nerve and nine tendons: the flexor pollicis longus (FPL), flexor digitorum superficialis (FDS, four), and flexor digitorum profundus (FDP, four).
   c. Median nerve branches of the hand.
    (1) The palmar cutaneous branch: Arises 5 cm proximal to the wrist crease.
    (2) The recurrent motor branch: Usually arises at or just beyond the distal edge of the TCL from the radiopalmar aspect of the nerve (many variants are described). **Kaplan's cardinal line** runs from the apex of the thumb/index web toward the hook of the hamate, parallel with the proximal palmar crease; the intersection of this line with the long finger localizes the recurrent motor branch.
    (3) Two common and three proper digital nerve branches: Arise distal to the TCL.
  3. Pathophysiology
   a. Vascular compromise: Leads to localized anoxia. Edema follows, resulting in further reduction of blood flow.

    b. Inflammation: A function of both ischemia and external repetitive stress; can cause synovial hypertrophy of the flexor tendons.

    c. Fibroblast proliferation: Interferes with nerve oxygenation and nutrition.

    d. Scarring and compression: Can tether the median nerve in the carpal canal, leading to traction injury.

    e. In general, the pathology is **progressive**. Stopping the compression earlier leads to quicker and more complete recovery.

4. Diagnosis

    a. History and physical examination

       (1) Pain and paresthesias of the palmar radial hand. Worse at night and with repetitive use.

       (2) Phalen's test and Tinel's signs may be positive; these support a CTS diagnosis but are not specific.

       (3) Advanced cases may demonstrate wasting of the thenar muscles.

    b. EMG findings

       (1) Distal motor latencies greater than 4.5 msec (or >1 msec difference between the hands).

       (2) Distal sensory latencies greater than 3.5 msec (or >0.5 msec difference between hands).

       (3) Conduction velocities less than 50 m/sec.

5. Nonoperative treatment

    a. Splint the wrist in neutral position. Have the patient wear the splint all the time or just at night, depending on the severity of symptoms.

    b. Antiinflammatory agents such as NSAIDs, to decrease inflammation.

    c. Control of systemic diseases (e.g., diabetes, rheumatoid arthritis).

    d. Steroid injections

       (1) Inject 1 cm proximal to the distal wrist crease between the palmaris longus (PL) and flexor carpi radialis (FCR) tendons.

       (2) Transient relief for 80% of patients, but few remain symptom free after 1 year.

       (3) Better results in milder cases of CTS, with symptoms present for less than 1 year.

       (4) Can be beneficial for debilitating CTS in pregnancy.

       (5) Response to steroids is also diagnostic, predictive of a good response to surgery.

6. Operative treatment: Carpal tunnel release (CTR)

    a. Objective: Release of the superficial (palmar) and deep (TCL) layers from the antebrachial fascia to the distal palmar crease.

    b. The standard open technique provides better exposure.

       (1) Incision is ulnar and parallel to the thenar crease, 2.0 to 2.5 cm long.

       (2) Do not need to cross the wrist crease with the incision.

       (3) Cut the TCL with care to avoid injury to the underlying nerve.

    c. Minimal-incision techniques require more blind dissection.

       (1) Incision is halfway between the distal wrist crease and a transverse line intersecting the base of first web space made in line with the radial border of the fourth ray, just ulnar to the thenar crease; 0.7 to 1.0 cm in length.

       (2) Use a scalpel to open the tensor fascia lata (TFL), then tenotomy scissors to divide the TCL first distally, then proximally.

       (3) The antebrachial fascia is divided blindly.

    d. Endoscopic techniques: Leave even smaller scars, but no superiority has been demonstrated over open methods.

    e. Synovectomy is only indicated in cases of proliferative or invasive tenosynovitis.

    f. Co-release of Guyon's canal is not indicated in isolated CTS.

    g. Postoperative splinting is optional; use for 1 week or less to minimize debilitation.

B. Pronator syndrome and anterior interosseous syndrome
1. **Sites of compression** (from proximal to distal)
   a. Supracondylar process of the humerus
   b. Ligament of Struthers (accessory origin of the pronator teres)
   c. Accessory bicipital aponeurosis
   d. Pronator arch: Between the humeral and ulnar heads of the pronator teres muscle (most common cause of these syndromes)
   e. Flexor digitorum superficialis arch
   f. Fibromuscular bands in the distal forearm
   g. Accessory/variant muscles; for example, Gantzer's muscle (accessory head of FPL)
   h. Post-traumatic (radius or ulna fractures)
2. **Diagnosis**
   a. **Pronator syndrome**
      (1) Forearm pain and paresthesias; hypesthesia in the cutaneous distribution of the median nerve, including the palmar cutaneous branch, which helps differentiate it from CTS. There can be a positive Tinel's sign in the proximal forearm and a negative Phalen's test.
      (2) Symptoms with isolated, resisted contraction of the biceps, pronator teres (PT), and/or FDS may indicate the site of compression.
      (3) Fewer than 50% of EMGs are diagnostic; EMG findings poorly predict the response to surgery.
      (4) Use three-view elbow films to look at the supracondylar process.
   b. **Anterior interosseous syndrome**
      (1) Weakness or loss of function of the FPL, index finger FDP, long finger FDP, and pronator quadratus (PQ).
      (2) No sensory symptoms.
      (3) Classic "pinch deformity": flexion of the interphalangeal (IP) joint of the thumb with key pinch (Froment's sign).
3. **Treatment**
   a. **Pronator syndrome**
      (1) Nonoperative (splinting and rest): 50% of patients will respond.
      (2) Operative: Only for failure of conservative therapy. Must explore above and below the elbow to remove all possible sites of compression (see previous list). Start movement after 5 days.
   b. **Anterior interosseous syndrome**
      (1) Obtain a baseline EMG after 3 weeks of weakness, then observe for 2 to 3 months.
      (2) If there is no improvement in the exam or the EMG, then surgery is indicated.
      (3) Operative intervention is the same as above. Neurolysis of the anterior interosseous nerve to above the elbow should be performed to eliminate fascicular constrictions.

III. Ulnar nerve
A. Cubital tunnel syndrome
1. **Sites of compression** (proximal to distal)
   a. Arcade of Struthers (8 cm above the elbow, between the triceps and the medial intermuscular septum)
   b. Medial intermuscular septum (from the medial epicondyle to the coracobrachialis muscle)
   c. Medial epicondyle
   d. Cubital tunnel retinaculum (also known as arcuate ligament of Osborne)
   e. Deep flexor-pronator aponeurosis (2–3 cm distal to cubital tunnel, between FDP and FDS muscles)
2. **Pathophysiology:** Work-related activities may aggravate the syndrome, but there are no data to support work as a risk factor.
3. **Diagnosis**
   a. **History and physical examination**

Table 39-3. Treatment of cubital tunnel syndrome

Grade	Compression	Findings	Treatment
1	Minimal	No motor weakness	Nonoperative trial
2	Intermediate	Muscle atrophy	Nerve transposition
3	Severe	Paralysis/clawing	Nerve transposition

      (1) Numbness of the small and ulnar half of ring fingers and the ulnar dorsal hand.

      (2) Weakness of grip and intrinsic wasting.

      (3) Positive Tinel's sign or pain at the medial elbow.

      (4) Ulnar nerve subluxation with elbow flexion.

      (5) Ulnar nerve paresthesias/numbness within 1 minute of full elbow flexion (Phalen's analogue).

   b. EMG findings

      (1) Ulnar nerve conduction across the elbow is less than 49 m/sec.

      (2) The first dorsal interosseous muscle is the most commonly affected, with evidence of denervation.

      (3) Abductor pollicis brevis (APB) should be normal (this excludes a C8/T1 nerve root or plexus lesion).

   c. Elbow x-rays: Especially useful if range of motion is abnormal or there is a history of trauma.

  4. The treatment algorithm was described by McGowan (Table 39-3).

  5. Operative treatment options

   a. *In situ* decompression: Only for mild and/or intermittent symptoms. Use in patients with a nonsubluxating ulnar nerve, normal bony anatomy, and absence of pain around the medial epicondyle.

   b. Subcutaneous anterior transposition: Indicated in most cases.

   c. Submuscular transposition: Preferred for very thin patients, reoperative cases, and cases of severe compression.

   d. Intramuscular transposition: Least popular surgical option.

   e. Medial epicondylectomy

      (1) Useful for post-traumatic cases with bony deformity.

      (2) Carries the risk of damaging the ulnar collateral ligament, resulting in elbow instability and pain.

B. Ulnar tunnel syndrome

  1. Anatomy

   a. Ulnar nerve analogue of the carpal tunnel. First described by Guyon in 1861; commonly referred to as **Guyon's canal.**

   b. Canal is 4.0 to 4.5 cm in length, extending from the proximal edge of the palmar carpal ligament to the fibrous arch of the origin of the hypothenar muscles.

  2. Pathophysiology (various compressive etiologies)

   a. Ganglia and soft tissue masses: Most common cause (33%–50% of all cases).

   b. Muscle anomalies: 10% to 15%.

   c. Thrombosis or pseudoaneurysm of the ulnar artery.

   d. Fracture of the hook of the hamate.

   e. Edema/scarring from burns.

   f. Inflammatory arthritis.

  3. Diagnosis

   a. History and physical examination

      (1) Pain in the wrist, with paresthesias radiating into the small and ring fingers; local tenderness.

      (2) Symptoms are exacerbated with sustained hyperextension or hyperflexion of the wrist.

        (3) Intrinsic muscle weakness (a late finding).

        (4) The ulnar palm is not affected, since compression is distal to the palmar (and dorsal) branches.

        (5) A bruit may be present. Check Doppler studies, Allen's test, Phalen's test, and Tinel's sign.

    b. EMG: Usually diagnostic.

    c. Computed tomographic scan: Helpful in detecting hook of the hamate fractures.

4. Nonoperative treatment

    a. Indicated if no identifiable lesion is present.

    b. Activity modifications.

    c. Splint the wrist in neutral position.

    d. NSAIDs.

5. Operative treatment

    a. Indications: An identifiable lesion or failure of nonoperative treatment.

    b. Operative technique.

        (1) Divide the volar carpal ligament and pisohamate ligament.

        (2) Divide the fibrous arch of the hypothenar muscle's origin.

        (3) Examine the floor of the canal for masses and fractures; examine the ulnar artery with the tourniquet up and then down.

    c. Postoperative care: Splint the wrist in slight extension for 3 weeks.

IV. Radial nerve

A. Posterior interosseous nerve (PIN) syndrome and radial tunnel syndrome

1. Anatomy

    a. PIN innervates the extensor carpi radialis brevis (ECRB), supinator, extensor carpi ulnaris (ECU), extensor digitorum communis (EDC), extensor indicis proprius (EIP), extensor digiti quinti (EDQ), abductor pollicis longus (APL), extensor pollicis longus (EPL), and extensor pollicis brevis (EPB; no sensory component).

    b. Radial tunnel: 5 cm long. It is bounded by the biceps tendon, ECRL, ECRB, brachioradialis, and radiocapitellar joint capsule. It ends at the proximal part of the supinator.

2. Sites of compression

    a. Thickened fascial tissue superficial to the radiocapitellar joint.

    b. "Leash" of vessels from the radial recurrent artery **(leash of Henry).**

    c. Fibrous edge of the ECRB muscle.

    d. Proximal edge of the supinator **(arcade of Frohse).**

    e. Distal edge of the supinator, or fibrous bands within the supinator.

    f. Entrapment or traction injury from proximal radius surgery.

3. Diagnosis

    a. PIN syndrome

        (1) Gradual weakness of finger and wrist extensors.

        (2) Acute onset following trauma.

        (3) Rheumatoid disease at the elbow can mimic symptoms, including radial head dislocation placing traction on the PIN.

        (4) Incomplete syndrome may be confused with tendon rupture (check tenodesis).

        (5) EMG is usually diagnostic.

        (6) Elbow x-rays to rule out radial head dislocation or fracture.

        (7) MRI or ultrasound to evaluate elbow masses (usually lipoma or ganglia).

    b. Radial tunnel syndrome

        (1) Chiefly a pain syndrome (weakness is secondary); sometimes night pain is significant.

        (2) Pain at the lateral elbow; exacerbated by resisted supination with the elbow extended.

        (3) Often seen in a work-related setting with a history of repetitive forceful elbow extension or forearm rotation.

      (4) Must differentiate from lateral epicondylitis: Tenderness is more distal with radial tunnel syndrome.

      (5) "Middle finger test": With elbow and fingers extended, press on the dorsum of the proximal phalanx of the middle finger. The test is positive if this produces pain at the edge of the ECRB in the proximal forearm.

      (6) EMG may not be useful.

      (7) Injection of local anesthetic into the radial tunnel that relieves pain and produces PIN palsy is diagnostic.

4. Nonoperative treatment

a. PIN syndrome

      (1) Selected patients may be observed for 2 to 3 months, provided there are no signs of progression. However, excessive delay can lead to permanent muscle weakness.

      (2) Rheumatoid patients may benefit from steroid injection.

      (3) Surgery is indicated if there is no improvement.

b. Radial tunnel syndrome

      (1) Nonoperative care should always be tried first (rest, splinting, NSAIDs).

      (2) No progression to muscle palsy has been documented.

5. Operative treatment

a. PIN syndrome

      (1) Indications: Failure of nonoperative treatment, known space-occupying lesion, post-traumatic or associated with open reduction and internal fixation (ORIF) of proximal radius.

      (2) Good or excellent results are obtained in 85% of patients, but may take up to 18 months.

b. Radial tunnel syndrome: Surgery is indicated for failure of conservative treatment.

B. Superficial radial nerve compression (Wartenberg) syndrome

1. Anatomy and pathophysiology

a. Described by Wartenberg in 1932. Sites of compression are as follows.

      (1) External compression (watch bands, handcuffs).

      (2) Overuse/repetitive activity (using a screwdriver, typing, writing) or wrist contusion.

      (3) Scissoring of ECRL and the brachioradialis tendons. May be worsened by nerve tethering in distal scar tissue.

b. The superficial branch of the radial nerve becomes subcutaneous about 9 cm proximal to the radial styloid. It may pierce the tendon of the brachioradialis.

2. Diagnosis

a. History and physical examination

      (1) Pain, numbness, and tingling over the dorsal radial hand, exacerbated by wrist movement, index-thumb pinch, or forceful pronation of the forearm (symptoms within 30–60 seconds).

      (2) May have a false-positive Finkelstein's sign (pain with ulnar deviation of the hand with the thumb grasped in palm).

      (3) Diagnosis can be confirmed by tracing Tinel's sign over the nerve or a diagnostic nerve block.

b. Electrodiagnostic studies are useful.

3. Nonoperative treatment: NSAIDs, splinting, local steroid injections, and activity alteration should be tried before operative intervention.

V. Thoracic outlet compression syndrome (TOCS)

A. Epidemiology and risk factors

1. Female gender: Four times more risk than men.

2. Age: Average age is 37.

3. Occupation involving awkward or static arm positioning at or above the shoulder level (e.g., painters, nurses, typists, etc.).

4. Insurance status: Private insurance more than Medicaid.

B. Anatomy and pathophysiology
   1. Sites of potential compression
      a. Interscalene triangle: Between the anterior and middle scalene and the first rib.
      b. Costoclavicular triangle: Between the clavicle and the first rib.
      c. Subcoracoid or pectoralis minor space.
      d. Cervical ribs: Present in 0.5% of the general population; 50% to 80% are bilateral.
   2. Wilbourn's classification: Based on the etiology of symptoms.
      a. Arterial (1%–2% of cases)
         (1) Major subtype is associated with obvious osseous anomalies.
         (2) Minor subtype is intermittent compression, usually at the pectoralis minor insertion.
         (3) 50% of arterial TOCS will have a fully developed cervical rib.
      b. Venous (2%–3% of cases)
         (1) Paget-Schroetter syndrome: Sudden, effort-induced thrombosis.
         (2) May also occur after prolonged malpositioning.
         (3) Less acute cases lead to large collateral development.
      c. "True" neurogenic (rare; only 1 in 1,000,000 patients)
         (1) Objective signs of chronic nerve compression: atrophy, weakness (usually C8-T1).
         (2) A bony anomaly is always present.
      d. "Disputed" neurogenic (97% of cases): Wide variety of complaints; no objective findings
C. Diagnosis
   1. History and physical examination
      a. Chronic pain of insidious onset (shoulder, upper back, neck) with upper extremity paresthesias.
      b. Easy fatigability and nighttime pain are common.
   2. Provocative tests: Looking for symptom reproduction and/or loss of the radial pulse.
      a. Adson's test (scalene test): With arm at the side, hyperextend the neck and turn the face toward the affected side and breathe deeply.
      b. Halstead maneuver (costoclavicular test; military brace test): With the arms at the sides, move the shoulder down and back with the chest out.
      c. Wright's hyperabduction maneuver: With the arm externally rotated and abducted 180 degrees, inhale deeply (look for symptoms within 1 minute).
      d. Roos' test (stick-up test): Hold arms abducted and externally rotated; pump hands open and closed quickly. Look for symptoms of rapid fatigue of the involved arm.
      e. Cervical rotation lateral flexion test: Rotate the head away, then flex toward the affected side. Look for bone blocking lateral flexion or bony asymmetry between the two sides.
   3. Other tests
      a. Doppler probe: Evaluate flow, bruits, etc.
      b. Diagnostic injection of the scalene(s) with lidocaine.
      c. Chest and cervical spine x-rays are part of the initial evaluation.
      d. Angiography and venography are the gold standards for vascular TOCS.
      e. MRI is generally not helpful: 10% false-positive rate and it is not very specific.
      f. EMG is recommended for routine workup of "disputed" cases, but is rarely helpful.
      g. Psychiatric workup or treatment may be helpful. Some insurers may require one.
D. Nonoperative treatment
   1. Should be the first course of therapy for all "disputed" neurogenic TOCS (97% of cases).

2. May be inpatient or outpatient.
3. Four stages
   a. Stage I: Identify and treat trigger points, spasm, tendonitis, and bursitis using medication and other therapies.
   b. Stage II: Restore normal mobility and posture with stretching, relaxation, and education (typically done concurrently with stage I).
   c. Stage III: Strengthen muscle and restore presymptomatic level of function.
   d. Stage IV: Establish a home program and return to work.
4. Success rates are 50% to 100% for "disputed" forms of TOCS.

E. Operative treatment
1. Principles of current treatment.
   a. Excision or release of any or all anomalous anatomy.
   b. Resection of the first rib.
   c. Release or excision of the anterior and middle scalene muscles.
   d. Neurolysis of the brachial plexus as indicated.
2. Indications
   a. Failure of conservative therapy.
   b. Intractable pain.
   c. Significant neurologic deficit ("true" neurogenic group).
   d. Impending or acute vascular catastrophe (vascular TOCS).
   e. For "disputed" cases, indications continue to be controversial.
3. Surgical techniques
   a. Transaxillary approach: Safest for routine decompression, but it is hard to see the posterior first rib, and access to the plexus is incomplete.
   b. Supraclavicular approach: Better for vascular TOCS operations, but retraction injury to the phrenic and long thoracic nerves is more common.
   c. Combined: Use both approaches.
4. Complications include brachial plexus injury (probably underreported), hemothorax, pneumothorax (up to 62% in reoperative cases), chylothorax, causalgia, and cutaneous nerve dysesthesias (usually resolve within 6 months, occasionally permanent).
5. Operative management is successful in 80% of cases (range 25%–100%).

Tendon Transfers

I. Principles
A. Definition: The relocation of a tendon from a functioning muscle to replace an injured or nonfunctional muscle-tendon unit.
B. Concept of a "muscle balance operation": Tendon transfer (TT) is a redistribution of power units from areas of lesser functional need to areas of greater functional need.
C. Loss of a single major nerve (i.e., ulnar/median/radial) is more amenable to TT; if two or three nerves are damaged, severe extremity impairment is inevitable.
D. Other important points
   1. Joints affected need to have a good passive range of motion; joint contractures need to be either prevented or released.
   2. Sensibility need not be perfect.
   3. In general, simpler procedures have better results. E.g., do not introduce more than one change of direction in a tendon.

II. Indications
A. Nerve injury: The most common indication. May be at the level of the spinal cord or in a major nerve trunk. Injuries to smaller branches are more likely to recover without the need for TTs.
B. Muscle/tendon destruction: May be from trauma or disease processes such as rheumatoid arthritis (however, most traumatic injuries do *not* require a TT).

C. Spastic disorders: A less common indication, in part because TTs are less beneficial to these patients.

III. Preoperative planning

A. Evaluation

1. Establish patient goals and needs.
2. Rank priority of the functions desired.
3. Assess expectations, making sure they are realistic.
4. Verify motivation and ability to follow through with rehabilitation.

B. Timing

1. **Factors in the recovery of nerve function**
   a. Children do better than adults, who do better than the elderly in recovering nerve function.
   b. Clean, sharp cuts recover better than large and/or contaminated wounds.
   c. Injuries close to the muscle have better functional recovery than those far from the target muscle.
2. **Immediate tendon transfer:** Only done if there is no chance of neurologic recovery (i.e., the muscle is destroyed or a large section of the nerve is missing and repair/regrowth is not feasible).
3. **Delayed tendon transfer:** Usually performed 9 to 12 months following injury to allow for potential regrowth of the nerve. The higher the nerve injury, the longer regrowth will take.

C. Wound site factors that must be addressed before a TT

1. The bony skeleton must be stabilized.
2. The wound must be closed.
3. Scars must be soft, or must be excised.
4. Adequate soft tissue must be present to protect the TT.
5. Joint mobility must be maximized for the best result.

D. Donor tendon/muscle evaluation

1. **Donor muscle assessment:** Inventory all muscles and rate their power on a scale of 0 to 5. Only donor muscles with power grades of 4 or 5 should be used for tendon transfer.
   a. 0: No active movement.
   b. 1: Can resist gravity.
   c. 2: Can overcome gravity, but too weak for tasks.
   d. 3: Weak but useful power.
   e. 4: Weaker than normal strength.
   f. 5: Normal strength.
2. **Control:** Tendons to be transferred should have independent power (e.g., the FDP tendon slips do not have independent function and therefore are poor donor choices).
3. **Excursion (amplitude)**
   a. Specific excursions.
      (1) Digits: 70 mm.
      (2) Wrist: 30 mm.
   b. Tenodesis can increase excursion by approximately 25 mm.
   c. Need to match the donor being transferred with the amount of excursion needed (e.g., a wrist flexor will not work well as a digit extensor).
4. **Need to match strength** (e.g., the FCU is too strong for use as a motor for the APB). Therapy can improve muscle strength, but not excursion.
5. **Location:** Reroute the donor tendon in as direct a line as possible; do not change direction of tendon more than once.
6. **Synergism:** If possible, use muscles that naturally work together (e.g., wrist extensors and finger flexors); this makes postoperative rehabilitation easier.
7. **Expendability:** Is tendon function worth giving up for the benefit gained at its new location?

E. Smith and Hastings' planning algorithm

1. What muscles are functional?

2. What muscles are available for transfer?
3. What transfers/functions are needed?
4. Match what is available with functional requirements.
5. What else needs to be done (arthrodeses, tenodeses, etc.)?
6. Protect transfers postoperatively with splinting.
7. Rehabilitate to protect transfers while maximizing function.

IV. Tendon transfers for specific nerve palsies

A. Radial nerve palsy

1. **Anatomy:** The radial nerve innervates the triceps, brachioradialis, and ECRL before branching into superficial and deep branches in the forearm. The superficial radial nerve is purely sensory, whereas the deep radial nerve innervates the ECRB, supinator, APL, and all finger extensors. It continues as the posterior interosseous nerve to innervate the dorsal wrist.

2. **Functional deficits**

   a. The radial nerve is mostly motor, and the return of function is often more complete than in median or ulnar nerve injuries.

      (1) Common radial nerve injury patterns include "Saturday night palsy" and humerus fracture palsies.

      (2) Such injuries generally recover without surgery on the nerve.

   b. Uncomplicated nerve repairs in the distal third of the arm should recover some function within 4 to 6 months (1 mm per day). Patients without recovery after 6 months should be considered for TT.

   c. **High radial nerve paralysis:** Wrist, thumb, and digit extension are lost, producing a wrist drop deformity. Loss of wrist extension weakens power grip strength. Over time, patients develop an adaptive functional pattern.

      (1) Patients use wrist flexion to assist with finger extension (i.e., the "tenodesis effect").

      (2) Wrist flexion may be difficult to overcome later with TTs.

      (3) Splints should be worn to force wrist extension and assist with finger extension; splints are cumbersome and often tolerated only at night, but are critical to the eventual outcome.

      (4) Alternatively, some surgeons advocate doing an end-to-side tendon transfer of the PT to the ECRB to facilitate grip strength during nerve recovery (termed an "internal splint" procedure).

   d. **Low radial nerve injury:** Greater radial wrist deviation than higher-level injury due to unopposed ECRL function with loss of other extensors.

3. **Common tendon transfers for radial nerve paralysis** (Table 39-4). Radial nerve palsy TTs require one tendon each for wrist, digit, and thumb extension.

B. Median nerve palsy

1. **Nerve function and anatomy**

   a. The median nerve enters the forearm through the pronator teres, and innervates the PT, FCR, PL, and FDS.

   b. The anterior interosseous nerve then branches off and innervates the FPL, PQ, and radial head of FDP.

   c. The main branch of the median nerve continues through the carpal tunnel and gives off sensory and motor branches.

   d. The thenar motor branch innervates the APB, opponens pollicis (OP), and (variably) flexor pollicis brevis (FPB) muscles.

   e. The common digital branches innervate the lumbricals to the long and index fingers.

2. **Functional deficits**

   a. **Low median nerve palsy:** Loss of nerve function at level of the wrist.

      (1) Loss of **thumb opposition** from paralysis of APB, OP, and superficial head of FPB.

      (2) Loss of the lumbricals to the index and middle fingers.

Table 39-4. Tendon transfers for radial nerve paralysis

Desired Function	Tendon Transfer	Comments
Wrist extension (high nerve palsies)	PT to ECRB	PT is the optimal donor for wrist extension. It may not be needed if the injury is below the level of ECRB innervation.
Wrist lateral deviation (low palsies)	ECRL to ECRB or ECU	Minimizes radial wrist deviation.
Digit extension (low and high palsies)	FCR to EDC; FCU to EDC	FCR is favored, because ulnar deviation is preserved. FCU has twice the force of FCR but less excursion. No independent digit extension is allowed with these TTs.
	FDS (MF, RF only) to EDC	For independent motion (Boyes' transfer).
Thumb extension (low and high palsies)	PL to EPL	PL is present in 80% of patients.
	FDS (MF) to EPL	FDS can be used if PL is not present (Boyes' transfer)
	BR to APL	APL tenodesis at the BR insertion at the radial styloid prevents flexion-adduction of the thumb metacarpal and compensatory MCP hyperextension and IP flexion.

APL, abductor pollicis longus: BR, brachioradialis; ECRB/ECRL, extensor carpi radialis brevis/longus; EDC, extensor digitorum communis; EPL, extensor pollicis longus; FCU, flexor carpi ulnaris; FDS, flexor digitorum superficialis; IP, interphalangeal joint; MCP, metacarpophalangeal joint; MF, middle finger; RF, ring finger; PL, palmaris longus; PT, pronator teres; TT, tendon transfer.

- **b. High median nerve palsy**
  - **(1)** In addition to the muscle losses listed, the anterior interosseous nerve is affected. Patients lose FPL, PQ, and FDP to index and middle fingers, resulting in loss of thumb and index flexion.
  - **(2)** Higher-level injuries will damage FCR and PT function, but these losses do not require tendon transfers.
- **3. Common tendon transfers for median nerve paralysis** (Table 39-5).
- **C. Ulnar nerve palsy**
  - **1. Nerve function and anatomy**
    - **a.** Enters the forearm between the two heads of the FCU, and innervates the FCU and the ulnar portion of the FDP (ring and little fingers).
    - **b.** Continues into the hand via Guyon's canal, and innervates the abductor digit minimi (ADM), flexor digiti minimi (FDM), and opponens digiti minimi (ODM) muscles (i.e., the hypothenar muscles) as well as the seven interosseous muscles, the adductor pollicis, and the ring and little finger lumbricals. The ulnar nerve may innervate part or all of the FPB.
  - **2. Functional deficits**
    - **a. Low ulnar nerve palsy**
      - **(1)** Paralysis of the AP, the deep head of FPB, all interossei, the hypothenar muscles, and the lumbricals to ring and little fingers.

Table 39-5. Transfers for median nerve paralysis

Desired Function	Tendon Transfer	Comments
Thumb opposition (low and high palsies)	EIP to APB	EIP is usually preferred to avoid using a tendon from the potentially scarred volar area.
	ADM to APB	The Huber procedure. Also used for thumb hypoplasia, combined nerve palsies, and trauma.
Thumb opposition (low palsy)	FDS (RF) to APB	FDS (RF) is routed through a loop of FCU at the wrist to approach the APB at the proper angle.
	PL to APB	The Camitz procedure. Used after long-standing CTS and can be performed at the time of CTR.
Thumb flexion (high palsy)	BR to FPL	Allows thumb IP flexion.
Index flexion (high palsy)	FDP (LF, RF) to FDP (MF, IF)	Tenorrhaphy (not transfer) allows DIP flexion of MF and IF.
	ECRL to FDP (IF)	Provides strength to index flexion.

ADM, abductor digiti minimi; APB/APL, abductor pollicis brevis/longus; BR, brachioradialis; CTR, carpal tunnel release; CTS, carpal tunnel syndrome; DIP, distal interphalangeal joint; ECRL, extensor carpi radialis longus; EIP, extensor indicis proprius; FCU, flexor carpi ulnaris; FDP/FDS, flexor digitorum profundus/superficialis; IF, index finger; IP, interphalangeal joint; LF, little finger; MCP, metacarpophalangeal joint; MF, middle finger; RF, ring finger; PL, palmaris longus.

- **(2)** Clawing of the hand: Specifically, metacarpophalangeal (MP) joint hyperextension and IP flexion in the ring and little fingers due to loss of intrinsic musculature in the setting of intact extrinsic function.
- **(3)** Weak key pinch: Due to denervation of the first dorsal interosseous and AP muscles. To compensate, patients use FPL flexion to stabilize the thumb and EPL to adduct the thumb. Exaggerated thumb IP flexion during key pinch is termed **Froment's sign.**
- **(4)** Little finger ulnar deviation occurs due to unbalanced extensors (EDC, EDM) to that digit **(Wartenberg's sign).**
- b. **High ulnar nerve palsy**
  - **(1)** Less clawing than with low ulnar palsies, because the paralysis of FCU and FDP to ring and little fingers decreases the deforming force.
  - **(2)** Reconstruction can improve the function of the hand, but normal function usually cannot be restored.
- 3. **Common tendon transfers for ulnar nerve paralysis** (Table 39-6).
- 4. **Additionally, static block procedures** can be done to prevent MP hyperextension, including MP arthrodesis, MP joint capsulodesis, or bone blocks on the dorsum of the MP head. These procedures can be used alone or in concert with TTs.
- V. **Tendon transfers for specific diseases**
  - A. **Rheumatoid arthritis**
    - 1. Rheumatoid patients often rupture extensor tendons due to synovial invasion of the tendon or to attrition from a subluxed ulnar head.

Table 39-6. Transfers for ulnar nerve paralysis

Desired Function	Tendon Transfer	Comments
Thumb, key pinch (low and high palsies)	ECRB to abductor tubercle of the thumb metacarpal	Abductorplasty through the second intermetacarpal space to attach to the abductor tubercle. A PL tendon graft is usually required.
	FDS (RF) to abductor tubercle of the first metacarpal	Abductorplasty. Use only the radial half of the RF FDS tendon. Palmar fascia acts as pulley. No tendon graft is needed.
Clawing (low palsy)	FDS (MF or RF) to LF, RF	Tendons are split, then sutured to lateral bands or to the proximal phalanx.
	FDS "lasso" to LF, RF A2 pulley	FDS (RF or MF) is divided and looped through the A2 pulley, and then sutured to itself, with half going to the LF and half going to the RF.
	EDC or BR to LF, RF LBs	Attached to the lateral bands. Stabilizes finger, but does not aid in power flexion.
	EIP or EDC (LF) to LF, RF LBs	Attached to the lateral bands through the intermetacarpal space.
Clawing (high palsy)	FDP (MF) to FDP (LF, RF)	Side-to-side tenorrhaphy.
Index abduction for key pinch (low and high palsies)	Slip of APL to first dorsal interosseous	Main part of the APL remains attached to thumb; may use tendon graft to augment.
	EIP or EPB to first dorsal interosseous	Alternatives used to restore IF abduction. Many variations, but all attach to the first interosseous.
Power digit flexion (low and high palsy)	ECRL to digits	Tendon grafts are used to extend the ECRL in two to four tails, which go under the TCL to attach to the digital lateral bands or to the A2 pulleys.
Little finger adduction (low palsy)	EDM to LF	Ulnar half of EDM is passed through the metacarpal space to attach to either bone or the A2 pulley.
Wrist flexion (high palsy)	FCR to FCU	Restores FCU function. Some authors feel this is not necessary.

APL, abductor pollicis longus: BR, brachioradialis; ECRB/ECRL, extensor carpi radialis brevis/longus; EDC, extensor digitorum communis; EDM, extensor digiti minimi; EIP, extensor indicis proprius; EPB, extensor pollicis brevis; FCR/FCU, flexor carpi radialis/ulnaris; FDP/FDS, flexor digitorum profundus/superficialis; IF, index finger; LB, lateral band; LF, little finger; MF, middle finger; RF, ring finger; PL, palmaris longus; TCL, tibial collateral ligament.

   2. EDM and little finger EDC are often the first affected; this manifests as difficulty extending the little finger at the MP joint.
   3. To repair, the distal EDC tendon from the little finger can be attached to the ring EDC. Alternatively, the EIP can be transferred to either the EDM or the little finger EDC.
   4. If both the ring and little finger EDC tendons have eroded, then either the EIP or the FDS from the ring or middle fingers can be used.
   5. An extensor tenosynovectomy and a Darrach procedure should be done to prevent additional extensor tendon loss.
B. Leprosy
   1. The most common deformity is clawing due to ulnar or combined ulnar/median nerve palsies.
   2. TTs are used to restore thumb opposition and key pinch activity.
   3. ECRL to intrinsic muscle tendon transfers can also be performed, using plantaris tendon graft(s).
C. Poliomyelitis
   1. The muscles weakened early in the disease course will often regain function.
   2. Wait until strength is stable (no progression of disease *and* no new recovery of function) for 6 months to a year before doing any tendon transfers.

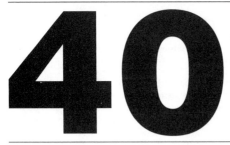

Rheumatoid Arthritis, Osteoarthritis, and Dupuytren's Contracture

Michelle S. Caird

Rheumatoid Arthritis

Rheumatoid Arthritis

I. General considerations
   A. Definition: Inflammatory arthritis characterized by morning stiffness, subcutaneous nodules, and lab abnormalities (positive rheumatoid factor in 70%).
   B. Typically involves: Cervical spine, shoulders, elbows, hands, hips, knees, and feet.
   C. Pathophysiology: Inflamed synovium (pannus) invades and destroys articular cartilage.
   D. Female-to-male ratio: 3:1.
   E. Treatment goals: Control synovitis, maintain joint function, and prevent deformity.
   F. Treatment overview.
      1. Maximize medical management: The patient should usually be under the care of a rheumatologist for at least 6 months before considering an operation.
      2. Physical therapy and occupational therapy: Critical to help with preoperative preparation and postoperative recovery.
      3. Surgery.
         a. Can be prophylactic, not just for late complications.
         b. Need to coordinate timing with the rheumatologist; maximize medical control.
         c. Preoperative cervical spine evaluation is essential.
         d. Generally, address joints from proximal to distal.

II. Hand findings
   A. Physical examination
      1. Ulnar drift at the metacarpophalangeal (MP) joints
      2. Caput ulna
      3. Swan-neck and boutonnière deformities (Fig. 40-1).
      4. Tendon ruptures
      5. Thumb deformities
      6. Radiocarpal collapse
   B. X-ray changes: Periarticular erosions and osteopenia

III. Ulnar drift at the metacarpophalangeal joints
   A. Mechanism of deformity.
      1. Synovitis at the MP joint causes capsule, ligament, and volar plate laxity.
      2. Radial sagittal band laxity causes ulnar deviation of the extensor tendons.
      3. Contraction of the ulnar intrinsics.
      4. Radial deviation of the wrist and metacarpals alters the direction of pull of the extensor tendons.
   B. Treatment depends on the degree of joint destruction.
      1. Address the wrist first.
      2. If no joint destruction: Synovectomy, soft tissue realignment, and ulnar intrinsic release.
      3. If joint destruction: Good results with MP implant arthroplasty (i.e., Swanson silicone implants).

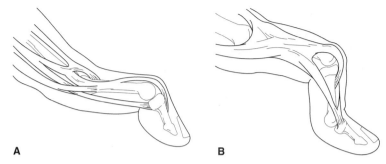

Fig. 40-1. A: Swan-neck deformity. **B:** Boutonnière deformity.

IV. Caput ulna
  A. Mechanism of deformity.
    1. Dorsal subluxation of the ulna due to distal radioulnar joint (DRUJ) synovitis and capsule stretch (piano key sign).
    2. Wrist supination and ulnar and volar translation result from extensor carpi ulnaris (ECU) subluxation ulnar and volar.
    3. Dorsal ulna subluxation can cause ischemic or attritional rupture of finger extensor tendons (Vaughn-Jackson syndrome).
  B. Nonoperative treatment.
    1. Optimize medical management.
    2. Splinting.
    3. Local steroid injections.
  C. Operative treatment (when nonoperative treatment fails) is indicated for pain relief with motion. These approaches require that the hand be under minimal load-bearing demands.
    1. Synovectomy of the DRUJ.
    2. Distal ulnar resection for unstable ulna (Darrach procedure).
    3. Distal ulnar pseudoarthrosis (Sauve-Kapandji procedure) preserves ulnocarpal joint if it is in good condition.
    4. Hemiresection arthroplasty of DRUJ preserves TFCC and ulnar length.
V. Swan-neck deformity (Fig. 40-1A)
  A. Hyperextension of the proximal interphalangeal (PIP) joint with distal interphalangeal (DIP) joint flexion.
  B. Three distinct mechanisms of deformity are possible:
    1. Synovitis at the DIP joint (or tenosynovitis) leads to rupture of distal extensor tendon, which leads to mallet deformity, which leads to extensor imbalance and volar plate laxity, which leads to PIP joint hyperextension.
    2. Synovitis at the PIP joint leads to volar plate laxity, which leads to PIP joint hyperextension, which leads to extensor imbalance, which leads to DIP joint flexion.
    3. Intrinsic tightness leads to MP joint subluxations, which lead to extensor imbalance, which leads to PIP joint hyperextension and DIP joint flexion.
  C. Correction of the deformity depends on PIP joint mobility and destruction.
    1. If passively correctable in all MP joint positions: Use PIP joint splint, DIP joint fusion, or retinacular ligament reconstruction.
    2. If flexion is limited by MP joint position: Fix MP joint subluxation or release tight intrinsics.
    3. If there is a fixed flexion deformity without joint destruction: Manipulation; lateral band mobilization; fix underlying deforming force.
    4. If there is a fixed flexion deformity with joint destruction: Arthrodesis versus arthroplasty of the PIP joints.
      a. Fuse joints where stability is most important.
        (1) Index (to maintain pinch): Fuse at 30 degrees.

(2) When necessary, can fuse middle finger at 35 degrees, ring finger at 40 degrees, and small finger at 45 degrees.
  b. Replace joint where motion is important—typically middle, ring, and small fingers (to maintain power grip).

VI. Boutonnière deformity (Fig. 40-1B)
  A. Flexion at the PIP joint with hyperextension at the DIP and MP joints.
  B. Mechanism of deformity.
   1. Synovitis at the PIP joint leads to attenuation of central slip, which leads to flexion at PIP joint, which leads to volar subluxation of the lateral bands.
   2. Shortened oblique retinacular ligaments lead to DIP joint hyperextension.
   3. Compensatory MP joint hyperextension.
  C. Correction of deformity.
   1. If passively correctable with mild deformity: Synovectomy and splinting with or without tenotomy of the terminal tendon.
   2. If passively correctable with moderate deformity: Synovectomy with central slip/lateral band reconstruction with or without tenotomy of the terminal tendon.
   3. If there is a fixed flexion deformity: Arthrodesis versus arthroplasty of the PIP joint (see "Swan-Neck Deformity," above).

VII. Tenosynovitis/tendon rupture
  A. Differentiate the cause of a sudden inability to extend a finger.
   1. Extensor tendon rupture from attrition: ($-$) active extension, ($-$) maintenance of extension, ($-$) tenodesis effect (passive finger extension with wrist flexion).
   2. Ulnar subluxation of an extensor tendon at the MP joint: ($-$) active extension, ($+$) maintenance of extension, ($+$) tenodesis effect.
   3. Posterior interosseous nerve palsy at the elbow from synovitis: ($-$) active extension, ($-$) maintenance of extension, ($+$) tenodesis effect.
   4. Palmar subluxation of the MP joint: Evident on x-ray and physical examination.
  B. Extensor tendon rupture.
   1. The extensor pollicis longus (EPL) is the most common extensor tendon to rupture.
   2. Vaughan-Jackson syndrome: The extensor digiti minimi (EDM), extensor digitorum communis (EDC) of the small finger, and the EDC of the ring finger usually rupture in sequence; may proceed to rupture more radial tendons.
   3. Treatment is tenosynovectomy, addressing caput ulna (Darrach procedure), and tendon grafts or transfers.
    a. EPL rupture: Transfer extensor indicis proprius (EIP), EDM, or extensor pollicis brevis (EPB).
    b. EDM rupture: Transfer EIP if necessary.
    c. Single EDC rupture (usually small finger): Cross-link to adjacent EDC (usually ring finger).
    d. Two EDC ruptures: Transfer EIP.
  C. Flexor pollicis longus (FPL) rupture (Mannerfelt's syndrome): Most common flexor tendon ruptured.
   1. Inability to flex the thumb interphalangeal (IP) joint.
   2. Causes: Synovitis, carpal osteophyte.
   3. Treatment is synovectomy, osteophyte resection, and tendon graft or transfer.

Osteoarthritis

I. Definition and epidemiology
  A. Arthritis characterized by cartilage changes, including increased water content and altered collagen and proteoglycans that lead to cartilage destruction.
  B. Females have a higher incidence than males; usually over 40 years of age.
  C. Possible genetic predisposition.
  D. Most common form of arthritis.

II. X-ray changes
A. Osteophytes, narrowed joint space, eburnation, and subchondral cysts.
B. Common sites include DIP joints and thumb carpometacarpal (CMC) joint; rare sites are PIP joints and scaphotrapeziotrapezoid (STT) joints.

III. Distal interphalangeal joints: Heberden's nodes
A. **Symptoms: Pain, deformity, and instability.**
   1. Rest, nonsteroidal antiinflammatory drugs (NSAIDs), rarely injection (painful)
   2. If not controlled with nonoperative trial, fusion of joint in 10 to 20 degrees of flexion.
B. **Mucous cyst or ganglion** communicates with the DIP joint due to underlying osteoarthritis.
   1. Thin skin can rupture, opening the DIP joint to environment.
   2. Can cause nail deformity due to pressure.
   3. Indications for surgery: Enlargement, rupture, pain, and nail deformity.
   4. Surgical treatment: Excision of cyst and osteophytes at the DIP joint; avoid disrupting the germinal matrix.

IV. Thumb carpometacarpal (CMC) joint
A. **Findings.**
   1. **Early symptoms:** Pain, swelling, crepitus, and weak pinch.
   2. **Late symptoms:** Metacarpal adduction and web contracture.
   3. **Signs:** Positive grind test (pain with axial loading of the thumb CMC).
B. **Mechanism of deformity:** Volar carpal (beak) ligament (from the volar-ulnar base of the first metacarpal to the trapezium) degenerates, which destabilizes the thumb CMC and leads to joint wear.
C. **X-rays:** Trapeziometacarpal arthritis or pantrapezial arthritis.
D. **Treatment.**
   1. Rest, splinting, NSAIDs, and steroid injection.
   2. **Surgical indications:** Persistent pain, instability, first web contracture, and decreased function despite nonsurgical measures.
   3. **Surgical options.**
      a. Arthrodesis.
         (1) Fuse at 30 to 40 degrees palmar abduction, 30 degrees radial abduction, and 15 degrees pronation.
         (2) Nonunion is a frequent complication.
      b. Trapezium excision with tendon interposition: Subsidence is a frequent complication.
      c. Trapezium excision with tendon interposition plus reconstruction of the volar beak ligament using flexor carpi radialis (FCR) and abductor pollicis longus (APL): Good pain relief and restoration of pinch.
      d. If MP hyperextension deformity exists, it should be treated.
         (1) Less than 30 degrees: Pinning.
         (2) Greater than 30 degrees: Volar plate advancement or arthrodesis (15 degrees flexion, 10 degrees pronation).

V. Proximal interphalangeal joints: Bouchard's nodes
A. **Symptoms:** Pain, deformity, instability, and decreased range of motion (ROM).
B. Less common than other conditions listed previously.
C. **Treatment.**
   1. Rest, NSAIDs, and (rarely) injection (painful).
   2. If not controlled with nonoperative measures, fusion of PIP (see "Swan-Neck Deformity," above).
   3. Arthroplasty is preferred in the ring and small fingers to maintain motion for power grip.

Other Common Arthritides

I. Systemic lupus erythematosus
A. Systemic autoimmune disease with characteristic malar rash and multiorgan involvement.

    B. Female-to-male ratio is 9:1; age of onset is late teens to early twenties.

    C. Hand findings are often passively correctable.

        1. Ulnar deviation and volar subluxation at the MP joints.

        2. Compensatory swan-neck deformities.

        3. Dorsal subluxation of the ulna.

        4. Extensor tendon attritional ruptures.

    D. X-ray changes: Joint deformity without destruction.

    E. Treatment.

        1. Medical management of systemic disease.

        2. Splinting of supple deformities.

        3. Distal ulnar resection for instability (Darrach procedure).

        4. MP joint implant arthroplasty or arthrodesis. Do not use soft tissue procedures for MP joint deformity, due to high recurrence rates.

II. Psoriatic arthritis

    A. Twenty percent of people with psoriasis develop arthritis; skin lesions appear first.

    B. Hand findings: Nail pitting, DIP joints affected, asymmetric involvement, arthritis mutilans, or telescoping of fingers.

    C. X-ray changes: Widened joint spaces or "pencil in cup" deformity (tapered proximal bone in a widened base).

    D. Control disease medically; surgery is indicated only if a functional limitation because of unstable or stiff fingers is present.

III. Crystalline arthropathies

    A. Gout (monosodium urate crystals)

        1. **Urate metabolism disorder** or high metabolic turnover diseases result in hyperuricemia and precipitation of crystals in the soft tissues and joints with a painful inflammatory response.

        2. **Men** are affected more than women.

        3. **Negatively birefringent crystals (yellow)** on microscopic examination of joint aspirate are required for diagnosis.

        4. **X-ray changes:** Soft tissue deposits (tophi) and punched-out periarticular erosions.

        5. **Acute attacks** are treated with colchicine and indomethacin; use allopurinol for chronic therapy.

    B. Pseudogout (calcium pyrophosphate dihydrate crystals)

        1. **Pyrophosphate metabolism disorder.**

        2. **Men and women** affected equally.

        3. **Positively birefringent crystals (blue).**

        4. **X-ray changes:** Calcification of fibrocartilage (triangular fibrocartilage complex in the wrist).

        5. **Acute attacks in the hand are rare;** treated with NSAIDs.

IV. Scleroderma

    A. Systemic sclerosis; possible small vessel and/or connective tissue disorder with fibrosis.

    B. Hand findings: Skin, PIP flexion contractures, compensatory MP hyperextension, thumb web contractures, Raynaud's phenomenon, and painful calcinosis.

    C. X-ray changes: Loss of tuft of distal phalanges, and soft tissue calcinosis.

    D. Treatment: Surgical excision of calcinosis, amputation of ulcerated fingertips, and PIP joint arthrodesis.

V. Septic arthritis: See Chapter 45, "Hand Infections, Compartment Syndrome, and High-Energy Injuries."

Dupuytren's Contracture

I. Definition

    A. Abnormal fibromatous tissue development in the palmar subcutaneous fibrous connective layer.

   B. Fibroblasts are involved in producing extracellular matrix proteins, which result in contraction.

   C. Nodules and cords on the palmar surface can cause flexion contractures.

II. Epidemiology

   A. Demographics

   1. Most commonly, people of Northern European ancestry are affected.

   2. Male-to-female ratio is 10:1.

   3. Rare before the age of 40.

   4. Inheritance pattern: Autosomal dominant with variable penetrance.

   5. Underlying cause is unknown; not occupational or traumatic.

   B. Location: Affects the palm and most commonly the ring and small fingers.

   C. Associated diseases

   1. Alcoholism

   2. Diabetes mellitus

   3. Epilepsy

   4. Human immunodeficiency virus infection

   5. Chronic obstructive pulmonary disease

   D. Dupuytren's diathesis: Presents aggressively, with early onset and early recurrence; may require more extensive treatment. Characterized by three classic findings:

   1. Knuckle pads

   2. Foot involvement (Ledderhose's disease)

   3. Penis involvement (Peyronie's disease)

III. Bands and cords

   A. Bands are normal digital and palmar subcutaneous fibrous connective tissue.

   1. Spiral band

   2. Lateral digital sheet

   3. Natatory ligament

   4. Pretendinous band

   5. Grayson's ligament: Palmar to the neurovascular (NV) bundle (see Fig.   )

   6. Cleland's ligament: Dorsal to the NV bundle; **does not** become diseased

   B. Cords are diseased tissue.

   1. Spiral cord: From diseased pretendinous band, spiral band, lateral digital sheet, and Grayson's ligament wraps around the neurovascular bundle.

   2. Lateral cord: Contributes to PIP joint contracture.

   3. Natatory cord: From diseased natatory ligament; causes web space contracture.

   4. Pretendinous cord: Cord in the palm from a diseased pretendinous band causes MP joint contracture.

   5. Central cord: Contributes to PIP joint contracture.

   6. Retrovascular cord: Causes DIP joint contracture.

IV. Indications for surgery

   A. MP joint contracture is usually correctible; operative release is indicated in the following cases.

   1. Contractures interfere significantly with daily activities (ask the patient).

   2. Arbitrary contracture angles are less important, but usually an operation is done if MP contracture is greater than 30 to 45 degrees.

   B. Any PIP joint contracture is difficult to fully correct, so early intervention is warranted.

   C. Contracture causing maceration or hygiene difficulties.

V. Nonoperative treatment

   A. Steroid injections may help painful palm nodules but do not prevent progression—they only delay it.

   B. Collagenase injections may have promise, but are not the current standard of care.

   C. Ultraviolet therapy: Role is unclear.

VI. Operative treatment

   A. Primary operations

    1. Subcutaneous fasciotomy.
      a. Not generally considered effective.
      b. Consider only for very sick or elderly patients.
    2. Limited fasciectomy: Resection of only diseased tissue.
    3. Regional fasciectomy: Resection of diseased tissue and a margin of nondiseased fascia (often advised in the palm).
    4. Extensive fasciectomy: Resection of diseased tissue and all potentially involved fascia (often advised in the fingers).
    5. Radical fasciectomy (dermofasciectomy): Consider in recurrent disease.
  B. Closure options
    1. Many skin incisions have been advocated.
      a. Palmar: Transverse incision in proximal palmar crease is preferred.
      b. Finger: Longitudinal incision, broken up by Z-plasties over creases, is preferred.
    2. Open palm technique (of McCash) heals well and prevents hematoma.
    3. Skin replacement (skin grafting) seems to prevent recurrence, even in cases where fascia excision is rather limited, although this is debated.
  C. Recurrent disease
    1. Repeat fasciectomy or dermofasciectomy with full-thickness skin grafting
    2. Joint arthrodesis
    3. Amputation in severely affected patients or for NV compromise
  D. Complications
    1. Hematoma formation
    2. Recurrence
    3. Nerve injury
    4. Vascular injury
    5. Stiffness (i.e., failure to correct contracture, especially at the PIP joint)
    6. Complex regional pain syndrome (CRPS, formerly known as reflex sympathetic dystrophy syndrome)
  E. Postoperative care
    1. Dressing changes if open palm technique was used.
    2. Early aggressive occupational therapy for active ROM.
    3. Splinting: Some variability of opinion exists.
      a. Some advocate nighttime extension splinting.
      b. Some advocate splinting in a position of function.

Pearls

---

1. The spiral cord pushes the neurovascular bundle volar, proximal, and midline. Beware.
2. The best predictors of neurovascular bundle displacement are PIP joint flexion contracture and interdigital nodule.
3. Do not combine fasciectomy with carpal tunnel release, because there is an increased chance of complex regional pain syndrome.
4. Surgery does not stop the underlying process in Dupuytren's contracture; it just addresses the deformity.
5. Mnemonic device for the structures that become the spiral cord in Dupuytren's contracture: **P**lastic **S**urgeons **L**ook **G**ood (**P**retendinous band, **S**piral band, **L**ateral sheet, and **G**rayson's ligament).

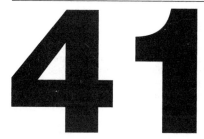

Hand Tumors

Sameer S. Jejurikar

I. Incidence
A. Benign tumors
1. **Most tumors of the hand are benign** (>90%), usually can be diagnosed clinically, and require no treatment. If lesions suddenly change in size, appearance, or aggressiveness, an appropriate workup (i.e., biopsy) must be done.
2. **The three most common hand masses** (in decreasing order of frequency) are as follows:
   a. Ganglion cyst (50% to 70% of all hand tumors).
   b. Giant cell tumor of tendon sheath.
   c. Epidermal inclusion cyst.
B. Malignant tumors
1. **Squamous cell carcinoma** is the most frequent primary malignancy of the hand; other malignancies are far less common.
2. **Malignant metastases** to bones of the hand are exceedingly rare.
3. A significant proportion of soft tissue sarcomas and melanomas occur in the upper extremity.

II. Ganglions
A. Ganglions are the most common benign tumor of the hand.
1. They consist of a mucin-filled cyst attached to tendon, tendon sheath, or joint capsule.
2. Most occur in the second through fourth decades of life.
3. Most occur at the dorsal wrist, followed by the volar wrist, flexor tendon sheath (volar retinacular), and distal interphalangeal (DIP) joint (also known as a DIP mucous cyst).
   a. These four sites make up more than 90% of the ganglions of the hand.
   b. Ganglions can also be seen with carpometacarpal bossing, at the PIP joint (similar to a DIP mucous cyst), and in association with extensor tendons.
B. Treatment
1. **Nonoperative**
   a. All nonsurgical methods have limited success.
   b. Lidocaine and corticosteroid injection can temporarily alleviate symptoms.
   c. Patient reassurance is an effective nonsurgical therapy.
2. **Operative**
   a. Should be excised in the operating room, under tourniquet control.
   b. No need to close the joint capsule after excision.
   c. Some surgeons apply a splint, but a light gauze dressing works as well.
C. Dorsal wrist ganglion
1. Make up 60% to 70% of all ganglions.
2. Usually arise directly over the scapholunate ligament.
3. Previously termed 'preacher's cyst', as treatment involved striking hand with a large book.
4. The ganglion is exposed through a transverse skin incision; excision includes a small portion of the underlying wrist capsule.
5. The ganglion usually appears between the third (extensor pollicis longus) and fourth (extensor digitorum communis) extensor compartments.

D. Volar wrist ganglion
1. Second most common site, making up 18% to 20% of all ganglion cysts.
2. Occurs over the distal edge of the radius (arising from the radiocarpal joint) or over the scaphoid tubercle (arising from the scaphotrapezial joint).
3. Usually arises adjacent to the radial artery; the patency of the radial and ulnar arteries should be tested preoperatively with an Allen's test, in the unlikely event of injury to the radial artery with excision.
4. The surgical technique is similar to that for a dorsal wrist ganglion.

E. Volar retinacular ganglion
1. Third most common, making up 10% to 12% of all ganglion cysts.
2. Arises from the A1 pulley.
3. Usually presents as a tender mass under the metacarpal flexion crease.
4. The cyst is attached to the tendon sheath and does not move (distinguishing it from a trigger finger).
5. Surgical exposure must allow for identification of the neurovascular bundles.
6. The ganglion should be excised with a small portion of the tendon sheath.

F. Mucous cyst
1. Ganglion of the DIP joint.
2. Most commonly occurs between the fifth and seventh decades of life.
3. Nail grooving may present before a mass does (due to impingement on the matrix).
4. X-rays may reveal arthritic osteophytes (Heberden's nodes), which should be removed at the time of surgery.
5. Must explore both sides of the extensor tendon to assess for occult cysts.

III. Giant cell tumor of the tendon sheath (Pigmented Villonodular Tenosynovitis)
A. Second most common tumor of the hand (after ganglions).
B. Usually presents as a firm, indolent, painless mass on the volar surface of the fingers or hand (no malignant potential).
1. Dorsal involvement occurs in approximately one-third of tumors.
2. Commonly occurs in the middle finger, index finger, or thumb.
3. Often occurs in the vicinity of the DIP joint.
C. Patients may have a sensory deficit secondary to digital nerve compression.
D. Radiographs may demonstrate a soft tissue mass.
1. May see pressure resorption of bone.
2. Invasion of bone suggests a more aggressive neoplasm.
3. Malignant transformation of this tumor has not been described.
E. Total surgical excision is the recommended therapy.
1. All discolored tissue and satellite lesions should be removed.
2. High risk of local recurrence (up to 50%).

IV. Epidermal inclusion cysts
A. Third most common tumor of the hand.
B. May be related to the embedment of epithelial cells into underlying tissue after local trauma.
1. Usually attached to the overlying skin.
2. Can be seen in bone, albeit rarely, following history of open injury.
C. Presents most often as a slow-growing mass on the fingertip.
1. Usually painless, but painful lesions have been described.
2. Occurs most often in the distal phalanx (volar surface).
   a. Metacarpal involvement is rare.
   b. No reported cases involve the carpal bones.
3. The lesion is usually well defined, compact, and minimally mobile.
4. The diagnosis is more difficult when the lesion involves bone.
   a. X-rays demonstrate a circumscribed lytic lesion.
   b. Can be confused with a primary malignancy.
D. Surgical therapy should involve excision of the entire epithelial sac to prevent recurrence.
1. Recurrence is rare.
2. Malignant transformation has not been described.

V. Skin cancers
A. Squamous cell carcinoma of the hand
1. **Most common malignancy of the hand.**
   a. Five-year mortality rate is 10%.
   b. Local recurrence and lymph node metastatic rates are 20% to 30%.
2. **Wide spectrum of presentation.**
   a. May arise *de novo*.
   b. May be seen in regions of previous actinic keratoses, burn injury, chronic wounds, and ultraviolet-injured or irradiated skin.
   c. Keratoacanthoma may be confused with squamous cell carcinoma.
3. **Bowen's disease**
   a. Squamous cell carcinoma *in situ*.
   b. Presents as a crusting brown plaque.
   c. Surgical therapy: Excision with 2–3 mm margins.
   d. If the nail matrix is involved, proper treatment is amputation at the DIP joint.
4. **Tumors less than 2.5 cm in diameter**
   a. Wide excision with 2- to 3-cm margins is the appropriate therapy.
   b. Treatment margins are more aggressive than in other body sites; this compensates for a delay in diagnosis, which is common for hand tumors.
5. **Tumors greater than 2.5 cm in diameter**
   a. High rate of local recurrence.
   b. Radical excision, including ray or segmental amputation, is appropriate.
   c. No benefit to prophylactic lymph node dissection.
6. **Recurrent tumors**
   a. High rate of lymph node metastases (60% to 70%).
   b. Lymphadenectomy is advised, even in the absence of palpable nodes.
B. Basal cell carcinoma
1. **Much less frequent** then squamous cell carcinoma.
2. Can present as a slow-growing, ulcerated lesion with a raised, pearly border.
   a. More frequently seen in fair-skinned individuals in sun-exposed areas.
   b. May invade deeper structures and cause significant tissue destruction.
   c. Rarely metastasizes.
   d. Recurrence is frequent in lesions with poorly defined borders.
3. **Surgical excision** should include a rim of normal appearing tissue (2–5 mm).
   a. Other treatment options include Mohs' surgery and radiation therapy.
   b. The best form of treatment has yet to be determined.
C. Melanoma (see Chapter 11, "Malignant Skin and Soft Tissue Lesions")
1. A large proportion (10% to 20%) of all melanomas involve the upper extremity.
2. **Subungual melanoma**
   a. Poor prognosis (30% 5-year survival) may be related to delayed diagnosis.
   b. Amputation is usually performed at the joint immediately proximal to lesion.
   c. May need more extensive resection depending on the extent of tumor invasion.
D. Merkel cell carcinoma (neuroendocrine carcinoma)
1. Very aggressive and rare lesion seen in the elderly population.
2. Bluish-red, painless, and fast-growing nodule.
3. Wide range in size on presentation (0.5–5.0 cm).
4. Treatment is radical excision with lymphadenectomy.
5. There may be a role for postoperative chemotherapy and XRT.
6. High incidence of local recurrence and distant metastasis.
7. Systemic spread of disease is always fatal.
E. Kaposi's sarcoma
1. Malignant vascular tumor.
2. Occurs in the hand, but is more common in lower extremities.

3. Whenever a patient presents with bluish-red skin nodules, one must consider a diagnosis of AIDS.
4. Highly radiosensitive tumor, though residual disease usually remains after aggressive XRT.

F. Malignant sweat gland tumors
1. This category includes clear cell carcinoma, aggressive digital papillary adenocarcinoma, and eccrine adenocarcinoma.
2. Like many other tumors of the hand, these tumors are painless and slow-growing nodules.
3. Most often occur in the elderly population.
4. Local recurrence and systemic spread are both very common.
5. Treatment is wide local excision and lymph node dissection for palpable nodes.
6. No role for XRT or chemotherapy.

G. Glomus tumors
1. Benign tumors of glomus cells as well as the tissue that composes the arteriovenous glomus body.
2. Classically occur in the subungual region.
3. Triad of symptoms (severe pain, cold sensitivity, and tenderness).
4. Can also see nail ridging and red to bluish discoloration.
5. Complete surgical excision is the appropriate therapy, with a low incidence of recurrence.

VI. Bony tumors
A. Benign bone tumors
  1. **Solitary enchondroma**
     a. The most common primary bone tumor of the hand.
     b. Occurs most frequently in the middle phalanx, and least frequently in the distal phalanx.
     c. Usually presents with a pathologic fracture.
     d. X-rays usually demonstrate a circumscribed lytic lesion.
     e. Treatment is curettage and possible cancellous bone grafting.
     f. Sarcomatous transformation is rare with solitary enchondromas.
  2. **Multiple enchondromatosis**
     a. **Ollier's disease.**
        (1) Multiple enchondromas in the bones of the hands and feet.
        (2) Enchondromas can be quite large and lead to significant functional impairment.
        (3) The rate of sarcomatous degeneration is as high as 30%.
        (4) Not an inherited condition.
     b. **Maffucci's syndrome.**
        (1) Similar to Ollier's disease, but predominantly affects the hands.
        (2) In addition to multiple enchondromas, patients have multiple hemangiomas.
        (3) Also has a high risk of sarcomatous degeneration.
  3. **Osteochondroma**
     a. Although the most common benign bony tumor of the body, it is quite rare in the hand.
     b. The tumor is an osseous mass with a hyaline cartilage cap thought to originate from the metaphysis.
     c. Most often seen at the distal portion of the proximal phalanx.
     d. Malignant transformation to chondrosarcoma is rare.
  4. **Unicameral bone cyst**
     a. Cystic lesion of unknown etiology that is rare in the hand and forearm.
     b. Presents as a pathologic fracture.
     c. No known risk of malignancy.
     d. Usually located in the distal third of the metacarpal.
  5. **Osteoid osteoma**
     a. Presents in second and third decades of life with nocturnal pain that is typically relieved by aspirin or nonsteroidal antiinflammatory agents.

b. Occurs most commonly in the proximal phalanx and carpal bones, as well as the distal radius.

c. X-ray shows a radiolucent nidus surrounded by cortical sclerosis.

d. Treatment is either en bloc surgical excision or curettage of the nidus.

e. Incomplete excision can lead to recurrence of the lesion.

6. Chondromyxoid fibroma

a. Rare cartilaginous bone tumor.

b. Arises in the metaphyseal region of the bone.

c. Tends to occur in males prior to the third decade of life.

d. Treatment is curettage and bone grafting.

7. Osteoblastoma

a. Rare tumor, usually greater than 2 cm in diameter.

b. Histologically similar to osteoid osteoma.

c. Must be distinguished from osteosarcoma.

d. Treatment is curettage and bone grafting, with high local recurrence rates (20% to 30%).

e. If recurrence occurs, may require wide excision and bony reconstruction.

8. Aneurysmal bone cyst

a. Most often occurs in the second decade of life.

b. Most commonly occurs in the metacarpals; carpal lesions are uncommon.

c. Radiographically similar to giant cell tumors.

d. Locally aggressive tumor, but does not metastasize.

e. Recurrence rate is as high as 60% after curettage and bone grafting.

f. Cryosurgery reduces the risk of local recurrence.

9. Giant cell tumor of bone

a. Rare tumors that are considered benign but are locally aggressive, with the potential for distant metastases.

b. Local recurrence rates are as high as 80% after curettage, even with adjuvant therapy with phenol.

c. Most commonly in the fourth decade of life.

d. Most common in the metacarpals and phalanges.

(1) Have been reported in the carpal bones, albeit rarely.

(2) Common site of occurrence is the distal radius.

e. X-rays show a lytic lesion without a matrix or clear borders, soft-tissue invasion, and cortical extension and destruction.

f. Curettage alone leads to unacceptably high rates of recurrence; the rate is improved with adjunctive cryotherapy.

g. Amputation or wide excision may be more appropriate surgical therapy.

B. Malignant bone tumors

1. Chondrosarcoma

a. Most common primary bone tumor of the hand.

b. Most often occurs in the proximal phalanges and metacarpals.

c. Tends to afflict patients over the age of 60.

d. Can present as slow-growing, hard, and painful mass.

e. X-rays demonstrate radiolucent regions with cortical destruction and stippled calcifications.

f. Most common site of metastasis is the lung.

g. Best treated by wide excision or ray amputation.

h. No role for chemotherapy or XRT.

i. Prognosis is generally good, although local or systemic recurrence can occur several years after treatment of the primary lesion.

2. Osteogenic sarcoma

a. Most common primary bone tumor in the first and second decade of life, but is very rare in the hand.

b. Presents as a rapidly growing, painful, hard mass.

c. Most often occurs in the proximal phalanges and metacarpals.

    d. X-rays demonstrate a destructive, sclerotic lesion.

    e. Treatment is wide excision or finger or ray amputation.

    f. Adjuvant chemotherapy improves survival.

    g. No role for XRT.

  3. Ewing's sarcoma

    a. Most commonly occurs in the first and second decades of life.

    b. Only rarely occurs in the hand; most commonly occurs in the metacarpals and phalanges.

    c. Presentation is similar to infection, with erythema, pain, and soft tissue swelling.

    d. X-rays show a destructive lytic lesion; magnetic resonance imaging is useful for demonstrating the extent of soft tissue invasion.

    e. Surgical therapy is wide excision or amputation.

    f. The tumor is radiosensitive, with adjuvant chemotherapy also having benefit.

    g. High rate of mortality, even with adjunctive therapy.

Pearls

1. More than 90% of all hand tumors are benign.
2. Ganglion cysts are the most common tumor of the hand, constituting 50% to 70% of all tumors.
3. Remember ABCD (**A**symmetry, irregular **B**order, irregular **C**olor, **D**iameter >6 mm) to assess nevi that are suggestive of melanoma.
4. Unlike most other regions of the body, in the upper extremity, basal cell carcinoma occurs far less frequently than does squamous cell carcinoma.
5. Perform a biopsy of any suspicious lesion because, although uncommon, malignancies of the upper extremity can be lethal.

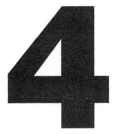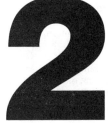

Congenital Anomalies of the Hand and Upper Extremity

Gregory H. Borschel

I. Epidemiology
  A. The overall incidence of congenital anomalies of the upper extremity is 1 in 600 births.
  B. The most frequent anomalies are syndactyly, polydactyly, and camptodactyly.
  C. Five percent of congenital upper extremity deformity is familial, and 95% is sporadic.

II. Hand development
  A. *In utero*
     1. **Patterns are determined by Hox A-D genes,** mediated by expressed proteins that include fibroblast growth factors (FGF), sonic hedgehog (Shh), and Wnt-7a.
     2. **Fourth week:** Limb buds appear (mesenchymal cells encased in ectoderm).
     3. **Fifth week:** Apical ectodermal ridge induces development longitudinally; hand plates form.
     4. **Sixth week:** Apoptosis results in digital separation.
     5. **Seventh week:** Mesenchymal differentiation; chondrogenesis and osteogenesis.
  B. **At birth:** Grasp reflex present.
  C. **3 months:** Power grip with ulnar digits.
  D. **5 months:** Finger grip with adducted thumb.
  E. **7 months:** Thumb opposition.
  F. **9 months:** Small object pinch.
  G. **10 months:** Fine pinch.
  H. **3 to 4 years:** Hand preference established.

III. Evaluation
  A. Initial discussion with family requires large amounts of time and patience.
  B. Families often feel guilty and anxious.
  C. It is important to formulate realistic expectations from the outset.
  D. Genetic counseling is indicated, especially if syndromic stigmata are present.

IV. General treatment goals
  A. Power grasp
  B. Precision pinch
  C. Maintenance of growth potential
  D. Cosmesis

V. American Society for Surgery of the Hand (ASSH) classification of congenital hand anomalies
  A. Failure of formation of parts (arrest of development)
  B. Failure of differentiation or separation of parts
  C. Duplications
  D. Overgrowth
  E. Undergrowth
  F. Constriction band syndrome
  G. Generalized skeletal abnormalities

VI. Failure of formation of parts

A. Transverse absence ("congenital amputation")
   1. May occur at any level.
   2. Commonly occurs below elbow or at wrist.
   3. Best treated with prosthesis at early age.

B. Longitudinal absence (phocomelia)
   1. **Presents with absence of the humerus.**
   2. **Usually caused by maternal use of thalidomide** (an antiemetic) during pregnancy.

C. Radial deficiency (so-called "radial clubhand")
   1. Present in 1 in 55,000 births.
   2. Usually unilateral.
   3. More often found on right side.
   4. More often in males.
   5. Linked to thalidomide use.
   6. **Presentation and anatomy**
      a. Radial deviation of wrist.
      b. Thumb hypoplasia.
      c. Variable degrees of deficiency, from minor to severe.
         (1) Type I: Short distal radius.
         (2) Type II: Hypoplastic radius with ulnar deformity.
         (3) Type III: Partial absence of the radius.
         (4) Type IV: Absent radius.
      d. The ulna is often short and curved.
      e. The preaxial bones, muscles, and tendons may coalesce into a fibrous anlage, resulting in stiffness.
      f. Preaxial vessels and nerves are often absent.
      g. The elbow joint is stiff.
   7. **Associated syndromes:** Many organ systems develop at the same time as the radius. Any child presenting with radial-sided congenital anomalies should undergo thorough evaluation for hematologic and cardiac anomalies, especially the following:
      a. **VATERR association**
         (1) **V**ertebral anomalies.
         (2) **A**nal atresia.
         (3) **T**racheo**e**sophageal atresia.
         (4) **R**enal anomalies.
         (5) **R**adial deficiency.
      b. **Holt-Oram syndrome:** Atrial septal defect (ASD) with radial deficiency.
      c. **Fanconi's anemia:** Radial deficiency with polydactyly, syndactyly, clinodactyly, ASD, and pancytopenia.
      d. **TAR syndrome: T**hrombocytopenia with **a**bsence of the **r**adius.
      e. **Nager's syndrome:** Radial deficiency and acrofacial dysostosis.
      f. **Goldenhar's syndrome:** Hemifacial microsomia with epibulbar dermoids.
      g. **Möbius' syndrome** (congenital facial paralysis): Limb abnormalities occur in 25% of cases.
      h. **Cleft lip/palate.**
      i. **Treacher-Collins syndrome.**
      j. **Klippel-Feil syndrome.**
   8. **Treatment**
      a. **Nonoperative therapy**
         (1) Physical therapy, including stretching, is used to decrease elbow and wrist stiffness.
         (2) Splinting is used to passively centralize the wrist preoperatively.
      b. **Surgical management**
         (1) Indications: Loss of function from carpal angulation, poor extensor excursion, cosmetic deformity.
         (2) Soft tissue release is performed early if passive centralization cannot be achieved with splinting.

(3) Distraction osteogenesis (Ilizarov technique) with or without wedge osteotomies can be used to lengthen and straighten the radius.

(4) Tendon transfers are used to maintain a centralized wrist position: Fused mass of flexor carpi radialis (FCR), extensor carpi radialis longus (ECRL), extensor carpi radialis brevis (ECRB), and brachioradialis is transferred to the extensor carpi ulnaris (ECU) to become an ulnar deviator, thus balancing the wrist.

(5) Pollicization.

(a) The thumb is usually hypoplastic.

(b) The index is often stiff, but still functions well after pollicization.

(c) Performed 6 months after wrist centralization.

D. **Thumb hypoplasia (Blauth classification; Table 42-1)**

1. **Type I:** All components are present, but the thumb is small.

2. **Type II:** Hypoplastic thenar muscles and web space adduction contracture are present; usually can be treated with web space deepening.

3. **Type III:** Intrinsic muscle aplasia, with extrinsic muscle hypoplasia (prevents extension/abduction of thumb). In **type IIIa** thumbs, the carpometacarpal (CMC) joint is stable, and the **thumb** can usually be managed with tendon transfers. In **IIIb thumbs,** the CMC is unstable, requiring index pollicization.

4. **Type IV:** *Pouce flottant,* or "floating thumb." Thumb remnant without any bony stability. Thumb must be amputated, with subsequent index pollicization.

5. **Type V:** Complete absence of thumb; requires amputation and index pollicization, if possible.

E. **Ulnar clubhand** (postaxial deficiency)

1. **Presentation**

a. Rare, compared with radial clubhand

b. Variable severity

c. Ulnar deviation

d. Wrist usually stable

e. Elbow flexion contracture

2. **Classification**

a. Type I: Ulnar hypoplasia

Table 42-1. Blauth classification of thumb hypoplasia

Type	Deformity	Treatment
Type I	Minor hypoplasia	If needed, web space deepening with Z-plasty
Type II	Adducted, hypoplastic thumb	Web space deepening MP stabilization Metacarpal lengthening Tendon transfer to restore opposition
Type IIIA	Severely adducted, hypoplastic thumb; CMC stable	As with type II, plus tendon transfers for extrinsic flexor/extensor function
Type IIIB	Severely adducted, hypoplastic thumb; CMC unstable	Index pollicization
Type IV	Floating thumb (*pouce flottant*)	Amputation of hypoplastic thumb, with index pollicization (skin from thumb is used in the web space)
Type V	Total thumb absence	Index pollicization

CMC, carpometacarpal joint; MP, metacarpophalangeal joint.

      b. Type II: Partial absence of the ulna

      c. Type III: Total absence of the ulna

      d. Type IV: Radiohumeral synostosis

  3. Associated syndromes: Fifty percent of ulnar deficiency patients have associated musculoskeletal dysplasias. It is very rare to find hematopoietic, cardiac, and vertebral anomalies.

  4. Treatment

      a. Splinting and soft tissue stretching therapy, beginning at birth.

      b. Soft tissue release if passive splinting fails to correct the deformity.

      c. Can consider fusing the proximal portion of the ulna to the distal radius to create a "one-bone forearm."

      d. Ilizarov distraction, with or without wedge osteotomy to correct length and angulation.

F. Cleft hand

  1. 1 in 25,000 births.

  2. Autosomal dominant.

  3. Often bilateral, with cleft feet.

  4. Middle ray alone may be absent.

  5. May extend to absence of index and ring rays.

  6. May present with border digit syndactyly requiring release, especially if the first web is involved.

  7. Treatment

      a. First web syndactyly release. This can be performed by transposing the index finger onto the base of the middle metacarpal. It also serves to simultaneously deepen the first web space.

      b. May need to deepen web space with Z-plasty.

      c. The Thumb may require an osteotomy or tendon transfers, depending on the degree of hypoplasia.

VII. Failure of differentiation or separation of parts

  A. Syndactyly

    1. Failure of normal sequence of apoptosis during the fourth to eighth week in utero, preventing digital separation.

    2. Epidemiology

      a. 1 in 1,400 births.

      b. Twice as common in males.

      c. 10% to 40% of cases are familial.

      d. Autosomal dominant with variable penetrance.

    3. Presentation

      a. Familial cases are often bilateral.

      b. Often associated with other disorders, including cleft hand and symbrachydactyly.

      c. The third web space is most commonly involved, followed by the fourth, second, and first web spaces.

      d. Syndactyly is classified as **complete versus incomplete.** Complete cases have fusion from the web space distally to the distal interphalangeal (DIP) joint, whereas incomplete cases do not.

      e. Syndactyly is also described as being **simple versus complex.** In complex syndactyly, bony fusion is present.

    4. Treatment

      a. Zigzag incisions are used to separate the syndactyly. These skin flaps interdigitate and cover the neurovascular bundles.

      b. A dorsal skin flap is used to cover the web space.

      c. A full-thickness skin graft is used to cover the remaining defect. Alternatively, a dorsally based island flap can be used for web space coverage, which may eliminate the need for skin grafting.

    5. Timing

      a. Early release is preferable for complete syndactyly, especially for the border digits (first operation at 1 year of age).

      b. Complex syndactyly warrants early intervention because of the potential for staged procedures.

    c. When multiple syndactylies are present (as in Apert's syndrome).
      (1) Release thumb at first stage.
      (2) Stage concurrent or subsequent releases to:
        (a) Minimize the number of operations.
        (b) Avoid operating on both the radial and ulnar side of any single digit at the same operation.

B. Symphalangism
1. Failure of interphalangeal joint differentiation, leading to ankylosis.
2. Usually PIP joints are affected.
3. Often associated with symbrachydactyly.
4. Treatment: Release of syndactyly, range of motion therapy.

C. Symbrachydactyly
1. Short fingers with small nails at fingertips.
2. Associated with Poland's syndrome.
3. Digital separation is more difficult.
4. Usually requires first web space deepening.

D. Congenital trigger thumb
1. IP joint held in flexion.
2. Can mimic clasped thumb (see below).
3. Presents with Notta's node (a palpable nodule in the flexor pollicis longus tendon).
4. Thirty percent of cases resolve spontaneously by 1 year of age.
5. If no resolution by 2 years of age, release of the A1 pulley is indicated.

E. Congenital clasped (clutched) thumb
1. Normal neonates clasp the thumb, which resolves at 3 to 4 months of age.
2. The male-to-female ratio is 2:1.
3. Specific anatomic lesion leads to the type of presentation.
    a. Extensor pollicis longus (EPL) absent: Flexed at the IP joint.
    b. Extensor pollicis brevis (EPB) absent: Flexed at the metacarpophalangeal (MP) joint.
    c. Abductor pollicis longus (APL) absent: Adducted across the palm.
4. Treatment: Early splinting, with web space deepening and tendon transfers if needed.

F. Camptodactyly
1. Camptodactyly is a congenital flexion contracture, usually at the PIP joint of the small finger.
2. Can be bilateral.
3. Treatment: Early splinting, with volar plate release or rarely arthroplasty.

G. Clinodactyly
1. Clinodactyly is a radial or ulnar deviation of the finger.
2. Most common at middle phalanx level.
3. Small finger clinodactyly is common in Down's syndrome.
4. Thumb clinodactyly is common in Apert's and Pfeiffer's syndromes.
5. Delta phalanx: Triangular phalanx with a C-shaped epiphysis.
6. Treatment: Usually not indicated. For severe deformity, osteotomy with grafting is indicated.

VIII. Duplications
  A. Polydactyly
    1. Caused by aberrant segmentation
    2. General types
      a. Type I: Extra soft tissue mass not attached to the skeleton.
      b. Type II: Extra digit (entire or part) articulating with a metacarpal or phalanx.
      c. Type III: Extra digit articulating with an extra metacarpal.
    3. Thumb duplication (radial or preaxial polydactyly)
      a. Wassel classification (Fig. 42-1).
      b. Represents one-third of all congenital hand abnormalities.
      c. Usually sporadic.
      d. Most common in Asians.
      e. Type IV is the most common form.

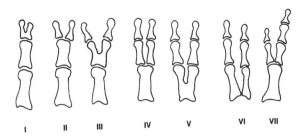

Fig. 42-1. Wassel classification of thumb duplication. (From Smith P and Laing H. Illustrated by Gault D Congenital hand deformity. In *Georgiade Plastic, Maxillofacial, and Reconstructive Surgery*, 3rd edition. Georgiade G, Riefkohl R, Levin S, (eds). Philadelphia, Williams & Wilkins, 1997. With permission.)

      f. Type VII (triphalangeal thumb) is the most complex and most difficult to treat. It is often inherited as an autosomal dominant trait, unlike the other polydactylies.

      g. Treatment

          (1) Type I/II: Resection of central duplicated halves with primary closure (Bilhaut-Cloquet closure).

          (2) Type III/IV: Ulnar thumb, with ulnar collateral ligament, is usually retained to maintain stability. Radial thumb soft tissue is used to augment function of the retained thumb.

          (3) Type V/VI: Radial digit may have better mobility than ulnar secondary to impingement of the ulnar thumb CMC on the index CMC; if so, the radial thumb base is retained, and the distal part of the ulnar thumb is transferred to the radial thumb base ("on-top-plasty").

          (4) Type VII (triphalangeal thumb): Complex, multistage reconstruction, often including on-top-plasty depending on the patient's anatomy.

   4. Central polydactyly

      a. Often autosomal dominant.

      b. May present with fused nail bed.

      c. Duplication may not be readily apparent within mass of fused digits.

      d. Treatment: Syndactyly release, when present, with ray resections.

   5. Small finger polydactyly (ulnar or postaxial polydactyly)

      a. Most common form of polydactyly.

      b. Most common in African Americans (1:300).

      c. Treatment

          (1) If only soft tissue involved, ligation at the bedside is performed.

          (2) Elliptical excision can also be performed for better cosmesis.

          (3) If bony involvement is present, the ulnar digit is usually removed, with reinsertion of muscles into the remaining small finger.

 B. Ulnar dimelia ("mirror hand")

   1. Extremely rare

   2. Duplicated ulna, with absence of the radius and thumb

   3. Total of six to eight fingers, with duplicated ulnar carpal bones

   4. Treatment: Elbow/wrist realignment, with digital ray resections and pollicization

IX. Overgrowth

 A. Macrodactyly

   1. True (primary) macrodactyly: Enlargement of all structures of a digit

   2. Very rare

   3. Not heritable; not associated with systemic syndromes

   4. 5% bilateral

   5. Treatment: Soft tissue and bony reduction

   B. Limb hypertrophy: Usually secondary overgrowth from vascular malformation or other cause

X. Undergrowth

   A. Brachysyndactyly (symbrachydactyly)

      1. Associated with Poland's syndrome

      2. Etiology is thought to involve subclavian artery stenosis

      3. Short, webbed fingers

      4. Treatment

         a. Consider removing nonfunctional stumps

         b. Syndactyly reconstruction

         c. Osteotomies and tendon transfers

         d. Distraction osteogenesis

         e. Phalangeal or free toe transfer

   B. Brachydactyly

      1. Short phalanges

      2. Treatment: As above, without syndactyly release

XI. Constriction band syndrome

   A. Also known as amniotic band syndrome or annular band syndrome.

   B. Caused by intrauterine focal necrosis. Unlike failures of growth or differentiation, proximal structures are usually intact, providing more reconstructive options.

   C. Broad spectrum of presentations.

      1. Partial banding: Treated with Z-plasty.

      2. Complete (circumferential) constriction: Treated with Z-plasty or local advancement flaps.

      3. Congenital lymphedema.

      4. Fusion of adjacent digits (acrosyndactyly).

      5. Amputation of affected parts: Treated with toe transfer or distraction.

   D. Urgent release may be indicated for acute, progressive edema distal to a band in a newborn.

XII. Generalized skeletal disorders

   A. Madelung's deformity: Palmar subluxation of the carpus with an overriding ulna

   B. Arthrogryposis multiplex congenita

      1. Multiple joint contractures at birth.

      2. Internally rotated shoulder, stiff elbow, flexed wrist with a ulnar deviation, adducted thumb, ulnar deviated fingers.

      3. Associated with spinal, renal, and cardiac anomalies, port wine stains (superficial capillary malformations), and Möbius' syndrome.

      4. Treatment: Early splinting and physical therapy, joint contracture release, and tendon transfers.

   C. Achondroplasia

   D. Marfan's syndrome

   E. Dyschondroplasia

   F. Diastrophic dwarfism

Pearls

1. Mnemonic device for the classification of congenital hand abnormalities: **F**ox **F**elt **D**ana **O**ver and **U**nder her **C**onstricting **G**enes (**F**ailure of formation, **F**ailure of **D**ifferentiation, **O**vergrowth, **U**ndergrowth, **C**onstriction bands, and **G**eneralized disorders).

2. Some polydactylies are best treated with ray amputation, resulting in a four-digit hand.

3. Many congenital hand anomalies do not fit into neat categories of diagnosis or treatment.

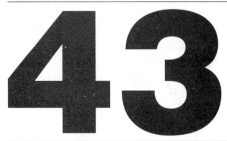

Thumb Reconstruction

Gregory H. Borschel

I. General
A. Goals of reconstruction
1. **Sensibility.**
   a. Protective sensibility prevents future injuries such as pressure ulcers from developing.
   b. Tactile perception is important; if not present, the patient will not use the thumb.
2. **Adequate length** should be provided to allow opposition with the other digits. However, length should not be preserved at the expense of mobility in most cases.
3. **Durable coverage** should protect underlying neural, vascular, and tendon reconstructions.
4. **Freedom from pain.**
5. **Cosmesis,** once the previously listed goals are met, is highly valued by patients. The hand, like the face, is often left uncovered in most interactions with other people.

B. Factors influencing choice of reconstruction
1. **Level of amputation:** The primary determining factor (Table 43-1).
2. **Age:** Young patients have more neural plasticity than older patients. For this reason, they are more able to adapt to pollicizations and neurovascular island flaps. In some adults, such transfers may never reach the point of feeling natural.
3. **Sex:** In female patients, cosmesis may play a larger role than in male patients. For this reason, some function may be sacrificed in order to provide a more cosmetic result.
4. **Functional demands** (vocation/avocation): Some reconstructions are more stable, whereas others provide more mobility. A heavy laborer has needs that are dramatically different from those of a clerk, for example.
5. **Patient preferences:** Some patients desire the most rapid reconstruction available, whereas others may be willing to undergo prolonged therapy to achieve a desired level of function.

II. Distal thumb reconstruction
A. General considerations
1. Decreased length, loss of soft tissue coverage, and cosmetic deformity all must be considered in order to formulate an optimal reconstructive plan.
2. Distal thumb injuries are often treated similarly to fingertip injuries (see Chapter 38, "Amputation, Replantation, and Fingertip and Nail Bed Injuries").
3. Attempt to preserve length, but not at the expense of durable, sensate coverage. Thumb function is usually acceptable without the length provided by the distal phalanx.

B. Volar advancement flap
1. **Moberg-type volar advancement**
   a. Indications: Pad defect of 2 cm or more.
   b. Need to put metacarpophalangeal (MP) and interphalangeal (IP) joints in flexion to achieve closure. It is safe to flex the IP joint to 45 degrees for closure.

Table 43-1. Thumb reconstructive options by amputation level

Injury Level	Preferred Treatment	Alternate Treatments
Distal thumb (IP to tip)	Local or regional flap (i.e., Moberg or FDMA)	Wraparound or trimmed great toe transfer
Distal midthumb (middle of proximal phalanx to IP)	Great toe transfer	Second toe or wraparound; local flaps
Proximal midthumb (distal metacarpal to middle of proximal phalanx)	Great toe transfer	Pollicization or distraction
Proximal thumb (proximal metacarpal)	Second toe transfer versus pollicization	If no adjacent digits are available, the second toe is preferred

FDMA, first dorsal metacarpal artery; IP, interphalangeal joint.

    2. Extended Moberg flap.
       a. If 2.5 cm of coverage is needed, the skin and subcutaneous tissue at the base of the flap can be released, making an island flap for advancement. A full-thickness skin graft is used to close the donor site.
       b. Place MP and IP joints in flexion.
       c. This flap cannot cover more than 2.5 cm.
  C. Cross-finger flap (Fig. 43-1)
    1. Indication: Avulsion of the entire volar thumb pad.
    2. Donor site: Dorsal surface of the proximal phalanx of the index finger.
    3. A full-thickness skin graft is applied to the donor site.
    4. The base of the flap is divided and inset at 3 weeks.
    5. Drawbacks.
       a. Only protective sensation is provided, since nonglabrous skin is transferred.
       b. Results in an aesthetic defect on the dorsum of index finger (usually well tolerated).
  D. Neurovascular island flap
    1. Indicated for loss of thumb digital nerves along with a thumb pad defect.
    2. Technically demanding: The neurovascular bundle is dissected from a fingertip down into the palm and swung over to the thumb.
    3. Use ulnar pad of the middle finger. If median nerve sensibility is lost, use the radial side of ring finger.
    4. Drawback: Produces a significant donor site deformity.
  E. Radial sensory cross-finger flap
    1. Indicated for loss of the entire thumb pad.
    2. Can resurface 4 cm of the volar thumb.
    3. Transfers a branch of the radial sensory nerve within an extended cross-finger flap taken from the dorsal MP joint to the proximal interphalangeal (PIP) joint of the index finger and transferred to the volar thumb.
    4. Results in significant donor site deformity that is greater than with a standard cross-finger flap.
  F. First dorsal metacarpal artery (FDMA) flap
    1. Indicated for large volar thumb defects up to 4 cm.
    2. The flap is raised distal to proximal as an island flap containing the FDMA, veins, branches of the radial nerve, fascia of the underlying interosseous muscle of the first web space, and skin overlying the MP joint and proximal phalanx of the index finger.
    3. The flap may then be transposed to cover the thumb.

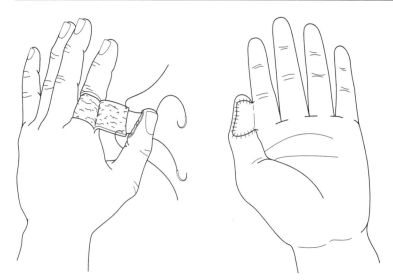

Fig. 43-1. Cross-finger flap for thumb pad coverage. Radial dissection of the flap stops dorsal to the neurovascular bundle, leaving it intact in the index finger. A full-thickness skin graft is used to cover the donor site defect. The base of the flap is divided at 3 weeks.

       4. Provides reliable and sensate coverage.
   G. Amputation
       1. Indicated only when stability and durable sensate coverage are not feasible.
       2. Patients with distal thumb loss usually retain good function despite loss of length at this level.
III. Midlevel thumb reconstruction
   A. General considerations
       1. Functional deficits of loss at this level include loss of fine pinch and strong grasp.
       2. There are three basic strategies for reconstruction at this level.
          a. Toe transfer (usually gives the best outcome).
          b. Web space deepening (alternative to toe transfer).
          c. Thumb lengthening (by distraction osteogenesis).
   B. Toe transfer
       1. General indications: Traumatic loss of midlevel thumb, and some congenital thumb deformities (see Chapter 42, "Congenital Anomalies of the Hand and Upper Extremity"). Toe transfers usually produce the best results compared with other reconstructive techniques at this level.
       2. Types of toe transfers (Table 43-1)
          a. Great toe: Good cosmesis and strength.
          b. Second toe: Allows more proximal reconstruction; not as strong or as aesthetically pleasing as the great toe.
          c. Wraparound great toe: Allows sensate coverage of the distal thumb when bony support is present.
       3. Foot donor site anatomy
          a. The great toe is 20% thicker than the thumb.
          b. The second toe is slightly thinner than the thumb, and the nail is usually shorter.

c. The first dorsal metatarsal artery supplies the great and second toes, and usually arises from the dorsalis pedis artery (although the dominant toe vessels can sometimes arise from the plantar surface via the deep plantar artery).

d. Venous drainage is by the superficial dorsal veins to the greater saphenous vein.

e. Volar digital nerves arise from the medial plantar nerve.

4. **Contraindications to toe transfer**
   a. Vascular disease.
   b. Other significant comorbidity precluding extended anesthesia time.
   c. Cultural footwear preferences (e.g., sandals in Asia).

5. **Advantages of toe transfers**
   a. Sensibility, both protective and tactile, is routinely restored.
   b. The transferred toe is reliably durable and mobile.
   c. Usually the best cosmetic option (allows a five-digit hand with nails).
   d. Single-stage reconstruction.
   e. Includes a viable growth plate in pediatric reconstructions.

6. **Disadvantages**
   a. Donor site morbidity is not insignificant. Delayed healing, chronic pain, and altered gait may result from toe harvest.
   b. Toe transfer is technically demanding and takes many hours.
   c. Extended postoperative monitoring and prolonged rehabilitation are necessary for optimal results.

7. **Timing**
   a. Usually done electively (in a delayed fashion) to allow patients to fully consider their functional deficits and decide if they are willing to sacrifice a toe.
   b. Urgent (within several days) wraparound toe transfer may be indicated if avulsion of soft tissue results in exposed phalanges.

C. **Alternatives to toe transfer in the distal midthumb**
   1. **Web space deepening by Z-plasty.**
      a. Indicated for amputation at the midshaft level of the proximal phalanx.
      b. Requires acceptable mobility of the carpometacarpal (CMC) and MP joints.
      c. Z-plasty is performed with the central limb lying along the first web to elongate and thus deepen the web space. The double opposing Z-plasty is an excellent choice in this location.
   2. **Web space deepening with other local flaps.**
      a. Indicated for severe adduction contracture.
      b. Dorsal rotational flap.
      c. Reverse radial forearm flap.
      d. First dorsal metatarsal artery flap.

D. **Alternatives to toe transfer in the proximal midthumb**
   1. **Heterotopic replantation, using "spare parts".**
      a. Indicated with concomitant amputation of another digit.
      b. If the thumb is not replantable, an amputated part from another finger may be replanted in this position to salvage function.
      c. With index finger amputation, index finger ray amputation results in web space deepening and improved function.
      d. In cases of thumb and index loss with middle finger injury, the middle finger can be transferred to the thumb position.
      e. Advantages of heterotopic replantation include the following:
         (1) A predictable outcome, with an acceptable functional result.
         (2) Removal of useless/hindering part.
   2. **Metacarpal distraction osteogenesis (DO):**
      a. Indicated for thumb amputations close to the MP joint. Also indicated if the patient does not want, or is not a candidate for, toe transfer or pollicization.
      b. Advantages.

        (1) Does not require sacrifice of a toe or an adjacent digit.

        (2) Can be aesthetically acceptable.

        (3) Can be effective in restoring length and function.

    c. Disadvantage: Patient must have the external distraction device in place for several weeks.

  3. Bone grafting with fasciocutaneous flap coverage, also known as osteoplastic reconstruction.

    a. Indications and requirements.

        (1) Thumb loss at the proximal midthumb.

        (2) If not a candidate for toe transfer or DO, and adjacent digits are too badly damaged or completely normal (i.e., not a candidate for heterotopic transplantation).

        (3) Adequate CMC joint mobility is a prerequisite.

    b. The bone graft is fixed to the metacarpal, and soft tissue coverage is achieved with local, regional, or distant flaps.

    c. Every effort should be made to reconstruct the pad with sensate tissue.

    d. Bone sources include the iliac crest, phalangeal remnants from the thumb or other digit, and the radius (included in a free or reverse radial forearm osteocutaneous flap).

    e. Soft tissue coverage.

        (1) Pedicled groin flap with subsequent pedicled neurovascular island flap (FDMA flap or pulp flap from the ulnar ring or long finger).

        (2) Reverse radial forearm osteocutaneous flap.

IV. Proximal thumb reconstruction

  A. General considerations

    1. Function is improved when 5 cm of length can be restored.

    2. Mobility may be limited at the basilar (CMC) joint.

    3. If the index or middle fingers are also injured, pollicization is preferred.

    4. If no other digits are injured, then pollicization and toe transfer are considered.

  B. Pollicization provides greater sensibility and fine motor control than toe transfer at this level.

  C. Toe transfer provides greater strength than pollicization, and in many cases the aesthetic result is superior.

Pearls

---

1. Involve the patient heavily in the decision-making process.

2. Perform the reconstruction in a delayed fashion. This allows patients to better appreciate their deficits, and allows them to weigh their reconstructive options.

3. Toe transfer is increasingly becoming the reconstruction of choice at all levels.

4. Some patients may not want any reconstruction even though it may be "indicated." Most of them will go on to do well. Allow patients to make decisions regarding their reconstruction in a fully informed manner. Only then will you accomplish what is truly in the patients' best interests and have satisfied patients.

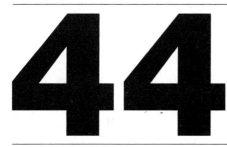

Brachial Plexus

Keith R. Lodhia and
Andrew S. Youkilis

I. Anatomy (Fig. 44-1)

A. Roots
  1. Ventral rami of C5–T1
  2. Scalene branches: C5–C8
  3. Long thoracic nerve: C5–C7

B. Trunks and divisions
  1. Superior trunk (C5–6)
    a. Direct branches: Dorsal scapular nerve (C4–5), nerve to subclavius.
    b. Anterior division: Merges into the lateral cord.
      (1) Suprascapular nerve (C5–6).
      (2) Lateral pectoral nerve.
    c. Posterior division: Merges into the posterior cord.
  2. Middle trunk (C7)
    a. Anterior division: Merges into the lateral cord.
    b. Posterior division: Merges into the posterior cord.
  3. Inferior trunk (C8–T1)
    a. Anterior division: Becomes medial cord; gives rise to the medial pectoral nerve.
    b. Posterior division: Merges into the posterior cord.

C. Cords
  1. Lateral cord: Becomes the musculocutaneous nerve; also provides sensory axons to the median nerve.
  2. Posterior cord: Becomes the axillary and radial nerves.
    a. Upper subscapular nerve (C5–7).
    b. Thoracodorsal nerve (C6–8).
    c. Lower subscapular nerve (C5–7).
  3. Medial cord: Becomes the ulnar nerve; also provides motor axons to the median nerve.
    a. Medial brachial cutaneous nerve.
    b. Medial antebrachial cutaneous nerve.

D. Branches
  1. Musculocutaneous nerve (C5–6): Supplies arm flexors.
  2. Median nerve (C5–T1): Supplies forearm/wrist flexors and pronators as well as LOAF muscles in hand (**l**umbricals of index and middle fingers, **o**pponens pollicis, **a**bductor pollicis longus, and **f**lexor pollicis brevis). Anterior interosseus nerve (purely motor) supplies the flexor digitorum profundus (FDP) of index and middle fingers, flexor pollicis longus (FPL), and pronator quadratus.
  3. Axillary nerve (C5–6): Supplies the deltoid and teres minor muscles.
  4. Radial nerve (C5–8): Supplies all of the extensors of the forearm and hand (synergistic). Posterior interosseous nerve (C7, 8): Supplies the extensors of the wrist, thumb, and fingers.
  5. Ulnar nerve (C8–T1): Supplies all of the intrinsic hand muscles except the LOAF muscles.

E. Pearls for memorization
  1. Rob **T**urner **D**rinks **C**old **B**eer (**r**oots, **t**runks, **d**ivisions, **c**ords, **b**ranches)
  2. 5–3–6–3–5 (palindrome).

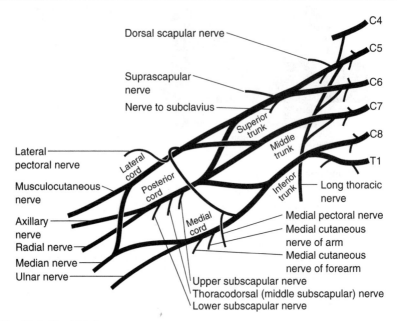

Fig. 44-1. Brachial plexus anatomy.

II. Pathology

A. Peripheral nerve injury classification (see Chapter 6, "Microsurgery")

B. Trauma

1. **Blunt trauma**

   a. **Duchenne-Erb palsy:** Upper plexus injury due to head/shoulder distraction. Most common in motorcycle accidents and shoulder dystocia.

   b. **Klumpke's palsy:** Lower brachial plexus injury, usually due to traction on an abducted arm. May include Horner's syndrome.

   c. **Obstetrical brachial plexus injury.**
      (1) Upper plexus injuries are more common than lower.
      (2) Approximately 90% of patients recover spontaneously. Repair is generally not considered until older than 6 months (see "Management").

   d. **Nerve root avulsions.**
      (1) Avulsions are more common with lesions in the upper brachial plexus due to nerve roots being bound down in bony "chutes" by connective tissue at C5–7.
      (2) Pseudomeningocele formation is visible on myelogram.

   e. **Fracture-related injuries.**
      (1) First rib fractures may cause lower trunk injuries.
      (2) Midhumeral fractures are often associated with radial nerve injuries.
      (3) Axillary artery and vein injuries are often associated with plexus injury.

2. **Penetrating trauma**

   a. **Lacerations.**

   b. **Gunshot wounds:** Injury is rarely due to actual division of nerves. Axonotmesis or neurotmesis is usually produced by the cavitation effect of the projectile.

3. **Thoracic outlet syndrome (TOS, chronic plexus compression)**
   a. Neurogenic (true or "classic" TOS): Associated with cervical rib or compressive band arising from the first rib. Compression of C8/T1 nerve roots as they arise out of the chest. May present with Gilliatt-Sumner hand (wasting of the thenar and hypothenar muscle groups).
   b. Vascular (disputed or "common" TOS): Pain or sensory symptoms predominate. Can elicit cessation of radial pulse with provocative maneuvers (e.g., Wright's test, Adson's test). Usually no cervical rib is present.

C. **Tumor**
   1. **Schwannomas** often have well-defined margins, allowing total resection.
   2. **Neurofibromas** are frequently associated with Von Recklinghausen's syndrome (NF-1); nerve and tumor margins are often indistinct.
   3. Other tumors (e.g., malignant peripheral nerve sheath tumor).

D. **Neuropathy**
   1. **Secondary to extrinsic compression from tumors** (e.g., Pancoast's syndrome); lesion usually at C8-T1. Workup should include apical lordotic chest x-ray to better visualize the upper lobe/apices of lungs.
   2. **Idiopathic brachial neuritis** (Parsonage-Turner syndrome): Acute onset of intense shoulder pain followed by weakness in the shoulder musculature (upper trunk often predominantly involved). Etiology is presumably immune mediated. Weakness is common and generally improves by 3 to 4 weeks after onset. The majority of cases improve spontaneously.
   3. **Post irradiation:** Classically seen following postmastectomy radiation, which causes fibrosis and edema of the brachial plexus. Commonly, sensory loss and/or pain without motor findings.
   4. **Viral** (e.g., herpes zoster): Not commonly a plexopathy per se; usually a sensory neuritis creating pain and hyperalgesia.
   5. **Diabetic:** Generally a distal symmetric sensory polyneuropathy with limited motor involvement; although can be asymmetric and truncal, mimicking brachial plexopathy.
   6. **Vasculitis:** Rare cause of brachial neuritis. Seen in some cases of allergic/hypersensitivity vasculitis.
   7. **Posttraumatic:** See above.
   8. **Inherited:** Rare (e.g., hereditary neuropathy with pressure palsies). The inheritance is autosomal dominant, producing painless brachial plexus palsies.

III. **Diagnosis**
A. **Physical examination** (Table 44-1)
   1. **Should be extremely detailed,** and performed with the assistance of a complete list of individual muscles and maneuvers to elicit isolated function. To determine the roots and/or peripheral nerves involved, have a standard dermatomal map available while performing the sensory (e.g. light touch, pin prick, and vibration) portion of the physical exam.
   2. **Horner's syndrome** (eyelid ptosis, miosis, and anhydrosis) suggests a lower plexus lesion.
   3. **"Waiter's tip" deformity** (shoulder internal rotation with elbow extension and wrist flexion) suggests an upper plexus lesion (C5, C6).
   4. **"Claw hand" (Klumpke's palsy)** suggests a lower plexus lesion; presents with metacarpophalangeal (MP) joints extended and interphalangeal (IP) joints flexed (C7, C8, T1). May include Horner's syndrome if T1 is involved (will disrupt sympathetic output to the superior cervical ganglion).
   5. **Thoracic outlet syndrome:** May present with "claw hand" with C8, T1 hypesthesia/radiculopathy on physical exam.
      a. Plain anteroposterior cervical spine x-ray can identify an offending cervical rib.
      b. Vasculogenic: Adson's test. Have the patient hyperextend their neck and rotate their head toward the affected side while gently tugging downward on their arms. They will have a loss of the radial pulse if positive.
      c. Wright's test: Have the patient hyperabduct their arm at the shoulder and externally rotate their hand. They will have a loss of the radial pulse if positive.

Table 44-1. Physical exam localization of a brachial plexus injury

Trunk or Cord	Roots	Nerve	Action and Test	Muscle	Sensory
	C5–7	Long thoracic	Outstretched arms against wall—"winged scapula" if deficit	Serratus anterior	
	C5	Dorsal scapular	Elevates scapula	Levator scapulae	
	C4,5	Dorsal scapular	Elevates and rotates scapula medially	Rhomboids	
Superior trunk	C4–6	Suprascapular	Initial shoulder abduction <90°	Supraspinatus	
	C5,6	Suprascapular	Externally rotates shoulder	Infraspinatus	
Posterior cord	C5–7	Subscapular	Internally rotates/adducts shoulder	Teres major, subscapularis	
	C5–7	Thoracodorsal	Adducts arms and internally rotates shoulder—"Superman pose" with hands on hips	Latissimus dorsi	
	C5,6	Axillary	Shoulder abduction >90°	Deltoid	Medial arm
	C5	Axillary	Externally rotates shoulder	Teres minor	
Medial cord	T1	Medial brachial cutaneous			
	C8, T1	Medial antebrachial cutaneous			Medial forearm
	C8, T1	Medial pectoral	Pectoralis minor—depresses scapula and shoulder and brings shoulder forward	Pectoralis minor and major	
	C5–7	Lateral pectoral	Pectoralis major—humeral/ shoulder adduction and internal/medial rotation	Pectoralis major	
	C5,6	MC	Flexes/supinates forearm—test with hand supinated to try to eliminate brachialis/ brachioradialis is	Biceps brachii	Lateral antebrachial cutaneous nerve—

Table 44-1. (Continued)

Trunk or Cord	Roots	Nerve	Action and Test	Muscle	Sensory
					branch of MC, supplies lateral forearm sensation
	C5,6	MC	Flexes forearm	Brachialis	
	C5,6	MC	Flexes/adducts arm	Coracobrachialis	
	C5–C8	Radial	Extends forearm	Triceps brachii	
	C5,6	Radial	Flexes forearm	Brachioradialis	
	C5,6	Radial	Extends hand	ECR	
	C6,7	Radial	Forearm supination	Supinator	
	C7,8	PIN—radial nerve branch	Abducts thumb—test by moving thumb perpendicular to palm	APL	
	C7,8	PIN	Interphalangeal joints of digits 2–5 extension	Extensor digitorum	
	C7,8	PIN	Ulnar hand extension	ECU	
	C7,8	PIN	Index finger extension and hand extension	Extensor indicis	
	C7,8	PIN	Thumb and radial wrist extension—test with "thumbs-up" sign	EPB and EPL	
	C7,8	Superficial branch of radial nerve			Sensation to the dorsum of the radial 3.5 digits
	C8	Ulnar			Sensation to ulnar 1.5 digits

(Continued)

Table 44-1. (Continued)

Trunk or Cord	Roots	Nerve	Action and Test	Muscle	Sensory
	C7–T1	Ulnar	Ulnar flexion of hand	Flexor carpi ulnaris	
	C7–T1	Ulnar	Flexion of DIP joint of RF, LF	Flexor digitorum profundus to Rf, and LF	
	C7,8	Ulnar	Flexes MPJ and extends DIPJ of RF, and LF	Lumbricals to RF, and LF	
	C7–T1	Ulnar	Flexes LF	Flexor digiti minimi brevis	
	C8, T1	Ulnar	Adducts thumb—test by grasping sheet of paper between straightened thumb and index finger ("key pinch")	Adductor pollicis	
	C7–T1	Ulnar	Opposition of LF—test by trying to touch tip of LF to thumb tip	Opponens digiti quinti	
	C7–T1	Ulnar	Abducts LF	Abductor digiti quinti	
	C8, T1	Ulnar	Adduct/abduct fingers and similar function as RF/LF lumbricals	Interossei	
Lateral cord "sensory head"	C5–7	Median			Palmar radial 3.5 digits
	C6,7	Median	Pronates forearm/hand	Pronator teres	
	C6,7	Median	Radial wrist flexion	Flexor carpi radialis	
	C7–T1	Median	Flexes wrist	Palmaris longus	
Medial cord "motor head"	C8, T1	Median	Flexes PIP joints; wrist flexion	Flexor digitorum superficialis	

Table 44-1. (Continued)

Trunk or Cord	Roots	Nerve	Action and Test	Muscle	Sensory
	C8, T1	Median		IF, MF lumbricals	
	C8, T1	Median	Thumb opposition—test by attempting to touch thumb tip to tip of LF	Opponens pollicis	
	C8, T1	Median	Abducts thumb at MCP joint	APB	
	C8, T1	Median	Flexes MCP joint of thumb	Flexor pollicis brevis	
	C7–T1	AIN— branch of median nerve	Flexes DIPJ of IF, MF—weak AIN if unable to touch tips of thumb and index finger to make "OK" gesture; instead makes "pinch sign"	Flexor digitorum profundus to IF, MF	No sensory
		AIN	Flexes DIPJ of thumb—"pinch sign" if weak	Flexor pollicis longus	
		AIN	Pronates hand—can test individually by pronating with elbow flexed (eliminates pronator teres)	Pronator quadratus	

AIN, anterior interosseous nerve; DIPJ, distal interphalangeal joint; ECR/ECU, extensor carpi radialis/ulnaris; MC, musculocutaneous, PTN, posterior interosseous nerve; PIPJ, proximal interphalangeal joint; IF, index finger; MF, middle finger; RF, ring finger; LF, little finger.

   d. Neurogenic (common): Roos' maneuver. Have the patient hyperabduct their arm at the shoulder and externally rotate their hand/shoulder. Concomitantly the patient should squeeze or pump their hand for 3 minutes or more. If this reproduces pain and/or sensory symptoms, the test is considered positive.

B. Imaging and electrodiagnostic studies

   1. Electromyography (EMG) and nerve conduction studies are best performed 3 weeks after injury, once Wallerian degeneration has occurred. EMG is useful for differentiating postganglionic from preganglionic injuries. Preganglionic injuries consist of nerve root avulsions from the spinal cord, proximal to the dorsal root ganglion, and therefore are not usually amenable to repair by nerve grafting. These injuries require neurotization procedures to regain distal nerve function.

   2. Magnetic resonance imaging (MRI): Best for identifying masses.

   3. Nerve action potentials (NAPs): Often used intraoperatively for determining nerve viability. More sensitive than a preoperative EMG for determining nerve potentials; often used for operative decision making (e.g., whether to perform neurolysis alone or resection of neuroma and grafting).

   4. Computed tomographic (CT) myelogram: Currently superior to MRI for identification of nerve root avulsion and/or pseudomeningocele formation. Important in evaluating patients with traumatic brachial plexopathy to preoperatively identify those patients who will likely require neurotization procedures.

   5. Ultrasonography: can be used to image portions of the brachial plexus, although it is not superior to other imaging methods. Occasionally used in anesthesia for guidance of needles in providing plexus/nerve blocks.

IV. Management (Fig. 44-2).

A. General principles

   1. Management is based on clinical observation, electrodiagnostic studies, mechanism of injury, and radiographic findings (e.g., nerve root avulsion).

   2. Generally, blunt trauma compression and/or traction injuries without continued insult should be followed for at least 3 to 4 months for clinical improvement. If no recovery is evident clinically and electrodiagnostically at 3 to 4 months, then exploration should be considered.

   3. Penetrating injuries, or those with associated vascular injury, require immediate exploration.

   4. Missile wounds to the brachial plexus should be treated conservatively because the nerve often remains in continuity. The nerve injury generally results from a concussive injury. Exploration and repair are indicated if there is no improvement clinically or electrodiagnostically in 6 months.

   5. Operations performed in the acute phase (before muscle fibers have atrophied) consist of neural operations, including nerve repairs, grafts, and nerve transfers. Operations performed later (after severe atrophy) consist of nonneural procedures, including tendon transfers, muscle flaps, and arthrodeses.

B. Special considerations in obstetric palsy

   1. Approximately 70% will have complete resolution without surgical intervention.

   2. Treatment is usually advocated at 6 months if there is significant and unimproved paresis. Some authors advocate delaying operative exploration for up to a year.

C. Nerve grafting procedures usually use sural, superficial radial, or medial antebrachial cutaneous nerves as donor grafts (see Chapter 6, "Microsurgery").

D. Common neurotization procedures

   1. For preganglionic plexus injuries, the descending cervical plexus or spinal accessory nerve can be transferred to the suprascapular nerve for upper trunk avulsion injuries (to restore shoulder abduction).

   2. Medial pectoral/thoracodorsal nerve to musculocutaneous or axillary nerves (to restore elbow flexion and/or shoulder abduction).

   3. Medial pectoral or intercostal nerve to musculocutaneous nerve (to restore elbow flexion).

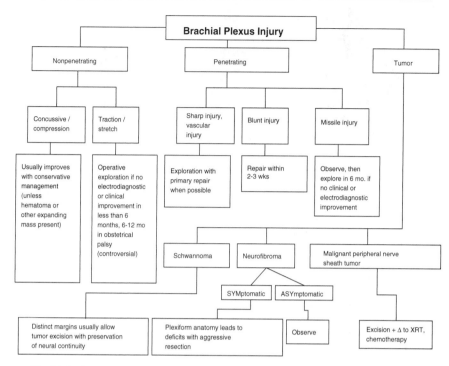

Fig. 44-2. Algorithm for management of brachial plexus injury.

E. Non-neural procedures

1. Tendon transfer techniques are often considered in cases of panbrachial plexus injury with global avulsions, wrist palsy, failed microsurgical brachial plexus reconstructions, and remote injuries.
2. Other procedures used in rehabilitation of long-standing brachial plexus injury include wrist fusion and functional muscle transfer techniques.
3. Upper extremity amputation followed by prosthesis has been used as an option for painful "flail arm."

Pearls

1. Plexus anatomy: Palindrome: 5-3-6-3-5. Mnemonic: Rob Turner Drinks Cold Beer.
2. The sensory roots of the median nerve come from C5–7.
3. The motor roots of the median nerve come from C8–T1.
4. Nerve root avulsion is more common in lower plexus injuries due to the nerve being bound down in connective tissue at C5–C7.
5. Peripheral nerve regeneration occurs at the rate of approximately 1 mm per day (roughly 1 inch per month).
6. Motor nerve regeneration must take place prior to atrophy of the target muscle.
7. Radial nerve repairs tend to do better due to the synergism of the muscle groups involved.
8. In general, brachial plexus repairs of C5–6 root injuries have better outcomes than C8–T1 or panbrachial plexus injuries.

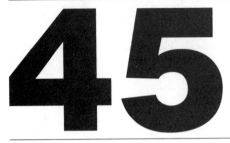

Hand Infections, Compartment Syndrome, and High-Energy Injuries

John C. Austin

Hand Infections

I. **General principles**
   A. **Risk factors**
      1. Diabetes mellitus
      2. Immune system compromise (AIDS, malignancy, steroids, transplant patients)
      3. Alcoholism and drug abuse
      4. Renal failure; liver failure
   B. **Mild infections:** May respond to oral antibiotics, elevation, and warm soaks.
   C. **Serious infections:** Require broad intravenous antibiotic coverage while awaiting culture results; often need operative irrigation and debridement (I&D).

II. **Paronychia**
   A. **Definition: Infection of the nail fold**, presenting with pain, erythema, and edema of the tissue s surrounding the nail. Represents the most common hand infection.
   B. **Acute paronychia**
      1. Etiology
         a. *Staphylococcus aureus* is the most common organism.
         b. 25% of cases of paronychia are caused by anaerobic flora.
         c. 50% are mixed aerobic and anaerobic infections.
      2. Treatment
         a. I&D, with partial or complete nail plate removal.
         b. Dressing changes, oral antibiotics.
         c. Stent eponychial fold open with a piece of foil or other material (suture pack foil works well), held in place with 5-0 chromic suture.
   C. **Chronic paronychia**
      1. Etiology: *Candida albicans* (70%–90%)
      2. Treatment
         a. Topical clotrimazole or tolnaftate.
         b. Eponychial marsupialization (opening the tissue and allowing it to drain as a sinus) may be necessary for infections resistant to conservative management.

III. **Felon**
   A. **Definition: Closed space infection of the volar fingertip pulp.**
   B. **Treatment:** I&D, intravenous antibiotics
      1. Use midlateral incisions: Ulnar for index, long, and ring fingers; radial for thumb and small finger.
      2. Must divide enough fingertip septa to allow decompression and drainage.

IV. **Flexor tenosynovitis**
   A. **Definition: Infection of flexor tendon sheath**
   B. **Clinical presentation: Kanavel's "cardinal signs"**
      1. Pain with passive digital extension, most severe at the proximal extent of the flexor sheath (earliest and most reliable sign).

    2. Tenderness over the flexor tendon sheath.

    3. Flexed digital posture.

    4. Fusiform swelling of the digit.

 C. Horseshoe abscess: Infection of the tendon sheath of both the thumb and small finger via proximal connection at Parona's space (a potential space between pronator quadratus and flexor digitorum profundus tendons).

 D. Treatment: Emergent I&D and intravenous antibiotics

    1. Many different incisions have been proposed.

    2. Limited proximal and distal incisions, with insertion of a catheter for continuous irrigation (left in >24–48 hours) may be the most effective.

V. Deep potential space infections

 A. Collar button abscess (web space infection)

    1. Presents with painful swelling of the involved web space and adjacent distal palm; adjacent fingers may assume an abducted posture.

    2. Treatment: I&D (volar and dorsal incisions, avoid incision in the web space) and intravenous antibiotics.

 B. Thenar space infection

    1. Presents with pain and swelling over the thenar eminence exacerbated by flexion of the thumb and index fingers.

    2. Treatment: I&D and intravenous antibiotics.

 C. Hypothenar space infection (rare): Analogous to thenar space infection.

 D. Midpalmar space infection (rare)

    1. Presents with volar pain with flexion of the long, ring, and small fingers.

    2. Treatment: I&D and intravenous antibiotics.

VI. Bone and joint infections

 A. Osteomyelitis

    1. Present in 1% to 6% of all hand infections.

    2. Treatment.

      a. Thorough I&D and intravenous antibiotics.

      b. All infected and necrotic bone must be removed.

      c. Amputation may be required in advanced cases.

 B. Septic arthritis

    1. Occurs most commonly following penetrating trauma.

    2. Common presentation: "Fight bite" (metacarpophalangeal joint infection after fist contact with teeth; see "Bites").

    3. Treatment: I&D and intravenous antibiotics; leave wound open to allow for drainage.

      a. Must explore the wound thoroughly to evaluate communication with joint space.

      b. Wounds through skin and tendon and joint capsule do not always line up, because the joint was in a different position at the time of injury.

VII. Infections requiring emergent surgery

 A. Necrotizing fasciitis

    1. Severe infection that is life and limb threatening.

    2. Mortality averages 30%; amputation is often required.

    3. Group A β-hemolytic streptococci are the most common organisms; necrotizing infections are often polymicrobial.

    4. Populations at greatest risk: Diabetics, immunocompromised patients, and elderly patients.

    5. Treatment

      a. Emergent radical debridement of all necrotic tissue (wounds left open).

      b. Broad-spectrum intravenous antibiotics (empiric coverage).

      c. Monitoring in the intensive care unit (ICU).

      d. Repeat I&D at 24- to 48-hour intervals until sepsis improves.

      e. Hyperbaric oxygen treatment is controversial in nonclostridial necrotizing infections.

B. Gas gangrene (clostridial myonecrosis)
   1. Severe necrotizing infection caused by *Clostridium* species (most commonly *Clostridium perfringens*) that develops in contaminated wounds with extensive tissue damage.
   2. Treatment: Similar to that for necrotizing fasciitis.
   3. Hyperbaric oxygen has been shown to be beneficial.

VIII. Bites
   A. Human bite
      1. Most commonly seen in ring and small finger metacarpophalangeal (MP) joints ("fight bite").
      2. Organisms: α-hemolytic streptococci, *Staphylococcus aureus*, and *Eikenella corrodens* (10%–30%).
      3. Treatment: I&D (mandatory if joint capsule or tendon sheath are penetrated) and intravenous antibiotics (e.g., ampicillin/sulbactam).
   B. Dog and cat bites
      1. Organisms: α-hemolytic streptococci, *Pasteurella multocida* (25%), *S. aureus* (15%), anaerobes (40%).
      2. Cat bites are frequently more severe than dog bites due to deeper penetration and more virulent oral flora.
      3. Treatment: Intravenous antibiotics (e.g., ampicillin/sulbactam) and often I&D.

IX. Herpetic whitlow
   A. Herpes simplex virus infection involving the finger or fingertip.
   B. Presents with intense pain and erythema; a small vesicular rash is often present.
   C. Common in dental and medical personnel.
   D. Self-limited; usually resolves in 3 to 4 weeks.
   E. Treatment: Supportive care (can mimic bacterial infection; avoid unnecessary I&D, which may lead to bacterial superinfection).

X. Fungal infections
   A. Most common in diabetic and immunocompromised patients.
   B. Cutaneous fungal infections
      1. Chronic paronychia (see "Chronic Paronychia").
      2. Onychomycosis: Destructive, deforming nail plate infection.
         a. *Trichophyton rubrum* is the most common organism.
         b. Treatment: Topical antifungals; resistant cases may require systemic antifungals (ketoconazole or griseofulvin).
   C. Subcutaneous fungal infections
      1. Commonly develop following penetrating injury while handling plants or soil.
      2. *Sporothrix schenckii* is the most common organism; associated with rose thorns.
      3. Papule initially seen at the puncture site, followed by erythematous lesions extending proximally along lymphatic channels.
      4. Treatment: Saturated potassium iodide solution irrigation once a day for 4 weeks.
   D. Deep fungal infections
      1. Infections include osteomyelitis, tenosynovitis, and septic arthritis.
      2. Multiple pathogens are possible. These infections include histoplasmosis, blastomycosis, and coccidioidomycosis; opportunistic infections include candidiasis, aspergillosis, and mucormycosis.
      3. Treatment: Surgical I&D and intravenous antifungals (amphotericin B or as dictated by fungal cultures).

XI. Atypical mycobacterial infections
   A. Rare, indolent infections that mimic other types of infection; difficult to diagnose and treat.
   B. Organisms: *Mycobacterium marinum* (fresh and saltwater), *M. kansasii* (soil), *M. terrae* (soil), *M. avium-intracellulare* (soil, water, poultry).
   C. Diagnosis: Biopsy (histopathology); successful culture requires incubation at 32°C for 6 weeks in Lowenstein-Jensen medium.

    D. Chest x-ray is necessary to evaluate for systemic spread.

    E. Treatment: Thorough I&D and oral antibiotics (rifampin, ethambutol, tetracycline).

Compartment Syndrome and High-Energy Injuries

I. Compartment syndrome

    A. Definition: Increased pressure in an enclosed fascial compartment that compromises circulation, eventually leading to tissue ischemia, necrosis, and death.

    B. Physical examination and diagnosis

        1. High index of suspicion is paramount.

        2. **P**ain with passive stretch of muscles in the affected compartment is the most sensitive test; affected compartments may feel tense.

        3. Other findings: **P**aresthesias, **p**allor, **p**aralysis, and **p**ulselessness (pulselessness is a late finding).

        4. Pain is persistent, progressive, and unrelieved by supportive measures.

        5. Diagnosis is confirmed with compartment pressures above 30 mm Hg or within 20 mm Hg of diastolic blood pressure.

           a. Have a low threshold for measurement.

           b. Can use a commercially available hand-held unit, or an arterial line setup (be sure to zero the setup prior to needle introduction, and enter tissues horizontally to obtain accurate readings).

    C. Etiologies

        1. Trauma (fractures, wringer injuries, crush injuries)

        2. Prolonged ischemia (arterial occlusion)

        3. Thermal and electrical burns

        4. Hemorrhage into compartment

        5. High-pressure injection injuries

        6. Snakebites

        7. Externally applied pressure (intoxication, tight casts, or dressings)

    D. Treatment

        1. Immediate therapeutic fasciotomy of all involved compartments (Fig. 45-1)

        2. Prophylactic fasciotomies are indicated in the following cases:

           a. Patients with equivocal findings and a high index of suspicion.

           b. Cases involving prolonged ischemia time (>4–6 hours).

           c. Electrocution injuries.

        3. Forearm compartment release.

           a. Three compartments.

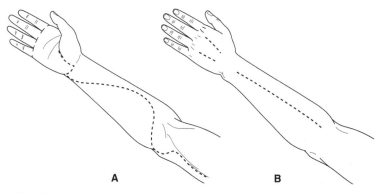

Fig. 45-1. Fasciotomy incisions of the hand and forearm. **A:** Volar. **B:** Dorsal.

          (1) Volar (largest muscle mass).
          (2) Dorsal.
          (3) Mobile wad (brachioradialis, extensor carpi radialis longus, and extensor carpi radialis brevis).
      b. Surgical approach: Many incisions have been described.
          (1) Should include carpal tunnel and Guyon canal releases.
          (2) Should include broad skin flaps to protect the median nerve at the wrist and the ulnar nerve at the elbow.
          (3) Usually a curvilinear volar incision is combined with a longitudinal dorsal incision to release all compartments.
          (4) Release the entire length of the fascia between compartments.
          (5) Preserve as many dorsal veins and cutaneous nerves as possible.
          (6) Use curved or transverse incisions when crossing flexion creases.
   4. Hand compartment release
      a. Ten compartments
          (1) Thenar
          (2) Hypothenar
          (3) Adductor pollicis
          (4) Dorsal interosseous (four)
          (5) Volar interosseous (three)
      b. Surgical approach
          (1) Longitudinal incisions over the dorsum of the index and ring metacarpals allow for release of the interossei and adductor pollicis compartments.
          (2) The hypothenar compartment is released via the ulnar aspect of the little finger metacarpal.
          (3) The thenar compartment is released via the radial side of the thumb metacarpal or incision placed in the first dorsal web space.
   5. Finger compartment syndrome
      a. Less common due to decreased muscle mass in the finger.
      b. Surgical approach: Midaxial incision with release of fascia between neurovascular bundles volarly and the flexor tendon sheath dorsally.
 E. Volkmann's ischemic contracture
   1. Follows untreated forearm compartment syndrome.
   2. Muscle fibrosis/death and neurovascular injury result in an insensate hand with contractures involving forearm pronation, wrist flexion, MP joint hyperextension, and interphalangeal joint flexion.
   3. Tendons with the longest excursion are often most severely affected (flexor digitorum profundus, flexor pollicis longus).
   4. Severity levels.
      a. Mild (wrist flexors involved): Dynamic splinting and tendon lengthening.
      b. Moderate (wrist and digital flexors involved): Necrotic muscle excision; tendon transfers as indicated.
      c. Severe (wrist and digital flexors and extensors involved): Necrotic muscle excision, neurolysis, and tendon transfers as indicated.

II. High-pressure injection injuries
 A. Etiology
   1. Variety of devices: Paint guns, power washers, grease guns, and diesel fuel injectors.
   2. Most common substances: Paint, grease, and water.
 B. Evaluation
   1. History: Inquire about timing, type of material injected, and force of injection (pounds per square inch, or PSI).
   2. Exam: Document neurovascular status; severity is easily underestimated.
      a. May have small puncture site and mild burning sensation initially.
      b. Swelling and pain worsen with time.
   3. Radiographs: Evaluate for radiopaque material such as lead paint.

C. Treatment
1. I&D: Emergent, thorough removal of all devitalized tissue and injected material; leave wounds open (for delayed primary closure or healing by secondary intention).
2. Broad-spectrum antibiotics.
3. Serial debridements are performed at 48- to 72-hour intervals.
4. Early range of motion with occupational therapy is instituted as soon as wound condition and pain tolerance allow.
5. Amputation may be necessary in severe injuries resulting in excessive tissue necrosis and/or ischemia and in late-presenting injuries.

D. Poor outcome is associated with the following.
1. Delay in presentation
2. Finger injuries (less potential space than hand injuries)
3. Greater injection pressure and larger injection volume
4. Oil-based solvents

III. Degloving injuries
A. Injuries involving extensive skin and soft tissue loss with variable amounts of contamination.
B. There may also be associated fractures and bone loss requiring extensive secondary reconstructive procedures.
C. Treatment
1. Tetanus prophylaxis and intravenous antibiotics.
2. Emergent, aggressive I&D in the operating room.
3. Repeat I&D every 48 hours until a healthy tissue bed (without further necrosis) is present.
4. Protect underlying structures (i.e., tendons, vessels) from desiccation.
5. Soft tissue coverage (local or distant flaps) is performed once the wound is clean.
6. Early, adequate debridement leads to earlier soft tissue coverage, which correlates with better long-term outcome.

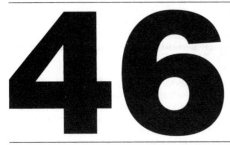

Thoracic and Abdominal Reconstruction

Andrew H. Rosenthal

General Principles

I. Define the defect
  A. Cause: Trauma, tumor resection, infection, congenital
  B. Size
  C. Location
  D. Layers involved: Skin, soft tissue, support
II. Define the patient
  A. Past medical history and risk factors: Can the patient tolerate a large reconstruction?
  B. Past surgical history
  C. Timing: Immediate versus delayed; single versus multiple stages
III. Define the goals of reconstruction
  A. Structure: Support, protection, and obliteration of dead space
  B. Function: Consider pulmonary dynamics and hernia prevention
  C. Durability: Fistula prevention, radiation tolerance, need for future procedures
  D. Aesthetics

Thoracic Reconstruction

I. Anatomy and physiology
  A. Rigid protection, with a flexible respiratory frame.
  B. Ribs articulate posteriorly with the spine and anteriorly with the sternum: They move like a bucket handle.
  C. Inspiratory muscles: Sternocleidomastoid, scalenes, and the diaphragm.
  D. Expiratory muscles: Rectus abdominis and the internal and external obliques.
II. Preparation for reconstruction
  A. Perform complete debridement of devitalized, infected, and/or radiation-damaged tissues. Inadequate debridement is the primary cause of reconstructive failure.
  B. Initiate appropriate antibiotic therapy, directed by tissue biopsy.
  C. Obtain a consultation from the thoracic and/or general surgery services as applicable.
  D. Maximize the patient's general medical condition.
    1. Nutrition: Maximize protein intake. Check nutrition laboratory values, including albumin, prealbumin, and transferrin (when appropriate).
    2. Oxygenation.
    3. Mobility.
    4. Avoid pressors, if at all possible.
III. Reconstruction of support
  A. Segmental resection of three or four ribs can be performed (depending on the location) without a significant impact on pulmonary mechanics (i.e., creation of a flail segment).

B. The irradiated chest wall becomes stiff and usually does not require reconstruction of support, even for very large defects.

C. For sternal reconstruction, it is usually not necessary to reapproximate the sternum (see below).

D. Options

1. **Split rib bone grafts** to bridge the defect: Rigid
   a. Pros: Autogenous tissue; replaces "like with like."
   b. Cons: Technically demanding; involves donor site morbidity, and fixation often fails due to motion with respiration.

2. **Acrylic** (e.g., polymethylmethacrylate): Rigid
   a. Pros: Technically straightforward.
   b. Cons: Complications associated with a foreign material (infection, erosion, etc.); strong exothermic reaction during curing can harm tissue if allowed to set up *in vivo*; difficult fixation to the chest wall.

3. **Fascia:** Semirigid
   a. Pros: Autogenous tissue; straightforward.
   b. Cons: Only semirigid; donor site morbidity; can tear; limited supply.

4. **Mesh:** Semirigid
   a. Pros: Straightforward.
   b. Cons: Foreign material; only semirigid.

5. **Composite mesh/methacrylate "sandwich":** Rigid repair with a flexible interface
   a. Pros: Straightforward; easier to secure in place.
   b. Cons: Foreign material.

IV. Dead space obliteration and coverage

A. Skin grafting
1. No filling of dead space
2. Poor durability
3. Poor coverage of irradiated tissues
4. Not a viable option with exposed bone, etc.

B. Regional flaps
1. **Pectoralis major:** Based on the thoracoacromial artery or inferior mesenteric artery (IMA) perforators.
2. **Latissimus dorsi:** Based on thoracodorsal artery or intercostals/lumbar perforators. Can be pedicled on the serratus branch if the thoracodorsal artery has been ligated.
3. **Serratus anterior:** Pedicled on the serratus branch of the thoracodorsal artery or the long thoracic artery.
4. **Trapezius:** Pedicled on descending branches of the transverse cervical artery.
5. **Rectus abdominis:** Pedicled on the superior epigastric artery. It can also be based on the eighth intercostal artery if the IMA was previously harvested.
6. **Omentum:** Pedicled on the right or left gastroepiploic artery.

C. Tissue expansion: Useful in delayed reconstruction.

V. Mediastinitis/sternal wound infection

A. Patients present with sternal instability and/or drainage from the wound.

B. The etiology can be mechanical or infectious. Both factors are important and synergistic.

C. More common following sacrifice of the IMA.

D. This complication previously resulted in high mortality rates. With aggressive debridement and muscle flap coverage, mortality is now quite low.

E. Radical debridement is essential.

F. The sternum is not rigidly fixed. Patients often complain of postoperative sternal instability and/or "clicking."

G. Late reconstruction has been described with plates or c-clamps in mechanical failures (not infected cases).

H. Workhorse flaps include the rectus abdominis, pectoralis major, and omentum (Table 46-1).

Table 46-1. Flap choice for thoracic reconstruction by location of defect

Location	First Choice	Second Choice
Midline, sternum	Pectoralis major, rectus abdominis	Omentum
Anterior chest	Latissimus dorsi, rectus abdominis	Omentum
Lateral chest	Latissimus dorsi	Rectus abdominis, omentum
Posterior chest	Latissimus dorsi	
Upper spinal/ paraspinal area	Trapezius	Latissimus dorsi, pectoralis major
Lower spinal/paraspinal	Latissimus dorsi, paraspinal muscles	

VI. Congenital defects
A. Poland's syndrome
1. Defined by a medical student in 1841.
2. **Incidence:** Males more than females; some familial tendency.
3. **Diagnosis:** The only true requirement for the diagnosis of Poland's syndrome is the congenital absence of the sternal head of the pectoralis major muscle. However, hypoplasia of other chest muscles is common. The breast often fails to develop fully, and upper extremity anomalies such as brachysyndactyly are common.
4. **Wide spectrum of severity:** The rib cage, scapula, serratus anterior, pectoralis minor, and latissimus dorsi can be affected.
5. **Reconstructive goals.**
   a. Creation of an anterior axillary fold.
   b. Symmetric breast mound and nipple-areolar complex.
   c. Chest wall symmetry.
6. **Options**
   a. **Custom chest wall prostheses.**
      (1) Pros: Straightforward, easily tailored.
      (2) Cons: Foreign body complications, migration or extrusion, and contour irregularities.
   b. **Latissimus transfer.**
      (1) The latissimus can be transposed to the anterior chest. This creates a new anterior axillary fold, while adding bulk to replace a missing or hypoplastic pectoralis muscle.
      (2) A tissue expander/breast implant can be placed under the muscle for breast reconstruction.
   c. **Contralateral breast reduction or mastopexy:** Commonly helps with symmetry.
B. Pectus excavatum ("funnel chest")
1. **Definition:** Involves a retrodisplaced sternum, starting at the angle of Louis.
2. **Side effects:** The deformity may cause abnormal pulmonary mechanics or cardiac irregularities.
3. **Incidence:** Male-to-female ratio is 4:1.
4. **Etiology:** Unknown; there is a familial tendency in some cases. The deformity may be due to an overgrowth of costal cartilage.
5. **Surgical options.**
   a. Sternal "turnover".
   b. Custom silicone implant.
   c. Cartilaginous wedge resections with or without an internal strut.
C. Pectus carinatum ("bird chest")
1. **Definition:** Convexity of the anterior chest.

2. **Incidence:** Much less common than pectus excavatum, but found in families with pectus excavatum.
3. **Repair:** With resection of costal cartilages and sternal osteotomies.

Abdominal Wall Reconstruction

I. **Anatomy and physiology**
   A. **Eight layers laterally**
      1. Skin.
      2. Subcutaneous tissue.
      3. Scarpa's fascia.
      4. External oblique muscle.
      5. Internal oblique muscle.
      6. Transversus abdominis muscle.
      7. Transversalis fascia.
      8. Peritoneum.
   B. **Centrally**
      1. Paired rectus muscles.
      2. Linea alba, in the midline. **Diastasis recti:** Thinning of the fascia in the midline, resulting in laterally displaced rectus muscles.
      3. Arcuate/semilunar line: Inferiorly, the only layer posterior to the rectus muscles is the transversalis fascia.
   C. **Goals of reconstruction**
      1. Protection for the abdominal viscera.
      2. Prevention of fluid losses.
      3. Fascial support.
      4. Muscle function, for pulmonary mechanics and stabilization of the trunk.
      5. Aesthetics.
II. **Preparation for reconstruction**
   A. Carefully outline the goals of the reconstruction.
   B. Obtain assistance from the general surgery service in planning, especially in relation to hernia reduction and entrance into the abdomen in reoperative cases.
   C. Consider the relationship between ostomy site(s) and reconstructive needs. For example, an ostomy already passing through the rectus abdominis may need to be repositioned, or a different reconstructive plan may need to be considered.
III. **Reconstruction of abdominal wall integrity**
   A. In some cases, abdominal wall reconstruction is not performed, in the interest of getting a closed, controlled wound (e.g., primary skin closure only, or skin grafting over exposed bowel).
   B. **Alloplastic materials**
      1. Polypropylene (Prolene, Marlex): Good incorporation; most common.
      2. PTFE (Gore-Tex): Lower foreign-body reaction and lower fistula rates.
      3. Polyester (Mersilene).
      4. Polygalactin (Vicryl): Can use in contaminated wounds, but only as a temporary solution, since it is biodegradable.
      5. Porcine intestinal submucosa (Surgisis): Role is still being defined.
   C. **Autogenous materials**
      1. **Grafts**
         a. Fascia lata
         b. Dermis
      2. **Regional flaps**
         a. **Tensor fascia lata**
            (1) Excellent for lower abdominal and suprapubic defects.
            (2) Pedicle: Ascending branch of the lateral circumflex femoral artery.

        (3) Enters 10 cm below the anterior superior iliac spine.
- **b. Rectus femoris:** A diminutive amount of tissue is available for abdominal coverage from this muscle.
- **c. "Separation of parts" or "component separation"**
  - **(1)** A powerful tool for abdominal reconstruction.
  - **(2)** Separation of the muscle/fascial layers of the abdominal wall with relaxing incisions to allow for differential advancement of the layers without hernia formation.
  - **(3)** Can be used in conjunction with mesh, as needed.

IV. Reconstruction of skin cover
- **A.** Skin grafting: Often unsightly, but simple.
- **B.** Separation of parts: The skin can be undermined and advanced with the abdominal wall layers.
- **C.** Tissue expansion.

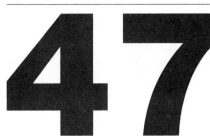

Pressure Sores

Douglas Sammer

General Information

I. **Definition**
   A. Necrosis or ulceration secondary to prolonged pressure.
   B. *Pressure sore* is the preferred term, because it correctly defines the etiology.
   C. Also known as bed sore, pressure ulcer, and decubitus ulcer.

II. **Epidemiology**
   A. Pressure sores occur in approximately 10% of hospitalized patients.
   B. Sixty percent of pressure sores occur in patients over the age of 70.
   C. Pressure sores cost over one billion dollars per year in the United States.

III. **Location**
   A. Supine patient
      1. The sacrum and heel are the most common locations.
      2. Less frequent: Ischium, trochanter, occiput, scapula, and elbows.
   B. Seated patient: Ischial and trochanteric sores are most common. Sacral sores can be seen with slightly reclined positioning.

IV. **Classification**
   A. National Pressure Ulcer Advisory Panel system (*Note:* the staging system is skewed toward early signs of ischemia, encouraging early detection and intervention.)
      1. Stage I: Nonblanchable erythema present greater than 1 hour after pressure relief; skin intact.
      2. Stage II: Partial-thickness skin loss.
      3. Stage III: Full-thickness skin loss into subcutaneous tissue, but not through fascia.
      4. Stage IV: Through fascia into muscle, bone, tendon, or joint.
   B. Caveats to staging
      1. If an eschar is present, the sore cannot be accurately staged until it is fully debrided.
      2. Skin erythema may be the only visible sign, even when underlying muscle necrosis has already occurred.

Etiology and Prevention

I. **Primary etiologic factors**
   A. Pressure
      1. Normal capillary pressure: 12 to 32 mm Hg.
      2. If tissue pressure is greater than 32 mm Hg, circulation decreases, leading to ischemia.
      3. There is an inverse time-to-pressure ratio: The greater the pressure, the less time is required to develop ischemia.
      4. Supine position: Tissue pressures of 40 to 60 mm Hg can be generated at the heels and sacrum.

5. Sitting position: Tissue pressures of 100 mm Hg can be generated at the ischial tuberosities.
6. Even though tissue pressure exceeds capillary pressure in the sitting and supine positions, periodic pressure relief can prevent pressure sores.
7. Underlying muscle necrosis may occur with minimal overlying skin changes, because muscle is more sensitive to ischemia than skin. Muscle necrosis occurs more quickly than skin necrosis when ischemia is induced.
8. Pressure gradient: Pressure is the highest in muscle overlying bone, and lower near the skin.

B. Shear: Stretches vessels, leading to thrombosis and ischemia.

C. Friction
1. Mechanical trauma to the epidermis.
2. Often occurs during patient transfer.

D. Moisture
1. Macerates skin.
2. Often due to incontinence and can be associated with local infection.
3. Pressure sore risk is increased in a moist environment.

II. Secondary etiologic factors
A. Malnutrition
1. Nutrition requirements are higher in patients with pressure sores.
2. Protein requirements: 1.5 to 3.0 gm/kg per day.
3. Nonprotein calories: 25 to 35 kcal/kg per day.
4. Vitamins A and C, zinc, and iron are essential to healing. Supplementation does not improve wound healing, however, unless the patient is deficient.

B. Sensory loss (with spinal cord injuries, etc.): The patient does not feel normal discomfort when high tissue pressure develops, and is therefore not prompted to shift positioning to relieve pressure.

C. Wound infection
1. All pressure sores are colonized with bacteria.
2. Colonization does not hinder and may actually aid healing.
3. Invasive infection with bacterial counts greater than 1×10^5 colony-forming units per gram (CFU/g) will impair healing.

D. Age: Older patients' skin has a decreased vascular supply and tensile strength.

E. Immobilization
1. Immobilized patients must usually rely on caregivers to relieve pressure.
2. Immobilization can lead to contractures, which cause uneven pressure distribution.

F. Systemic issues: Diabetes, vascular disease, smoking, etc.

III. Prevention
A. Pressure sores are preventable.
B. Modify the primary risk factors: pressure, moisture, shear, and friction.
1. **Pressure relief**
   a. **Turn** supine patients every 2 hours.
   b. **Lift** sitting patients from their chair for more than 10 seconds every 10 minutes.
   c. **Use specialized mattress or wheelchair cushions** for patients at high risk.
      (1) Low air-loss mattresses maintain tissue pressure below 25 mm Hg.
      (2) Air-fluidized mattresses can lower tissue pressures even more.
      (3) Specialized wheelchair cushions decrease pressure, but not below capillary pressure.
2. **Minimize moisture** by frequent changing of linens and clothing.
3. **Minimize shear** by appropriate positioning and support.
4. **Minimize friction** by careful transferring.

C. Modify secondary risk factors.
1. Treat infection.
2. Optimize nutrition to meet increased requirements. Monitor nutrition state with albumin and short-turnover protein levels (transferrin, prealbumin, etc.).

3. Treat contractures with physical therapy and muscle relaxants, with surgical release as a last resort.
4. Smoking cessation.
5. Maintain tight glucose control in diabetic patients.
6. Treat vascular disease.

Management of Established Pressure Sores

I. **Partial thickness (Stages I and II)**
   A. **Pressure relief** by frequent repositioning is usually adequate.
   B. **Reduce moisture, shear, friction, and other risk factors.**
   C. **Wound dressings**
      1. **DuoDerm or a semipermeable transparent dressing** protects the wound and prevents desiccation. Their use should be avoided if signs of invasive infection are present.
      2. **Xeroform or petroleum gauze.**
      3. **Silver sulfadiazine** dressing changes protect the wound and prevent desiccation, as well as providing antimicrobial activity.
   D. Most stage I and II pressure sores can heal within 2 to 3 weeks.
II. **Full thickness (Stages III and IV)**
   A. Pressure relief by repositioning is sometimes adequate, but often a specialty mattress or wheelchair cushion is required.
   B. Reduce moisture, shear, friction, and other risk factors.
   C. **Debridement**
      1. Excision of all nonviable tissue can often be adequately performed at the bedside or in clinic. Debridements may be staged to prevent unacceptable acute blood loss.
      2. Aided by dressing changes.
   D. **Dressings**
      1. **Wet-to-moist dressings**
         a. The wound surface should be kept moist to promote the growth of fibroblasts and keratinocytes.
         b. There is no role for true wet-to-dry dressings: These desiccate the wound and prevent healing.
      2. **Debriding dressings**
         a. **Collagenase** dressings can soften tough, devitalized tissues.
         b. Alternate with wet-to-moist dressings.
         c. These types of dressings can damage healthy tissues. Their use should be limited (1–2 weeks).
         d. Significant amounts of necrotic material should be surgically debrided.
      3. **Antimicrobial dressings**
         a. **Silver sulfadiazine:** Antimicrobial; prevents desiccation
            (1) Avoid in patients with sulfa allergies.
            (2) Can cause neutropenia.
         b. **Oxychlorosene** (Dakin's solution; dilute bleach) wet-to-moist dressing changes: The antimicrobial effect is especially useful in cases of suspected *Pseudomonas* infection.
         c. Many antimicrobials damage healthy tissue, as well as promote resistant colonization. Once the wound is clean, other dressings should be used.
      4. **Occlusive dressings:** For debrided, noninfected wounds.
         a. **Hydrocolloids:** Mix with the wound exudate to form a gel that keeps the wound moist and promotes granulation. They are changed every few days.
         b. **Alginate or absorbant foam:** Used for wounds that have significant drainage or discharge.

5. **Growth factors**
   a. **Recombinant platelet derived growth factor (rPDGF, Regranex)** helps decrease the wound size and accelerate healing.
   b. The wound must be debrided and noninfected prior to use.
   c. Should be used for 4 to 6 weeks to see results.
E. **Treatment of soft tissue infection**
   1. **Signs of a wound infection**
      a. Local: Surrounding erythema, foul odor, and purulent discharge.
      b. Systemic: Fever, leukocytosis, and sepsis.
   2. **Obtain tissue biopsy** (after debridement) for quantitative counts, culture, and sensitivities.
      a. Counts greater than 1×10^5 CFU/g indicate an invasive infection.
      b. The antimicrobial choice should be based on culture results.
      c. *Staphylococcus, Streptococcus, Escherichia coli,* and *Pseudomonas* are the most common organisms.
      d. Mixed aerobic/anaerobic infections are also common.
   3. Treat with adequate debridement, drainage, and antibiotics.
F. **Osteomyelitis**
   1. **If bone is exposed,** osteomyelitis should be presumed until disproved.
      a. **Bone biopsy is the gold standard** for diagnosis.
         (1) Can usually be obtained at bedside with a rongeur.
         (2) Should be done only after thorough debridement.
         (3) Permanent pathologic analysis confirms the presence of osteo-myelitis.
         (4) Culture and sensitivities determine the offending organism(s) and guide antimicrobial administration.
      b. **Bone scans** can be helpful if a bone biopsy is unable to be obtained (which is rarely the case).
         (1) A negative bone scan can rule out osteomyelitis.
         (2) However, if the bone scan is positive, a bone biopsy is needed to make a definitive diagnosis. Bone scans are not specific, and can be positive due to local or regional inflammation or increased bone turnover (present in all wounds of this type).
      c. **Magnetic resonance imaging**
         (1) Useful for defining the extent of bone involvement, particularly in pelvic osteomyelitis.
         (2) 98% sensitive and 90% specific.
   2. Osteomyelitis requires aggressive debridement of devitalized and infected bone and usually at least 6 weeks of intravenous antibiotics for treatment.
   3. Occasionally, osteomyelitis is so extensive that complete debridement is not possible.
      a. The patient will require chronic suppressive antibiotics.
      b. Wound care should consist of appropriate debridement and dressing changes indefinitely.

Flap Closure

I. **Preoperative preparation for flap closure**
   A. Preoperative preparation is the most important factor for maintaining a healed wound after flap closure.
   B. Medical management should be maximized preoperatively: pressure relief protocols and surfaces, control of diabetes, nutrition optimization, spasticity, and so forth.
   C. Physical medicine and rehabilitation services should be involved.
   D. Adequate home and social support must be present.
   E. Patients must demonstrate a history of compliance and motivation.

F. The wound must begin to show evidence of spontaneous healing. If the patient cannot demonstrate the ability to initiate healing, then a flap closure will likely be a futile exercise.

G. The wound must be thoroughly débrided and free from infection prior to flap closure.

    1. Debride all necrotic or devitalized tissue, including bone, until healthy bleeding tissue is observed.

    2. Obtain adequate biopsies.

        a. Always complete debridement prior to obtaining soft tissue or bone biopsies.

        b. The patient should be off systemic antibiotics for 7 days prior to biopsy to improve the accuracy of culture results.

H. Osteomyelitis must be eradicated prior to surgical closure.

II. General considerations in flap closure

A. Tissue requirements

    1. Muscle and musculocutaneous flaps provide well-vascularized tissue for fill of dead space, but can impair lower extremity function in nonparalyzed patients.

    2. Fasciocutaneous flaps are also well vascularized, are more durable than muscle flaps, and have less effect on function, but provide less tissue bulk.

    3. Cutaneous flaps do not provide significant volume, and generally have less reliable vascular supplies.

B. Future flaps

    1. The possibility of needing a repeat flap in the future due to flap failure or development of other pressure sores must always be considered. Do not burn any bridges.

    2. Rotation and V-Y advancement flaps are advantageous because readvancement is relatively easy.

C. Patient characteristics

    1. Sensation: It is sometimes possible to move sensate tissue into the wound, thereby decreasing the likelihood of recurrence.

    2. Nonparalyzed patients: If a patient has the potential to ambulate in the future, a flap that does not limit ambulation should be chosen.

III. Sacral closure

A. Gluteal flaps (gluteus maximus)

    1. Anatomy.

        a. Type III vascular supply.

        b. The superior and inferior gluteal arteries arise from the internal iliac artery's posterior and anterior divisions and pass superior and inferior to the piriformis, respectively, before entering the gluteus maximus.

    2. The superior or inferior segment alone can be used to preserve ambulation.

    3. The flap can be designed as a rotation-advancement or as a V-Y advancement musculocutaneous flap.

B. Lumbosacral transverse back flap

    1. Anatomy.

        a. A fasciocutaneous flap utilizing the fascia of the paraspinous muscles

        b. Based on perforators from lumbar and posterior intercostal arteries

    2. Transverse flap: Crosses the midline, with perforators at the base on the contralateral side; transposed to a sacral defect.

    3. Requires skin grafting of the donor site.

IV. Ischial closure

A. Gluteal flaps

    1. Can be used as a rotation-advancement musculocutaneous flap of the entire gluteus maximus, or the inferior segment can be rotated alone.

    2. It can also be used as an inferior segment island flap or inferior segment muscle transposition flap, requiring a skin graft.

B. V-Y hamstring flap

    1. Anatomy.

  a. Biceps femoris with or without the semitendinosus and semimembra-nosus muscles.
  b. Type II vascular supply.
  c. The dominant pedicle is the first branch of the profunda femoris artery.
  2. It is designed as a musculocutaneous V-Y advancement flap.
C. **Posterior/gluteal thigh flap**
  1. Fasciocutaneous.
  2. Based on the descending branch of the inferior gluteal artery.
  3. Rotated into an ischial defect.

V. **Trochanteric closure**
  A. **Tensor fascia lata flap**
    1. **Anatomy.**
      a. Type I vascular supply.
      b. Based on the ascending branch of the lateral circumflex femoral artery.
    2. **Advances as a V-Y flap** or rotates as a transposition flap.
  B. **Vastus lateralis flap**
    1. Type I vascular supply.
    2. Based on the descending branch of the lateral circumflex femoral artery.
    3. Designed as a muscle flap that requires split-thickness skin graft coverage.
  C. **Gluteal thigh flap** (described above)

VI. **Postoperative care**
  A. Maximized nutrition
  B. Appropriate specialty mattress
  C. Frequent turning and pressure relief
  D. Control of spasm
  E. Bowel/bladder elimination control program
  F. Drainage of surgical site with closed-suction drains
  G. Sitting advancement
    1. No sitting for 4 to 6 weeks after flap closure.
    2. Advance sitting duration over 1 to 2 weeks.
    3. Begin with 30 minutes of sitting twice per day, with at least 1 hour rest in between.
    4. Advance by 15 minutes per day until 2 hours' length is reached.
    5. Evaluate the flap after each sitting session.
      a. Check for signs of ischemia or breakdown and adjust the schedule accordingly.
      b. Sitting cannot be resumed until any erythema is resolved.
      c. Do not increase sitting time if erythema lasts more than 30 minutes after a sitting session.
    6. During each sitting session, the patient must be lifted for more than 10 seconds every 10 minutes for pressure relief.

Pearls

1. The physical medicine and rehabilitation service should be consulted for any patient with a new pressure sore.
2. Whether or not a patient heals a pressure sore is largely dependent on the patient's home and social support.
3. Optimize all associated medical conditions and ensure patient compliance and motivation prior to attempts at operative closure.
4. Many pressure sores recur, usually within 1 year of operation.
5. Patient selection is critical for success of operative closure.

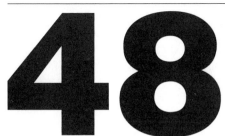

Lower Extremity Reconstruction

Steven C. Haase

Reconstruction for Trauma

I. Goals
  A. Preserve function: Three components
  1. Stability: Weight bearing.
  2. Sensation and proprioception: Especially on the plantar surface.
  3. Mobility: Ankle and knee.
  B. Preserve form: Structure, body image, etc. However, form without function is not a satisfactory outcome.
  C. Amputation may result in a more functional limb in some cases (e.g., quicker return to activity, work, and ambulation; improved mobility). Some amputees climb mountains, run marathons, play tennis, and so forth.

II. Anatomy
  A. Bones
  1. Femur.
  2. Patella.
  3. Tibia: Bears 85% of the weight through the lower leg. It has no muscle coverage on its anteromedial surface.
  4. Fibula: Its primary function is for muscle attachment. Its midportion can be sacrificed without significant morbidity.
  5. Tarsals: Calcaneus, cuboid, navicular, and cuneiforms (medial, intermediate, and lateral).
  6. Metatarsals (5).
  7. Phalanges (14).
  B. Thigh musculature and innervation (Table 48-1)
  C. Lower leg musculature and innervation (Fig. 48-1 and Table 48-2). *Note:* There is no such structure as the "posterior" tibial nerve.
  D. Plantar foot musculature and innervation: Four layers (Table 48-3)
  E. Nerves: Sensory distribution (Fig. 48-2)

III. Evaluation
  A. Trauma evaluation: ABCs
  B. History
  1. Ascertain when, where, and how the injury occurred, including possible contamination source (farm soil or equipment, marine exposure, etc.).
  2. Exact mechanism of injury: Get a sense of severity and potential zone of injury, which can directly affect treatment choice.
  3. Tobacco use.
  C. Physical examination
  1. Document neurovascular status.
  2. Joint range of motion (ROM), stability: At least one joint on either side of the fracture.
  3. "Fracture + laceration = open fracture" in most instances.
  D. Wound assessment
  1. What is missing? (skin, subcutaneous tissue, muscle, bone).
  2. What is affected and/or exposed? (nerves, vessels, bone, joint, hardware).

Table 48-1. Thigh musculature and innervation

Muscle	Function	Innervation
Tensor fasciae latae	Extends knee, stabilizes leg with standing	Superior gluteal nerve
Sartorius	Extensor group	Femoral nerve
Quadriceps		
Rectus femoris		
Vastus lateralis		
Vastus medialis		
Vastus intermedius		
Pectineus (lateral)		
Pectineus (medial)	Adductor group	Obturator nerve
Adductor longus		
Adductor brevis		
Adductor magnus		
Obturator externus		
Gracilis		
Biceps femoris	Flexor group	Sciatic nerve
Semimembranosus		
Semitendinosus		

    3. What is the level of contamination or infection? (chronicity, cultures, debridements).

    4. Are there any "spare parts" available? (skin grafts, fillet flaps).

    5. Expectations of the patient versus realistic goals of potential treatment options.

  E. Gustilo classification of lower extremity fractures and associated soft tissue injury (Table 48-4)

  F. Osteomyelitis

    1. Two broad categories

      a. Acute: Early infection without significant devitalized bone (sequestrum) that can potentially be cured with antibiotics

      b. Chronic: Long-standing infection, typically involving a sequestrum

    2. Diagnostic tests

      a. Erythrocyte sedimentation rate (ESR): Can help rule out osteomyelitis if normal.

      b. Bone culture: To identify the organism.

      c. Bone biopsy: Confirms osteomyelitis pathologically.

      d. Adjunctive tests (generally not needed)

        (1) X-ray: Findings lag behind the progression of the disease.

        (2) Technetium 99 (^{99}Tc): False negatives are possible if blood flow to the area is poor.

        (3) Gallium: False positives are secondary to soft tissue inflammation.

        (4) Magnetic resonance imaging (MRI): T1 images show decreased signal in infected bone. Hardware may interfere with images, however.

      e. The most reliable diagnostic measures are bone biopsy/culture, MRI, and ESR.

    3. Treatment

      a. Thorough debridement of any and all nonviable tissue.

      b. Definitive reconstruction as indicated.

      c. Long-term intravenous antibiotics (approximately 6 weeks). Consider infectious disease consultation.

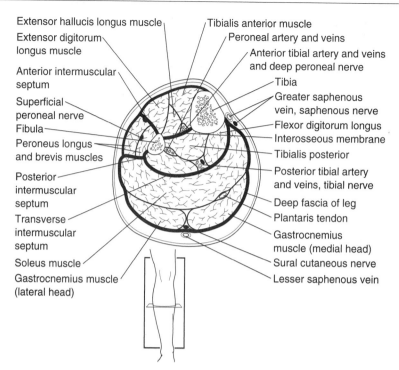

Fig. 48-1. Anatomy of the leg in cross-section.

G. Compartment syndrome

1. Can occur with any crush injury to a closed compartment.
2. Occurs in 5% to 10% of open tibia fractures.
3. **Pathophysiology**
   a. Increased pressure within a closed osteofascial compartment rises above capillary pressure (about 30 mm Hg), leading to decreased perfusion and eventually to muscle and nerve necrosis.
   b. Dying muscle releases myoglobin into the bloodstream, which is toxic to the kidney and precipitates in the tubules.
   c. Renal toxicity is minimized by alkalinizing the urine.
      (1) Add bicarbonate to the i.v. fluids.
      (2) Dip urine to maintain the pH $\geq$ 8.
4. **Key signs and symptoms**
   a. Pain out of proportion to the injury.
   b. Pain on passive flexion or extension of muscles within the compartment.
   c. Palpably swollen or tense compartments.
   d. Paresthesias.
   e. Loss of pulses (a **late** sign).
5. **Definitive diagnosis:** Measure pressure within the compartment, a procedure that is straightforward, simple, and quick to perform, with low morbidity. A compartment syndrome should never be suspected without monitoring the compartment. Generally, pressure above 30 mm Hg is an indication for fasciotomy.
   a. Stryker pressure monitoring instrument.
   b. Arterial line setup with a large-bore needle.

Table 48-2. Lower leg anatomy

Compartment	Muscle	Function	Innervation
Anterior	Tibialis anterior	Dorsiflex foot, invert foot	Deep peroneal nerve
	Extensor digitorum longus	Extend toes II–V, dorsiflex foot	
	Extensor hallucis longus	Extend great toe, dorsiflex foot	
	Peroneus tertius	Dorsiflex foot, evert foot	
Lateral	Peroneus longus	Plantar flex foot, evert foot	Superficial peroneal nerve
	Peroneus brevis	Plantar flex foot, evert foot	
Superficial posterior	Gastrocnemius	Plantar flex foot, flex knee	Tibial nerve
	Soleus	Plantar flex foot	
	Plantaris	Plantar flex foot	
	Popliteus	Flex knee, rotate tibia	
Deep posterior	Flexor hallucis longus	Flex great toe, flex foot	Tibial nerve
	Flexor digitorum longus	Flex toes II–V, flex foot	
	Tibialis posterior	Plantar flex foot, invert foot	

Table 48-3. Plantar foot anatomy

Layer	Muscles	Innervation
1 (Superficial)	Flexor digitorum brevis	Medial plantar
	Abductor hallucis	Medial plantar
	Abductor digiti minimi	Lateral plantar
2	(FHL tendon)	
	(FDL tendon)	
	Lumbricals	1: Medial plantar
		2–5: Lateral plantar
	Flexor digitorum accessorius (quadratus plantae)	Lateral plantar
3	Flexor hallucis brevis	Medial plantar
	Flexor digiti minimi brevis	Lateral plantar
	Adductor hallucis	Lateral plantar
4 (Deep)	(Tibialis posterior tendon)	
	(Peroneus longus tendon)	
	Interossei	Lateral plantar

FDL, flexor digitorum longus; FHL, flexor hallucis longus.

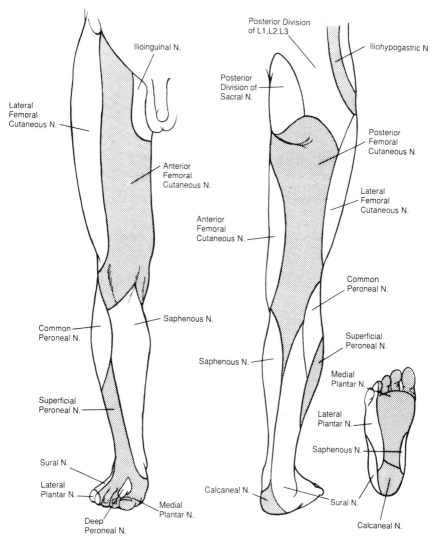

Fig. 48-2. Cutaneous innervation of the lower extremity. (From Attinger. Foot and ankle preservation. In *Grabb and Smith's Plastic Surgery*, 5th ed. Aston SJ, Beasley RW, Thorne CH, Philadelphia, Lippincott-Raven Publishers, 1997. With permission.)

H. Contraindications to reconstruction
1. Absolute
a. **Unsalvageable limb:** Less functional than the outcome anticipated with an amputation. This decision must also take into account the long-term effects.

b. **Threat to life, unstable patient:** "Life before limb."
2. Relative
a. Laceration of the tibial nerve (no plantar sensation)

Table 48-4. Gustilo classification of open tibial fractures

Type	Description
I	Open fracture with wound < 1 cm
II	Open fracture with wound > 1 cm without extensive soft tissue damage
III	Open fracture with extensive soft tissue damage
IIIA	III, with adequate soft tissue coverage
IIIB	III, with soft tissue loss with periosteal stripping and bone exposure
IIIC	III, with arterial injury requiring repair

      b. Devascularization with major soft tissue injury and/or open fractures.

      c. Concomitant diaphyseal and major joint fractures.

      d. Massive burns with an open long-bone fracture.

IV. Primary reconstruction

A. Timing

1. Immediate coverage is indicated for clean wounds with exposed vital structures.
2. Early coverage (within 1 week) has been associated with fewer complications.
3. The wound must be clean prior to any attempts at closure.

B. Debridement

1. **Serial debridements** are often required.
   a. Allows time for marginal tissue to declare itself and zone of injury to become more apparent.
   b. Allows time for dressing changes to clear away debris and bacteria.
   c. Interval of 1 to 2 days between debridements is probably ideal.
   d. Consider tobramycin-impregnated cement beads as local antibiotic therapy.
2. **Quantitative cultures** should be taken after débridement for the following reasons.
   a. To gauge contamination levels and the need for further debridement, antibiotics, and/or dressing changes.
   b. To gauge the success of closure: Fewer than 10^5 colony-forming units per gram of tissue is associated with higher closure success rates.
3. **Avulsion/degloving injuries**
   a. Damage to the avulsion flap is often underestimated acutely, and progressive necrosis over the week following injury is common.
   b. Consider debriding avulsed flaps and harvesting the skin for use as a skin graft.
4. **Inadequate debridement** *will* lead to an infected reconstruction.
5. **A fully debrided wound** should appear much like a fresh or acute surgical wound.

C. Bony stabilization

1. **Bone healing requirements**
   a. Immobilization.
   b. Blood supply via periosteal and nutrient arteries. Therefore, periosteal stripping should be minimized.
2. **Techniques**
   a. Traction.
   b. Cast immobilization.
   c. Open reduction and internal fixation (ORIF): Intramedullary nail or a plate-and-screws fixation.
      (1) Increasingly common, even in open fractures.
      (2) Early, stable coverage is important.
   d. External fixation.

D. Revascularization

1. Fracture reduction may resolve spasm and kinking of the vessels.
2. Consider temporary vascular shunts if the stabilization process will be prolonged and the limb is ischemic.
3. Usually only one infrapopliteal vessel is necessary for adequate perfusion of the lower limb.
4. Saphenous vein is a common source for vein graft for this application.
5. Consider fasciotomies after revascularization.

E. Soft tissue coverage

1. **Use the reconstructive ladder,** progressing from simple to more complex options. However, many of the lower rungs on the ladder may not be viable options in complex lower extremity wounds, necessitating use of the **"reconstructive elevator,"** moving up to use the most optimal, albeit more complex, reconstructive option.
2. **Observation and dressing changes**
   a. Not an option if any critical structures are exposed.
   b. The vacuum-assisted closure (VAC) device can be used to encourage granulation tissue formation and to clean up dirty wounds.
3. **Primary closure**
   a. Need healthy tissue.
   b. Must be free of tension.
4. **Skin graft**
   a. Provides poor durability coverage on weight-bearing regions (e.g., the heel).
   b. Will not survive on top of bare tendon, bone, or hardware.
5. **Tissue expansion:** Poor results in the lower extremity, with complication rates greater than 75%.
6. **Local flaps** (see below)
   a. Pedicled tissue adjacent to the wound.
   b. May include skin, fascia, muscle, or bone in nearly any combination.
7. **Regional flaps**
   a. Pedicled tissue separated from the immediate vicinity of the wound.
   b. Cross-leg versions of many flaps have been described.
8. **Free flaps** (free tissue transfer)
   a. Especially valuable in wounds complicated by osteomyelitis, radiation therapy, and recurrent nonunions.
   b. Their contour improves with time as the bulky muscle flap atrophies due to denervation and disuse (usually about 50%).
   c. Use vein grafts as needed to locate the anastomosis outside the zone of injury, avoiding areas of subtle vessel damage.
   d. Use end-to-side anastomosis when possible in the leg to permit runoff.
   e. Contraindications: No flap available, no vessel available, no microsurgeon available.
9. **Flap classification systems** (see Chapter 4, "Flaps")
   a. Muscle flaps: Mathes and Nahai classification.
   b. Fasciocutaneous flaps.

V. Regional reconstruction options

A. Thigh

1. There is usually abundant muscle present around the femur.
2. Skin grafting is usually the only coverage required.
3. Local muscle flaps may be used for coverage of exposed bone or neurovascular structures.
4. Distant or free flaps are rarely indicated.
5. Thigh flaps are listed in Table 48-5.

B. Knee

1. Skin grafting is OK if the joint capsule is intact, but this type of coverage can be unstable over the knee joint.
2. The gastrocnemius is the flap of choice in this area. The medial head has a longer reach, but either head can be used.

Table 48-5. Thigh flaps

Flap	Class	Pedicle	Comments
Fasciocutaneous			
Posterior thigh	B	Descending inferior gluteal artery	Good for perineal wounds; can be raised as sensate flap with posterior femoral cutaneous nerve
Anterior lateral thigh	B and C	Branches (septocutaneous and musculocutaneous) of descending branch of lateral circumflex femoral artery	
Muscle and musculocutaneous			
Rectus abdominis	III	Superior and inferior epigastric arteries	Reliable, large skin paddle; good free flap.
Vastus lateralis	II	Lateral femoral circumflex artery	Good for infected hip wounds; good for middle and lower thigh; skin paddle rarely used
Vastus medialis	II	Profunda femoris branch	Good for middle and lower thigh; skin paddle rarely used
Rectus femoris	I	Medial femoral circumflex and distal segmentals	Must reconstruct quadriceps/patellar tendon after harvest
Gracilis	II	Medial femoral circumflex artery and SFA segmentals	Reliable skin paddle; good for perineal wounds; good free flap
Sartorius	IV	8–10 segmental pedicles from superficial femoral vessels	Flap of choice for small anterior defects, exposed groin vessels
Tensor fasciae latae	I	Terminal branch of lateral femoral circumflex artery	Flap of choice for posterior defects; reliable skin paddle to 10 cm above knee; can be raised as a sensate flap with lateral femoral cutaneous nerve

SFA, Superficial femoral artery.

3. Alternates: Distally based gracilis (delayed) and sartorius flaps have been described, but are risky alternatives.
4. Consider a free flap if the gastrocnemius is not available or the defect is extensive.

C. **Reconstruction of the lower leg is divided into thirds.**
   1. **Proximal third**
      a. First choice: Gastrocnemius muscle flap covered with a skin graft.
      b. A cross-leg flap may be used, but a free flap should be considered in this instance.
   2. **Middle third**
      a. First choice: Soleus muscle flap with a skin graft.
      b. Alternates or adjuncts: Gastrocnemius, tibialis anterior, and flexor digitorum longus muscle flaps.

Table 48-6. Lower leg flaps

Flap	Class	Pedicle	Comments
Fasciocutaneous			
Medial calf flap	A	Perforators from saphenous artery, medial geniculate artery and posterior tibial artery	Unsightly donor site; requires skin graft
Retrograde peroneal flap	C	Retrograde peroneal artery	Depends on distal communication between peroneal and anterior and/or posterior tibial arteries
Reverse superficial sural artery flap	B	Retrograde superficial sural artery, via peroneal artery	Can cover nearly any ankle or proximal foot defect
Muscle and musculocutaneous			
Gastrocnemius: medial (larger) & lateral heads	I	Paired (medial/lateral) sural branches of the popliteal artery	Pedicle enters just below knee joint; skin paddle can extend to 5 cm above medial malleolus; ugly donor defect when skin taken
Soleus: medial & lateral heads	II	Medial portion: posterior tibial and popliteal arteries; lateral portion: peroneal artery	Delicate muscle; harder to elevate than gastrocnemius; distal end unreliable
Tibialis anterior	IV	Anterior tibial artery	Not expendable; raise as bipedicled flap or "book flap" for middle or distal third
Extensor digitorum longus	IV	Anterior tibial artery	Not expendable; must preserve function
Flexor digitorum longus	IV	Posterior tibial artery	Used with soleus for small tibial defects
Peroneus longus	II	Peroneal artery	Can be used for small middle-third defects
Extensor hallucis longus	IV	Anterior and posterior tibial arteries	For small defects in distal one-third
Peroneus brevis	II	Peroneal artery	For small defects in distal one-third
Any			
Cross-leg flap	N/A	Varies	Rarely used; can be fasciocutaneous, musculocutaneous, or muscle alone

  c. May need a free flap for large defects.
3. Distal third
  a. Most challenging; a free flap is usually required.
  b. If a free flap is contraindicated, the following can be used.
    (1) Local muscle flaps: Soleus, peroneus brevis, extensor digitorum longus, extensor hallucis longus, and tibialis anterior can provide piecemeal coverage.
    (2) Local fasciocutaneous flaps.
      (a) Random, multiply delayed flaps.
      (b) Reverse superficial sural artery flap: A relatively new flap with great promise.
      (c) Dorsalis pedis flap.
4. Lower leg flaps are listed in Table 48-6.
D. Foot
  1. Dorsal
    a. Need thin coverage for shoe wear.
    b. Local flaps for small defects: Rotation or transposition flaps.
    c. Free flaps for larger defects: Temporoparietal fascia, radial forearm, or latissimus dorsi (in children).
  2. Plantar
    a. Skin grafts can be used if adequate padding is present and the wound is less than one-third of the weight-bearing surface.
    b. Several local flaps are available; free flaps are needed for large wounds (greater than two-thirds of surface).
  3. Foot flaps are listed in Table 48-7.
E. Free flaps: See Chapter 4, "Flaps."
VI. Secondary reconstruction
  A. Nerve repair
    1. Results of nerve repair in the lower extremity are poor in adults, but somewhat better in children.
    2. Most patients require lifetime splinting or tendon transfers.
    3. The sural nerve is a common source for nerve graft.
      a. Minimal donor deficit: Numbness of the lateral foot and ankle.
      b. The nerve courses from the midline of the posterior leg to travel with the lesser saphenous vein in a groove between the lateral malleolus and the Achilles tendon.
      c. Since nerve graft supply is limited, use of the sural nerve as a donor is usually limited to high-yield situations (i.e., clean, closed wounds).
  B. Bone gaps
    1. Bone grafting is typically postponed until 6 to 12 weeks after the soft tissues have healed.
      a. Nonvascularized cancellous bone grafts: For nonunions or small gaps (<3 cm).
      b. Ilizarov bone lengthening: For intermediate gaps (4–8 cm).
      c. Vascularized bone grafts: For larger gaps.
    2. Fibula graft: Can be used as a pedicled local flap or as a free flap.
      a. Up to 25 cm of length can be harvested from the average adult.
      b. The proximal and distal 4 to 6 cm of the fibula should be preserved for knee and ankle function.
      c. The fibula is supplied by the peroneal artery, which enters the bone at its midportion as the nutrient artery. The other main blood supply is periosteal.
      d. The skin paddle overlying the fibula on the lateral surface of the leg can be included with the flap.
VII. Amputation principles
  A. Preserve length.
    1. A below-knee amputation (BKA) greatly reduces the work of ambulation relative to an above-knee amputation (AKA).
    2. The quality of life is also significantly better for patients with a BKA versus an AKA.

Table 48-7. Foot flaps

Flap	Pedicle	Comments
Skin/Subcutaneous		
Reversed dermis flap	Dermal/subdermal plexus	Turn-over flap of dermis to cover adjacent wound; may be useful for Achilles coverage
Fillet of toe flap	Digital artery	Sensate flap via deep peroneal nerve or digital nerves
Lateral calcaneal artery skin flap	Lateral calcaneal artery (branch of peroneal artery)	Can cover Achilles tendon and posterior heel
Suprafascial rotational flap	Proximal subcutaneous vascular plexus via dorsalis pedis and medial calcaneal arteries	Sensate flap via medial calcaneal nerve
Cross-foot flap (also cross-thigh and cross-groin flaps)	Multiple musculocutaneous perforators	Seldom used; can transfer plantar skin to opposite foot in theory
Medial plantar flap	Cutaneous branch of medial plantar artery	Versatile; can elevate abductor hallucis brevis muscle with flap
Fasciocutaneous		
Flexor digiti minimi brevis	Lateral plantar artery	Can reach proximal fifth metacarpal
Muscle		
Abductor digiti minimi	Lateral plantar artery enters near origin	Can reach lateral heel and beneath lateral malleolus
Flexor digitorum longus	Perforators from posterior tibial artery	May reach distal-third anteromedial ankle wounds
Flexor hallucis brevis	Medial plantar artery and first plantar metatarsal artery	Can reach around to dorsum of foot; often used in combination flaps
Extensor digitorum brevis	Dorsalis pedis artery via lateral tarsal artery	Thin; OK for local defects of dorsum
Abductor hallucis brevis flap (with skin = medial plantar flap)	Medial plantar artery enters on lateral side	Can reach to posterior heel; sensate flap if medial plantar nerve preserved
Muscle or musculocutaneous		
Flexor digitorum brevis (with skin = plantar artery-skin-fascia flap)	Dominant: lateral plantar artery enters undersurface of the proximal one-third of muscle; Minor: reverse flow via plantar arch	Can reach to heel and Achilles tendon if dominant pedicle divided (risky); harvest results in loss of arch support

    3. Midfoot amputations (Chopart, Symes) have little functional advantage over a BKA.
  B. Conserve "spare parts" from the amputation specimen and use them as necessary in the reconstruction, without additional donor site morbidity.
    1. Fillet flaps (typically fasciocutaneous flaps) can be used as free tissue transfer.
    2. Full- or split-thickness skin grafts can be obtained from the amputated part.

The Diabetic Foot

I. Etiology
  A. Neuropathy (the most critical factor)
   1. Origin: Multifactorial
      a. High glucose levels lead to altered neuron metabolism. Glucose is converted to sorbitol, which builds up in the perifascicular connective tissue and swells, causing intraneural compression.
      b. Antegrade axoplasmic flow is slowed, leading to decreased nerve repair mechanisms.
      c. The above two mechanisms set up a situation ripe for the double-crush phenomenon: Any additional site of compression (e.g., the cubital tunnel or the tarsal tunnel) can significantly worsen symptoms of neuropathy.
   2. Sensory neuropathy: Leads to the inability to detect injuries or prevent new ones.
   3. Diagnostic threshold: 5.07 Semmes-Weinstein filament (10 g of pressure).
   4. Autonomic neuropathy: Anhydrosis and arteriovenous shunting lead to dry, cracked skin.
   5. Motor neuropathy: Intrinsic denervation leads to altered mechanics and clawing of the toes.
  B. Ischemia: Due to diabetic macrovascular and microvascular disease.
   1. Ankle-brachial indexes are often invalid (falsely high) due to vessel incompressibility secondary to calcification.
   2. The usual pattern of disease is the "trashed trifurcation": Most of the disease is infrapopliteal.
   3. The foot vessels are often spared from extensive involvement.
  C. Immune system dysfunction
   1. Both cellular (polymorphonuclear neutrophils, lymphocytes) and humeral (antibody) immunity are compromised in diabetic patients.
   2. Superficial infections are usually caused by gram-positive cocci.
   3. Deeper infections are usually polymicrobial, including anaerobes.
  D. Mechanical
   1. Charcot foot: Collapse of the midfoot bones (present in 1 of 800 diabetic patients).
   2. The Achilles tendon shortens due to loss of collagen elasticity.
II. Evaluation
  A. Note ulcer characteristics.
   1. Location and size.
   2. Presence of surrounding cellulitis or fungal infection.
   3. Presence of exposed bone (almost always indicates osteomyelitis).
  B. Examine the rest of the foot.
   1. Joint deformities (e.g., talipes equines, Charcot foot).
   2. X-rays to evaluate the following.
      a. Joint damage.
      b. Midfoot collapse.
      c. Signs of osteomyelitis.
      d. Soft tissues; presence of gas.
III. Treatment
  A. Superficial and/or no cellulitis
   1. Pressure relief: Off-loading orthotics or shoe inserts.
   2. Topical antibiotics only.
  B. Cellulitis
   1. Requires antibiotics: Start with oral, and switch to intravenous if improvement is not shortly forthcoming.
   2. Therapy should be guided by **tissue cultures.** Swab cultures are meaningless. Send a tissue biopsy specimen from the wound to the microbiology lab.
   3. Consider treatment for tinea pedis (a fungal infection) in cases of persistent or atypical cellulitis.

C. Deep ulcers
1. Probe to determine if there is any exposed bone within the wound.
2. Bone biopsy is the best way to prove or disprove the presence of osteomyelitis.
3. Thorough debridement of all devitalized bone (sequestrum) should be performed.
4. Following debridement, osteomyelitis should be treated with at least 6 weeks of intravenous antibiotics.
5. A clean, thoroughly debrided wound can be closed with a variety of flaps (see above).

IV. Practical considerations
A. Debridement of necrotic tissue and fastidious off-loading will allow most ulcers to heal.
B. Osteomyelitis that requires extensive debridement usually occurs in patients who are poor candidates for local flaps or complicated reconstructions. In these situations, some level of amputation is often ultimately required.

Pearls

1. Know the contents of the four compartments (Fig. 48-1) and the sensory innervation (Fig. 48-2) of the lower leg.
2. Always document the patient's neurovascular status on examination.
3. Don't forget about the potential for use of spare parts and fillet flaps in cases of unsalvageable amputations.
4. Best choices for lower leg reconstruction: Proximal third = gastrocnemius; middle third = soleus; distal third = free flap.
5. Debridement is the key to success.

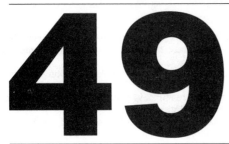

Necrotizing Soft Tissue Infections

Andrew P. Trussler

Introduction

The keys to successful management of necrotizing soft tissue infections are early recognition and prompt surgical debridement. These lesions may present with few external manifestations. Diffuse internal inflammation may progress rapidly, with significant underlying deep tissue destruction. A 24-hour delay in diagnosis and treatment may result in a mortality rate of 50%.

General Information

I. **History**
   A. 1883: Fournier described a necrotizing infection of the scrotum (Fournier's gangrene).
   B. 1924: Meleney reported streptococcal gangrene associated with bacterial synergism (Meleney's synergistic gangrene).
   C. 1952: Wilson described necrotizing fasciitis.
   D. 1983: Greenberg reported necrotizing fasciitis with group A streptococci and toxic shock syndrome (TSS).

II. **Etiology**
   A. **Monomicrobial infections:** Caused by three broad classes of organisms.
      1. **Bacteria**
         a. *Streptococcus pyogenes.*
         b. *Clostridium perfringens.*
         c. Rarely, Gram-negative aerobes such as *Pseudomonas aeruginosa* or Fungi *vibrio vulnificus* may be involved.
      2. **Fungus** (e.g., *Mucor*): Can invade deeply, bypassing fascial planes.
      3. **Protozoa:** Rarely cause necrotizing infections (e.g., *Entamoeba histolytica, Trichinella, Toxocara* spp.). Meleney's synergistic gangrene is thought to be caused by *Entamoeba* infection.
   B. **Polymicrobial infections:** Much more common than monomicrobial necrotizing infections.
      1. **Bacterial synergism:** Allows one organism to potentiate the growth of another.
      2. **Gram-positive aerobes** (*S. pyogenes, Staphylococcus aureus,* or *Enterococcus faecalis*) **plus Gram-negative aerobes** (*Escherichia coli, Pseudomonas* spp., *Clostridium* spp., *Bacteroides* spp., or *Peptostreptococcus*).

III. **Risk factors**
   A. **Impaired host defense mechanisms:** Extremes of age, immunosuppression (transplant patient or infection with human immunodeficiency virus), extremity lymphedema, or chronic systemic illnesses (cancer, chronic renal failure, alcoholism, diabetes mellitus, and peripheral vascular disease).
   B. **History of trauma, burns, wound contamination, or foreign body.**

IV. Pathogenesis
   A. A microaerobic wound environment promotes the growth of bacteria, leading to a local decrease in oxygen, producing a permissive environment for anaerobic bacteria.
   B. The presence of proteolytic enzymes enhances the rate and extent of spread of infection.
   C. Thrombosis of nutrient blood vessels to the skin and subcutaneous tissues produces more ischemic tissue, creating a vicious cycle.

V. Presentation
   A. Necrotizing soft tissue infections are characterized by sudden presentation and rapid progression.
   B. The extent of infection is often diffuse, with deeper tissues more affected than superficial ones.
   C. Early signs
   1. Presence of edema beyond the extent of erythema
   2. Crepitus
   3. Skin vesicles or bullae
   4. Fever and early sepsis
   5. Grayish watery drainage ("dishwater pus")
   6. Coppery hue of the skin
   D. Late signs
   1. Cutaneous anesthesia
   2. Focal skin gangrene
   3. Shock, coagulopathy, and multiorgan failure

Classification

I. Clostridial necrotizing infections
   A. Caused by multiple species of *Clostridia*, most commonly *C. perfringens* (80%), *C. novyi* (20%), and *C. septicum*, which are common contaminants of traumatic wounds.
   B. A decrease in local oxygen tension results in spore activation.
   C. Production of multiple exotoxins: Most common is alpha toxin (lecithinase), which causes cell membrane breakdown.
   D. The diagnosis of gas gangrene is made clinically. Necrotizing cellulitis has early local signs with moderate pain and involvement of superficial tissue. Myonecrosis presents with severe pain and involvement of deep tissues.
   E. A Gram stain of wound fluid reveals gram-positive rods without inflammatory cells.

II. Nonclostridial necrotizing infections
   A. Streptococcal gangrene
   1. Caused by hemolytic streptococci.
   2. Presents with rapid development of erythema over 24 hours, with progression to blue discolored bullae and then superficial gangrene in 4 to 5 days.
   B. Necrotizing fasciitis
   1. Typically has a slower onset of symptoms compared with streptococcal gangrene.
   2. Bacterial synergy between aerobic and anaerobic bacteria occurs when lytic toxins enhance the spread of anaerobic bacteria.
   3. **Two main bacteriologic types**
      a. Type I: Enterobacteriaceae/non-group A β-hemolytic streptococci and anaerobic cocci/*Bacteroides;* more common than type II.
      b. Type II: Group A streptococci and staphylococci.
   4. **Meleney's synergistic gangrene:** Occurs postoperatively in surgical wounds, typically either thoracic or abdominal.
   5. **Variant causes**
      a. *Vibrio vulnificus:* Puncture wounds exposed to seawater; rapid onset.
      b. Phycomycosis: More insidious; differentiated only by histology.

C. **Necrotizing fasciitis with streptococcal toxic shock syndrome**
   1. "Flesh-eating bacteria": Caused by *Streptococcus pyogenes*.
   2. Systemic pathogenesis is related to superantigens, M proteins, and induction of monokines (tumor necrosis factor, interleukins 1 and 6).
   3. Rapid presentation of pain, edema, fever, shock, and organ failure.
   4. Clindamycin impairs M-protein synthesis and exotoxin production.
D. **Idiopathic scrotal gangrene**
   1. Fournier's gangrene: Perineal gram-negative synergistic necrotizing cellulitis.
   2. Causative organisms: Anaerobic streptococci.
   3. Presentation: Sudden onset of fever and rapid development of scrotal gangrene and skin sloughing (24–30 hours).

Management

I. **Early diagnosis**
   A. **Primarily based on clinical suspicion**, but may be assisted with laboratory studies that include a complete blood count, serum electrolyte levels, and lactate levels.
   B. **Soft tissue x-rays** (soft tissue gas), computed tomographic scan, or magnetic resonance imaging with gadolinium.
   C. **Early tissue biopsy** may facilitate early recognition of phycomycoses.
II. **Radical surgical debridement**
   A. **Debridement of all necrotic tissues should be performed, with intraoperative quantitative culture** and collection of biopsy specimens. Gram staining of wound fluid should be performed.
   B. **Debridement should extend to viable tissue,** with possible extremity amputation in clostridial gangrene, debridement of abdominal wall in Meleney's synergistic postoperative gangrene, and creation of a testicular thigh pouch in Fournier's gangrene.
   C. **Postoperative intensive care** is usually required, with invasive monitoring, aggressive resuscitation, immobilization and elevation of involved extremities, and initiation of dressing changes (topical antimicrobial versus moist gauze).
   D. **Repeat exploration in 24 to 48 hours** is performed, and remaining infected tissue is excised.
III. **Antibiotic coverage**
   A. **Broad coverage** should be used until microbiologic analysis of the wound is available. Penicillin, ampicillin, and beta-lactams are effective for *Clostridia*, enterococci, and *Peptostreptococcus*. Clindamycin is excellent for anaerobes, and gentamicin is effective against most *Enterobacter* and gram-negative species.
   B. **Single-agent,** broad-spectrum drug therapy may be initiated.
   C. **Amphotericin B** should be started for demonstrated phycomycoses.
   D. **Third-generation cephalosporins and doxycycline or fluoroquinolones** should be used for *Vibrio vulnificus* infection.
   E. **Human immunoglobulin** should be given to patients with streptococcal TSS.
   F. **Antibiotic treatment alone is not enough.** Surgical debridement of all devitalized tissues is required.
IV. **Hyperbaric oxygen therapy**
   A. Can be used for clostridial necrotizing infections in conjunction with the previously listed treatments.
   B. There is no proven efficacy in nonclostridial infections.

Brown Recluse Spider Bites

I. **Entomology**
   A. *Loxosceles reclusa* is identified by a violin-shaped mark on the dorsal cephalothorax.

B. The spider measures 1 to 3 cm in size, and is often found indoors or outdoors in debris piles.

II. Clinical presentation

A. The bite presents with superficial erythema with surrounding purplish discoloration (6–24 hours).

B. Progression to full-thickness skin necrosis often ensues (over >48 hours).

C. Systemic symptoms may include fever, myalgia, malaise, and/or gastrointestinal upset (beginning at 12–24 hours).

III. Pathophysiology

A. The spider's venom is cytotoxic, with protease, hyaluronidase, esterase, and sphingomyelinase components.

B. There is potentiation of the local neutrophil-mediated immune response, with development of dermatonecrosis and systemic lymphokine response.

C. Histologic polymorphonuclear neutrophil perivasculitis with local hemorrhage also occurs.

IV. Treatment

A. Correct identification of the lesion can be difficult, and is often delayed.

B. Evaluate for other causes and monitor for systemic symptoms.

C. Initial irrigation, local cold therapy, tetanus prophylaxis, and elevation of the affected extremity are helpful.

D. Closely observe for 72 hours.

E. Dapsone (a leukocyte inhibitor) should be initiated orally if a brown recluse spider bite is suspected. Dapsone is continued until the skin lesion resolves.

F. Surgical debridement with skin grafting is indicated if medical therapy fails and the lesion is well demarcated.

G. Failure of grafting is high—around 15%.

Pearls

---

1. Necrotizing fasciitis is a surgical disease.

2. Biopsies of tissue for culture are mandatory, as is a "second look" operation in 24 hours.

3. Hyperbaric oxygen therapy may be helpful in the treatment of clostridial infections.

4. Dapsone can reduce the need for surgical treatment of wounds from brown recluse spider bites.

5. Skin grafting of brown recluse spider bites is associated with high failure rates.

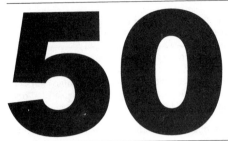

Hypospadias

Brent K. Hollenbeck
and Caleb P. Nelson

I. Biology and development
   A. The urethra normally coalesces at the raphe in the midline, from proximal to distal (from perineum to glans). Hypospadias results from failure of the urethral folds to fuse completely. This leaves the meatus located along the ventral aspect of the penis.
   B. Testosterone influences the development of the genitals by induction of virilization of indifferent external genitalia.
   C. Potential causes of hypospadias.
      1. Abnormal androgen production.
      2. Varying degrees of androgen receptor sensitivity in pertinent tissues (e.g., the genital tubercle).
      3. Environmental estrogens (controversial).

II. Characterization
   A. Incidence: 1 in 300 live births.
   B. Common triad: Hypospadias, chordee, and a dorsal hood.
      1. Chordee
         a. Ventral curvature of the penis.
         b. Historically was thought to be due to a band of fibrous tissue along the course of the urethral plate, the dorsal half of the hypoplastic urethra.
         c. The true etiology is currently unclear.
         d. The artificial erection test (see "Pertinent Principles in Hypospadias Repairs") is useful to gauge the severity of the curvature and to measure the adequacy of correction.
      2. Dorsal hood: In the presence of hypospadias, the dorsal foreskin is termed the dorsal hood, and is often quite noticeable due to the relative absence of ventral tissue.
   C. Associated congenital anomalies
      1. Other urinary tract anomalies are not typically associated with isolated hypospadias. Therefore, reserve urinary tract imaging for those patients with other congenital anomalies (e.g., imperforate anus).
      2. Enlarged prostatic utricle (Müllerian remnant): Present in 10% to 15% of hypospadias patients; can lead to difficult urethral catheterization.
      3. Cryptorchidism: Present in 9%; may be associated with intersex (ambiguous genitalia).
      4. Intersex conditions: More likely to be associated with proximal (e.g., perineal) hypospadias or cryptorchidism.
         a. Reserve intensive evaluation (e.g., karyotyping) for such patients.
         b. Mixed gonadal dysgenesis is the most common intersex variant in this population.
   D. Location of meatus
      1. Determines the type of repair to some degree; may be related to degree and timing of the androgen insult.
      2. Incidence according to the location *after* the correction of chordee.
         a. Anterior hypospadias (50%): Glanular, coronal, and subcoronal.
         b. Middle hypospadias (30%): Distal penile, midshaft, and proximal Penile.
         c. Posterior hypospadias (20%): Penoscrotal, scrotal, and perineal.

III. Surgical repair
A. Best performed between 6 and 18 months of age.
1. Minimizes anesthetic risk (after 3 months of age).
2. Limits psychological impact of surgery.
3. Avoids feeling of being "different" (e.g., sitting to urinate).
4. Limits the potential impact on toilet training.

B. Goals of repair
1. **Create a functionally straight phallus:** Verified by the artificial erection test.
2. **Establish a functional urethra:** Allows for a directed stream and micturition while standing; can be objectively followed by uroflowmetry.
3. **Provide a normal appearance:** Critical goal. One-third of adult patients are dissatisfied with their cosmetic result due to scarring, redundant skin (from preserving skin for possible secondary procedures), and reduced penile length (a consequence of dorsal plication).

C. Pertinent principles in hypospadias repair
1. **Optical magnification** ($2.5\times$ to $3.5\times$ operating loupes).
2. **Subcutaneous injection of epinephrine** along planned incision lines facilitates hemostasis.
3. **Correct the chordee first.** Use the artificial erection test: Insert a small-gauge butterfly needle into the corpora through the glans (to avoid penetrating Buck's fascia) and inject saline while having a tourniquet (e.g., a rubber drain) around the base of the penis to prevent outflow.
4. **Formation of a watertight neourethra** is essential.
5. **Tension-free skin and neourethral repairs,** as well as delicate tissue handling, are essential for optimal wound healing.
6. **Closure is performed in multiple layers** using a Dartos or tunica vaginalis flap.

D. Types of repair
1. **Chordee correction**
   a. Excision of the urethral plate.
   b. Dorsal plication of the corpora.
      (1) Plication stitches are placed laterally to avoid the neurovascular bundles in the dorsal midline.
      (2) It is unclear if early repair predisposes to recurrence during puberty, the period of corporal growth.
      (3) Potential exists for penile shortening.
   c. Elevation of the urethral plate.
   d. Recurrence rates are variable (up to 40%).
2. **Meatal advancement and glansplasty (MAGPI)**
   a. Initially described in 1981.
   b. Indicated for glanular and coronal variants only; results are largely dependent on patient selection.
   c. Meatal regression, the most troublesome complication, may be minimized by careful approximation of the glans ventrally.
   d. Urinary diversion with a catheter is not necessary.
   e. Complication rate: 1%.
3. **Parameatal-based flap** (e.g., Mathieu)
   a. For slightly more proximal variants.
   b. Flap cannot contain hair-bearing skin.
   c. Complications: 6%.
4. **Onlay island flap**
   a. Flap from the inner preputial skin of the dorsal hood.
   b. Useful for midshaft variants.
   c. Onlay onto the urethral plate; must tailor to the appropriate size to prevent formation of a urethral diverticulum.
   d. Complications: 6%.
5. **Tubularized flap** (e.g., transverse preputial island flap)
   a. Same flap as an onlay island flap, except completely tubularized.

       b. Intended for longer gaps; can use even if the urethral plate has been excised.

       c. There is potential for stricture formation at the proximal anastomosis.

       d. Complications: 10% to 15%.

    6. Tubularized incised plate (e.g., Snodgrass repair)

       a. Useful for most variants.

       b. Has essentially supplanted other techniques as the procedure of choice for "middle" hypospadias variants and possibly others.

       c. Direct incision and subsequent tubularization of the urethral plate.

    7. Grafts (e.g., buccal mucosa, bladder mucosa) can be performed as onlay or tubular grafts.

E. Staged repairs

    1. Generally reserved for more proximal (posterior) variants or very small phalluses (to allow for growth).

    2. Second stage is usually performed 6 to 12 months after the initial procedure.

IV. Outcomes

  A. The more proximal the meatus, the more likely are complications.

  B. Potential complications of hypospadias reconstruction.

    1. Urethrocutaneous fistula: Occurs in 5% to 10% of one-stage repairs. Excision and closure of the fistula can be performed at 6 months, provided no distal obstruction is present.

    2. Other complications include meatal stenosis (which may lead to urethrocutaneous fistula), urethral stricture, inadvertent transfer of hair-bearing skin, recurrent chordee, and urethral diverticula.

Pearls

---

1. Correct the chordee first. Once the penis is adequately straight, the best technique for hypospadias repair can be determined.
2. Do not rush to fix a fistula. Wait at least 6 months, and make sure that there is no distal urethral obstruction.
3. Proximal/posterior hypospadias and any variant associated with undescended testes warrant an intersex evaluation.
4. Never use skin that will eventually be hair-bearing.
5. Most successful repairs have multilayer flap coverage.

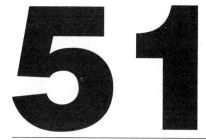

Penile and Vaginal Reconstruction and Gender Identity Disorder

Andrew H. Rosenthal

Anatomy and Embryology

I. Male anatomy
- **A. Layers of the penis**, from superficial to deep
  1. Skin.
  2. Superficial (Dartos') fascia.
  3. Deep (Buck's) fascia.
  4. Neurovascular bundle: Deep dorsal vein, dorsal artery, and paired dorsal nerves.
  5. Tunica albuginea: Surrounds each corpus individually.
  6. Erectile tissue: Paired corpora cavernosa and the corpora spongiosum.
- **B. Arterial supply**
  1. **Internal pudendal artery.**
     - **a. Perineal artery:** Supplies the perineum and the scrotum.
     - **b. Common penile artery:** Three branches to the penis.
       - **(1)** Bulbourethral artery.
       - **(2)** Dorsal artery.
       - **(3)** Deep (cavernosal) artery.
  2. **Testicular arteries:** Branch high off of the aorta, due to the testes developing intraabdominally.
- **C. Urethral segments**
  1. **Posterior:** Proximal to the bulb; prostatic and membranous portions.
  2. **Anterior:** Distal to the bulb; contained within the corpus spongiosum (bulbar and penile/pendulous portions, fossa navicularis).
- **D. Size**
  1. **Normal term neonates:** 35 ± 7 mm stretched length, 11 ± 2 mm width.
  2. **Adult:** The average erect penis ranges from 10 to 17 cm in length.

II. Female anatomy
- **A.** Female anatomy has many analogues to male anatomy.
- **B.** The urethra is shorter and less convoluted.
- **C.** Feminization of the external genitalia is due to absence of, or insensitivity to, androgens.
- **D.** Differentiation at 8 weeks: Preferential growth of the paramesonephric ducts.
- **E.** Vaginal plate (from the urogenital sinus) eventually canalizes into the vaginal vault (by the fifth month).
- **F.** Clitoris: Formed as the phallus turns caudal and has abbreviated growth.
- **G.** Labioscrotal swellings do not fuse in the midline; they fold in to become the labia.

III. Embryology
- **A. Gender-indifferent stage**
  1. **Development during weeks 1 to 7** of gestation is the same for either sex.
  2. **Critical structures and sequences**
     - **a.** The genital tubercle is present by the end of week 5.

       b. Germ cells (gonad precursors) migrate into the region.

       c. Mesonephric (Wolffian) ducts develop.

       d. Paramesonephric (Müllerian) ducts develop.

B. Male differentiation

    1. **The histocompatibility Y (H-Y) antigen** causes maturation of the gonads into testes.

    2. **Functional fetal testes determine and influence the male phenotype via the following.**

       a. Müllerian-inhibiting substance: From Sertoli cells; inhibits the development of müllerian structures.

       b. Androgenic steroids.

          (1) Testosterone: Causes the Wolffian duct system to develop into male structures.

          (2) Dihydrotestosterone (a testosterone metabolite): Induces the development of the prostate and male external genitalia (the genital tubercle becomes the phallus).

       c. Paired urethral folds fuse ventrally, in a proximal-to-distal direction, to form the penile urethra.

       d. Distally, the lateral glans rolls medially to envelop the advancing urethra, bringing the dorsal foreskin around ventrally.

       e. The hallmark of male differentiation is midline fusion of the foreskin, penile urethra, and scrotum in the median raphe.

C. Female differentiation

    1. Female differentiation is the "default" (occurring when no H-Y antigen is present).

    2. If the testes are dysfunctional, differing degrees of feminization will develop.

    3. In the absence of testicular-produced androgens, the müllerian ducts mature into the internal female structures.

    4. The vagina forms when the central cells of the vaginal plate degenerate, creating the vaginal vault.

    5. This process is completed by the fifth month of gestation.

Penile Reconstruction

I. Indications

  A. Congenital abnormalities

  B. Acquired defects

    1. **Peyronie's disease:** Angulation of the penis secondary to connective tissue fibrosis of the penile fascia.

    2. **Trauma.**

    3. **Fournier's gangrene:** Perineal tissue necrosis secondary to (poly)microbial infection, usually in immune-suppressed patients (e.g., diabetes mellitus).

  C. Gender identity disorder (see below).

II. Reconstruction

  A. First, identify missing or altered structures.

    1. Urethra.

    2. Penis.

    3. Glans.

    4. Scrotum.

  B. Methods of reconstruction are the same as for gender identity disorder (see below), and are altered depending on intact structures.

  C. For genetic males, if the congenital defect is significant, consider female organ reconstruction with rearing as a female due to the relative difficulty of functional male urogenital reconstruction.

Vaginal Reconstruction

I. **Indications**
  A. **Congenital abnormalities**
  B. **Acquired defects**
    1. Cancer
    2. Trauma
  C. **Gender identity disorder**
II. **Reconstruction**
  A. **First, identify missing or altered structures.**
    1. Urethra
    2. Vagina
    3. Vulva/labia
  B. **Vaginal reconstruction**
    1. Nonoperative: Graduated dilatation. Effective even in complete agenesis but requires a motivated patient.
    2. Skin grafts: Tendency to contract.
    3. Intestinal substitution (see "Gender Identity Disorder").
    4. Medial thigh skin flaps.
    5. Labial flaps.
    6. Pudendal thigh flaps (Singapore flap): Based on the terminal branches of the internal pudendal artery.
    7. Superficial inferior epigastric artery (SIEA) flap: The pedicle is inconsistent.
    8. Gracilis myocutaneous flap.
    9. Rectus abdominis myocutaneous flap.
    10. Free flaps: Usually reserved for cases of local flap failure.
  C. **Vulvar reconstruction**
    1. Skin grafts
    2. Fasciocutaneous medial thigh flap
    3. Gracilis myocutaneous V-Y advancement flap

Gender Identity Disorder (Gender Dysphoria)

I. **Diagnostic criteria**
  A. The desire to live and be accepted as a member of the opposite sex.
  B. Transsexual identity has been present persistently for at least 2 years.
  C. Not a symptom of another mental disorder or chromosomal abnormality.
II. **Surgical candidates**
  A. **The Harry Benjamin International Gender Dysphoria Association** has created standards of care and internationally accepted guidelines for treatment.
  B. Potential candidates should be evaluated by a multidisciplinary team.
  C. **Sequence of treatment**
    1. Real life experiences
    2. Hormone therapy
    3. Surgical therapy
  D. **Goal of surgical therapy:** To create body congruity with the preferred sexual identity.
  E. **Often patients undergo lesser or nongenital surgery** to assist in their gender integration before genital reassignment.
    1. Breast implants or reduction mammoplasty
    2. Facial surgery: Rhinoplasty, blepharoplasty, and facial bone contouring
    3. Thyroid cartilage reduction
    4. Vocal cord surgery
    5. Liposuction

III. Contraindications to surgical treatment
  A. Sexual ambiguity
  B. Prior to age of consent
  C. Paranoid or emotionally disturbed
  D. Lack of group support
  E. Unrealistic expectations
  F. Medical issues precluding surgery
IV. Male-to-female genital surgery (vaginoplasty)
  A. Goals
   1. Single stage
   2. Aesthetically appealing
   3. Erogenous sensibility
   4. Low complication risk (*Note:* All methods for reconstruction risk rectal damage during dissection to create the neovagina in the plane just ventral to the rectum.)
   5. Adequate depth and diameter to accommodate intercourse
  B. Skin grafts
   1. Use penile or nongenital skin for vagina in association with orchiectomy, penectomy, and urethral reconstruction.
   2. Simple.
   3. Requires prolonged dilation due to the tendency for contracture over time.
   4. No natural lubrication.
  C. Intestinal substitution
   1. A segment of the rectosigmoid is mobilized for vaginal reconstruction.
   2. Performed with orchiectomy, penectomy, and urethral reconstruction.
   3. More complicated; requires a gastrointestinal anastomosis; produces excess odor and mucus; fragile mucosa often bleeds during intercourse.
  D. Penile inversion
   1. Uses inverted penile skin for reconstruction of a new vagina with a posteriorly based triangular skin flap for the posterior vault.
   2. The neoclitoris can be created from an island flap of the glans.
   3. Performed in association with orchiectomy, penectomy (once the penis is degloved), and urethral reconstruction.
   4. The labia are reconstructed from the scrotum.
   5. Uses existing parts to recreate like structures; good sensibility; no donor site morbidity; high success rate; responds well to dilation to increase size.
   6. No natural lubrication.
V. Female-to-male genital surgery
  A. Phalloplasty
   1. Goals
     a. Single stage
     b. Aesthetically appealing
     c. Erogenous sensibility
     d. Ability to have sexual intercourse
     e. Ability to void while standing, with a stream from the tip of the penis
     f. Appropriate size, shape, and location
     g. Minimal donor site morbidity
   2. Pedicled flaps
     a. Bipedicled abdominal flap
     b. Single-pedicled infraumbilical flap
     c. Groin flaps
     d. Thigh flaps
     e. SIEA flap
     f. Gracilis or rectus abdominis flaps
   3. Free flaps
     a. Radial forearm
     b. Lateral arm

4. **Metaidoioplasty**
   a. Transfer of the urethra to the enlarged clitoris (after hormone therapy)
   b. Results in a much smaller neophallus than with other methods
5. **Urethral lengthening**
   a. Vaginal flaps are the workhorse.
   b. Mucosal, skin, intestinal, and other local flaps are also options.
B. **Glansplasty:** Local flaps are used to sculpt the glans for the neophallus.
C. **Neoscrotum construction**
   1. Local perineal advancement flaps
   2. Labia majora flaps
   3. Testicular prosthesis

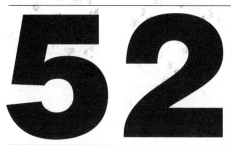

Acute Burns

Salvatore Pacella

I. Pathophysiology

A. **The severity of the burn** is determined by temperature and length of exposure to the heat source.

B. **Skin has a large water content;** therefore, it overheats slowly and cools slowly.

C. **Heat continues to penetrate** deeper tissue layers even after the external heat source is removed. Immediate cooling may reduce underlying tissue temperature, but it has a limited role in large burns because it may reduce the patient's core temperature.

D. **Three areas of injury**
1. **Central "zone of coagulation":** Nonviable, irreversibly injured tissue.
2. **Middle "zone of stasis":** Initially characterized by dilated blood vessels and capillary diffusion. After 24 to 48 hours, dilated capillaries become occluded, with resulting conversion of this zone of tissue to coagulation. Injury in this zone may be reversible with appropriate treatment (cooling, fluid resuscitation, critical care).
3. **Outer "zone of hyperemia":** Composed mostly of viable, edematous tissue.

E. **Progressive changes in microcirculation**
1. There is an initial, sudden decrease in blood flow.
2. Arteriolar vasodilation follows.
3. Increased capillary permeability leads to edema formation, which is greatest at 8 to 12 hours.
4. Endogenous mediators (histamine, serotonin, kinins) increase capillary permeability, leaking protein into the interstitial space.
5. Hypoproteinemia decreases intravascular oncotic pressure, resulting in a shift of fluid into the interstitium (i.e., "third spacing").

II. Initial management

A. **History**
1. **Identify the source:** Hot liquid, chemicals, flame, superheated air/steam, explosion, etc.
2. **Duration and location of exposure:** Closed space; potential for smoke inhalation
3. **Concomitant drug or alcohol ingestion**
4. **Associated injury mechanism:** Explosion, jump/fall, motor vehicle crash, etc.

B. **Airway and breathing** (see also "Inhalation Injury")
1. **Early intubation**
   a. Frequently necessary to prevent airway obstruction due to progressive airway edema.
   b. Most patients with extensive (>50%) burns require intubation.
   c. Use humidified oxygen.
2. **Chest and abdominal wall burns** can severely limit chest wall excursion and impair ventilation. Escharotomies may be necessary (see "Circumferential Burns and Escharotomy").

C. Circulation

1. **Intravenous access:** Ideally, several peripheral large-bore intravenous lines (e.g., 14 gauge) should be placed through nonburned tissues. Central lines are the next best option.

2. **Intravenous fluid administration** (see also "Fluid Resuscitation")

   a. Isotonic salt solutions are used for resuscitation and maintenance.

   b. Glucose should be avoided. Burn patients are frequently glucose intolerant and hyperglycemic due to the stress response. The resulting osmotic diuresis can lead to spuriously high urine output.

D. Disability: A rapid, thorough baseline neurologic examination should be performed. This is especially important in the setting of blunt trauma, head injury, carbon monoxide exposure, and/or the need for sedation.

E. Initial wound care

1. **Stop the burning process.**

   a. Flame burns: Smoldering or burning materials must be extinguished and removed, since they can retain heat and exacerbate the burn injury. Irrigate the wounds with normal saline if any foreign material remains.

   b. Chemical burns: Remove all clothing and begin gentle, copious irrigation with warm normal saline. Avoid the use of neutralizing solutions.

2. **Cover:** Clean, dry, nonadherent dressings are used to protect the wound and prevent hypothermia.

3. **Analgesia.**

4. **Tetanus prophylaxis.**

5. **Prophylactic intravenous antibiotics are *not* indicated.**

6. **Criteria for admission to a burn center.**

   a. If 10 to 40 years old: Greater than 15% total body surface area (TBSA) second-degree burns or greater than 3% TBSA third-degree burns should be treated on an inpatient basis.

   b. If younger than 10 years or older than 40 years: Greater than 10% TBSA second- or third-degree burns.

   c. Burns involving the face, hands, feet and/or perineum.

   d. Circumferential extremity burns.

   e. Electrical burns.

III. Inhalation injury

A. Etiology

1. **Chemical irritants** in smoke affect the distal airways, resulting in an intense inflammatory response, which can lead to adult respiratory distress syndrome (ARDS) and/or systemic inflammatory response syndrome (SIRS).

2. **Direct thermal injury:** Inhalation of superheated air or water vapor can cause a thermal burn to the airway mucosa.

3. **Oropharyngeal and supraglottic edema** caused by thermal injury can progress to airway obstruction.

B. Evaluation

1. **Maintain a high index of suspicion.**

2. **Signs and symptoms.**

   a. History of burn in a closed space.

   b. Presence of facial burns and/or oral carbon deposits.

   c. Singed facial hair/nares, hoarseness, or wheezing.

   d. Unconsciousness.

3. **Nasopharyngoscopy:** Can be used to directly evaluate the larynx and vocal cords for injury.

4. **Bronchoscopy:** Via the endotracheal tube, if symptoms warrant.

C. Treatment

1. **Intubation, mechanical ventilation**

   a. Early intubation is essential. Patients with inhalation injury often present as conscious, awake, and comfortable initially. Upper airway edema can progress rapidly to complete airway obstruction.

       b. Ventilator management goals: Maximize oxygenation while avoiding oxygen toxicity (keep FiO_2 <0.7) and barotrauma.

    2. Bronchodilators: Useful in treating bronchospasm associated with smoke inhalation.

    3. Steroids: Have not been shown to be beneficial in avoiding pulmonary complications with burns.

  D. Carbon monoxide (CO) poisoning

    1. CO is generated by fire. When inhaled and absorbed, it preferentially binds with hemoglobin, displacing oxygen and blocking oxygen binding sites, causing a substantial reduction in oxygen delivery.

    2. Signs and symptoms

      a. Pulse oximetry is unreliable.

      b. Cherry red skin.

      c. Hypoxemia.

      d. Mental status changes or a history of a loss of consciousness.

      e. Persistent acidosis in the presence of normovolemia.

    3. CO level

      a. May be normal or minimally elevated, even with significant exposure.

      b. 20% to 40%: Associated with severe neurologic symptoms.

      c. Greater than 60%: Commonly fatal.

    4. Treatment

      a. 100% oxygen administration: Displaces CO from hemoglobin.

      b. Hyperbaric therapy: Consider if the patient is at risk for CO exposure and has mental status changes.

IV. Burn wound assessment

  A. Area

    1. Patient's palm is approximately 1% of TBSA.

    2. Adults: Rule of 9's.

      a. Arm, anterior/posterior legs, head = 9% each.

      b. Anterior/posterior torso = 18% each.

    3. Children: The head has a proportionately larger surface area.

  B. Depth: Initial estimates may be inaccurate, since the depth of the burn can progress over time.

    1. Superficial—first degree

      a. Example: sunburn.

      b. Confined to the epidermis.

      c. Skin: Mildly erythematous.

      d. Pain: Resolves in 48 to 72 hours.

      e. No scarring.

    2. Partial thickness—second degree

      a. Entire epidermis and variable thickness of dermis.

      b. Skin: Painful, red, edematous, blistered.

      c. Superficial: Dermal appendages intact; heals in less than 3 weeks, usually with minimal to no scarring.

      d. Deep: Less pain; heals in weeks to months with scarring.

      e. The most important distinction is between superficial and deep partial-thickness burns, since excision and grafting is performed for deep partial-thickness burns and usually not for superficial partial-thickness injuries.

    3. Full thickness—third degree

      a. The epidermis and dermis are destroyed, no dermal appendages remain, and there is no possibility of spontaneous regeneration.

      b. Skin: Not painful. It has a leathery, waxy, charred appearance with thrombosis of vessels.

V. Fluid resuscitation

  A. No formula uniformly predicts fluid requirements accurately for every patient. The physician must repeatedly assess each patient's ongoing fluid requirement to maintain an adequate circulatory volume. All resuscitative endpoints (e.g., physical examination, distal perfusion, urine output, central wedge pressure) are important.

B. Modified Brooke (Parkland) formula
   1. First 24 hours' requirement = 4 cc × %TBSA × patient's weight (kg).
   2. Administer half of the above volume during the first 8 hours (calculated from the time of injury, not the time of hospital admission), and the other half over the next 16 hours.
   3. The adequacy of resuscitation is best judged by hourly urine output (30–50 cc/hr in adults, or 1 mL/kg/hr in children).
   4. High-voltage electrical burns or deep tissue burns: There is a high risk for myoglobin-induced acute tubular necrosis.
      a. Maintain urine output at 2 mg/kg/hr.
      b. Alkalinize the urine: Add bicarbonate to intravenous fluid (50 mEq/L).
      c. Monitor urine myoglobin levels.
C. Colloid administration: Not recommended in the first 24 hours after a burn. Increased capillary leak causes the colloid to become trapped in the interstitial space, increasing third spacing and edema.
D. Hyponatremia and hyperkalemia are common: Follow serial electrolyte levels.
VI. Burn wound care
A. Infection
   1. Bronchopneumonia is the leading cause of death.
   2. Burn wound sepsis, septic thrombophlebitis, and bacterial endocarditis are also common infections in the burn patient.
   3. *Pseudomonas, Enterococcus,* and methicillin-resistant *Staphylococcus* are the main offending organisms.
B. Topical antimicrobial agents
   1. Silvadene (1% silver sulfadiazine)
      a. Widely available.
      b. Broad gram-negative and gram-positive coverage.
      c. Moderate wound penetration.
      d. Can damage the cornea.
      e. May cause **leukopenia.**
   2. Sulfamylon (10% mafenide acetate)
      a. Broad-spectrum coverage.
      b. Excellent wound penetration.
      c. The best topical agent for exposed cartilage (e.g., the ear and nose).
      d. Painful.
      e. Can cause **acidosis** due to carbonic anhydrase inhibition. Its use should be avoided in burns greater than 20% TBSA.
   3. Silver nitrate (0.5% solution)
      a. Broad-spectrum coverage.
      b. Poor eschar penetration.
      c. Costly, messy.
      d. Can cause **hyponatremia.**
   4. Bacitracin zinc ointment
      a. Effective against gram-positive organisms only.
      b. Does not penetrate burn eschar.
      c. Commonly used for facial burns.
C. Excision and grafting
   1. Tangential burn wound excision and skin graft coverage is performed following hemodynamic stabilization, often beginning within 2 to 4 days of injury.
   2. Tangential excision
      a. Thin-layer sequential excision of all nonviable tissue until a viable tissue level is reached.
      b. Skin grafting on fat can be tenuous due to its poor blood supply and difficulty in delineating a healthy level.
      c. Delayed grafting
         (1) Performed in cases of inadequate donor sites for graft harvest.
         (2) Cover wounds first with cadaveric allograft or a nonbiologic dressing to protect against fluid losses and burn wound infection.

   d. Operative blood loss can be considerable. The recommended limit for excision in a single session is approximately 10% to 20% TBSA or less than 10 units of packed red blood cells transfusion.
   3. Grafting techniques (see Chapter 3, "Grafts")
   a. Graft thickness: Generally 12 to 14/1000th inch. The thinner the graft, the more likely the take, but more significant is the degree of secondary contraction. Use 16 to 20/1000th-inch thickness for the face, if possible.
   b. Meshing: Usually at a 1:1.5 ratio. Meshing the graft increases the surface area that can be covered, and can decrease hematoma and seroma collection beneath the graft. Higher mesh ratios can be used, as necessary (e.g., 1:2, 1:3, or 1:4).
   c. Unmeshed "sheet" grafts are typically used on cosmetic or functional areas, such as the face, breast, and hands.
   4. Graft failure
   a. Inadequate wound debridement prior to graft application is the primary cause.
   b. Infection (see "Infection").
   c. Seroma, hematoma.
   d. Lack of moisture.
   e. Shear: Improper padding, dressing, or patient positioning.
   f. Poor nutritional or overall physiologic status (e.g., poor visceral protein levels or sepsis).
VII. Circumferential burns and escharotomy
   A. Circumferential burns: Result in limited ability for expansion of tissues with edema. This can cause supraphysiologic pressures to develop, causing tissue ischemia and necrosis.
   B. Physical signs are often obscured by the burn injury or tissue edema. Doppler examination is unreliable in estimating tissue perfusion.
   C. Burned extremities should be elevated.
   D. Escharotomy: Incision of burned skin to relieve constriction.
      1. Electrocautery incision is the method of choice, and can be performed at the bedside because the burned skin is anesthetic.
      2. Arms and legs: Medial and lateral incisions; may include digits.
      3. Chest and upper abdomen: Bilateral midaxillary releases can be connected with a horizontal incision to form an H.
VIII. Burns of the face, eyes, and ears
   A. The central face has deeper skin appendages, resulting in a greater healing capacity.
   B. Use unmeshed sheet grafts, applied by aesthetic units.
   C. Attempt to perform facial grafting less than 2 weeks from the time of injury to decrease scarring.
   D. Eyes: Lid edema usually protects the eyes in the early stages. As edema subsides and wound contraction occurs, keratitis and corneal abrasion are common risks. Temporary tarsorrhaphy and/or surgical release may be required.
   E. Ears: Twice per day sulfamylon application is the treatment of choice. Avoid any external pressure to the ear. Suppurative chondritis requires urgent debridement.
IX. Burns of the hands and feet
   A. Always perform a complete hand examination.
   B. Maintain a low threshold for escharotomies and fasciotomies, as these procedures save extremities.
   C. Superficial burns: Elevation, topical antimicrobials, and passive range of motion for each joint twice per day.
   D. Appropriate splinting is crucial to prevent contractures.
   E. Deep partial- and full-thickness burns: Early excision and sheet grafting are preferred. Immobilize for 5 days, then start occupational therapy.
   F. Palmar skin is thick. Only 20% of palmar burns ultimately require resurfacing. A conservative approach is recommended to preserve thick fascial attachments.

G. Burns of the feet are managed similarly to hand burns.

X. Genital burns

A. Place burned foreskin into its normal position to prevent paraphimosis.

B. Topical antibiotic therapy may be instituted for several weeks as needed. Any remaining open wounds should then be sheet grafted.

C. Catheters should be removed as soon as possible.

XI. Nutrition

A. **A hypermetabolic response** is common with all large burns.

1. The metabolic rate is proportional to the size of the burn, up to 60% TBSA, remaining constant thereafter.

2. This response begins soon after injury, reaching a plateau by the end of the first week. Most burns of more than 30% TBSA require intensive nutritional support until wound healing is complete.

3. Energy expenditure is unpredictable.

4. **Harris-Benedict equation**

   a. 24-hour caloric requirement = (25 kcal × kg body weight) + (40 kcal × %TBSA).

   b. Frequently undercalculates the real metabolic needs.

B. **Protein:** 2.5 to 3 g/kg per day are recommended. In children, requirements are 3 to 4 g/kg per day.

C. **Intestinal feeding** should be performed early.

D. **Prealbumin levels** are drawn to monitor adequate nutritional progress in patients with large burns.

XII. Electrical injuries

A. **Low-voltage injuries** can be locally destructive without systemic sequelae.

B. **High-voltage injuries** (>1,000 volts): Can result in extensive internal destruction.

1. Entrance and exit wounds: Usually less than 10% to 15% TBSA.

2. Deep tissue injury is caused by the passage of current through tissues. The damage is analogous to a massive crush injury with intact skin.

3. Injury is proportional to tissue resistance: Bone > muscle > nerve.

4. A full trauma workup is paramount. Associated injuries from a fall or tetanic contraction of muscles (paravertebral) are common.

C. **Significant cardiac damage is extremely rare.** Cardiac monitoring should be instituted during the first 24 to 48 hours.

D. **Muscle damage**

1. Should be suspected with myoglobinuria and/or pigmenturia.

2. Maintain a high urine output.

3. Apply Sulfamylon for eschar penetration.

4. Compartment syndrome.

   a. Continually reevaluate the peripheral circulation.

   b. Measure compartment pressures with a Stryker instrument or arterial line setup with a large-bore needle (normal: <15 mm Hg; abnormal: >30 mm Hg).

   c. Fasciotomy: Perform in the operating room.

XIII. Chemical burns

A. Usually deeper than they appear.

B. Injury is due to a chemical reaction rather than thermal injury.

C. In general, dilution, not neutralization, is the key to management.

D. Specific agents.

1. **Hydrofluoric acid**

   a. Liquefaction necrosis in subcutaneous tissues and deeper.

   b. 10% calcium gluconate: Infiltrate subcutaneously after topical dilution with water if pain persists. It is also available as a topical gel.

2. **Phenol**

   a. Poorly soluble in water.

   b. Has an analgesic effect.

   c. Some systemic absorption is possible, causing arrhythmias.

   d. Wash with polyethylene glycol if available.

3. White phosphorus
  a. Chemical and thermal burns.
  b. Copper sulfate: Facilitates removal of the particles (following copious water lavage).

Pearls

1. Use formulas only as a guide to fluid replacement. Monitor fluid status on an ongoing basis via urine output and other measures.
2. Be wary of inhalation injury and have a low threshold for early endotracheal intubation.
3. Have a low threshold for obtaining an ophthalmologic evaluation for burns involving the face.
4. Watch for myoglobinuria and renal failure in electrical burns.
5. Look for circumferential burns and consider early escharotomies.

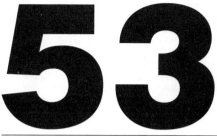

Frostbite, Toxic Epidermal Necrolysis, Staphylococcal Scalded Skin Syndrome, and Meningococcemia

Anil Mungara

Frostbite

I. **Pathophysiology**
   A. **Frostbite is most common in unconscious persons** (from accidents or alcohol intoxication). The severity of injury is exacerbated by wet clothing and peripheral vascular disease. It usually involves the hands, feet, nose, and ears.
   B. **Freezing**
      1. **Rapid freezing** causes **intracellular** ice crystallization, leading to architectural damage and cell death.
      2. **Slow freezing** causes **extracellular** ice crystallization, leading to intracellular dehydration from osmotic fluid shift out of cells.
   C. **Thawing**
      1. Causes capillary leak and microvascular occlusion, which lead to edema of the affected part.
      2. Edema results in tissue ischemia, which exacerbates microvascular occlusion. This results in a vicious cycle of edema and local ischemia.
II. **Classification**
   A. **First degree**
      1. Superficial freezing of the epidermis (i.e., "frostnip").
      2. Presents with hyperemia and mild edema.
      3. Vesicles/blisters do not form.
   B. **Second degree**
      1. Partial-thickness skin injury.
      2. Presents with hyperemia and edema; pain and paresthesias are present.
      3. Vesicles form.
   C. **Third degree**
      1. Necrosis of the entire skin thickness and variable depths of the subcutaneous tissue. There is typically less pain than in milder degrees of frostbite.
      2. Vesicles are usually smaller than in a second-degree injury.
   D. **Fourth degree:** Necrosis extends to deeper tissues (i.e., muscle and bone).
III. **Treatment**
   A. **Rewarming**
      1. Remove cold clothing, and wrap the patient in warm blankets.
      2. Immerse any frozen part(s) in a moving water bath heated to 40°C.
      3. Dry heat (such as fire) is less effective and dangerous.
   B. **Protection of the affected part**
      1. Avoid friction.
      2. Keep the injured part elevated and at room temperature.
      3. Avoid refreezing. If this is a possibility, avoid thawing until at an appropriate facility.
   C. **Anti-infective measures**
      1. Protect vesicles from physical contact.
      2. Antibiotics may be required for established infections.

   3. There is no role for prophylactic antibiotics.
   4. Tetanus prophylaxis should be administered, based on the patient's immunization history.
IV. Surgery
   A. Tissue necrosis may be superficial, with underlying viable tissue. Therefore, amputation should not be considered until complete tissue loss is established. Complete demarcation usually takes several weeks.
   B. Early regional sympathectomy to prevent sequelae of frostbite is controversial.
V. Prognosis
   A. Complete recovery can often be expected.
   B. The affected part may exhibit cold intolerance and an increased susceptibility to cold injury.

Toxic Epidermal Necrolysis (TEN)

I. Etiology
   A. Usually a reaction to antigenic material that causes a split in the epidermis, with necrosis of the superficial portion of the epidermis.
   B. Often drug induced (e.g., ampicillin, allopurinol, and sulfonamides).
   C. TEN can also be caused by staphylococcal infections in immunocompromised patients.
II. Treatment
   A. The skin injury should be treated like a burn.
   B. Mortality rates are significant and, like burns, correlate with comorbidities and age of the patient.

Staphylococcal Scalded Skin Syndrome (SSSS)

I. Etiology
   A. A reaction to staphylococcal toxin causes separation of the granular layer of the epidermis.
   B. This results in desquamation: separation and loss of the epidermis over wide areas.
II. Diagnosis
   A. The clinical presentation of SSSS is similar to that of TEN.
   B. The mucous membranes and conjunctiva are spared in SSSS, in contrast to TEN.
III. Treatment
   A. A detailed search for the focus of a staphylococcal infection should be initiated while systemic antibiotics are started.
   B. The superficial wounds heal quickly if desiccation and superinfection are prevented.

Meningococcemia

I. Clinical Presentation
   A. Fever, headaches, rash, and arthralgias.
   B. A petechial rash starts distally and extends to the trunk.
   C. Fulminant meningococcemia (Waterhouse-Friderichsen syndrome): Results in mental changes and vascular collapse, and can lead to skin necrosis secondary to thrombosis of small vessels in the dermis.

II. Diagnosis

A. Blood cultures prior to the start of antibiotics are positive in 50% of cases. Culture results drop to 5% after the initiation of antibiotics.

B. Gram stains of skin lesions are diagnostic in 70% of cases.

III. Treatment

A. Intravenous penicillin-G or ceftriaxone is used for 7 days to treat the acute infection.

B. Necrotic skin lesions should be debrided and dressed as needed. Once the acute sepsis has resolved and the patient's nutritional status is adequate, skin grafting alone is usually sufficient to reconstruct the cutaneous defects.

Pearls

---

1. Frostbite victims are often homeless and have impaired healing abilities secondary to malnutrition.
2. Avoid friction and/or shear of the frostbitten region. Keep injured parts elevated and protected.
3. Administer tetanus prophylaxis.
4. Avoid amputation for severely frostbitten extremities until complete demarcation is established.
5. Most cases of frostbite result in complete recovery, but the affected area may have an increased susceptibility to repeat cold injury.

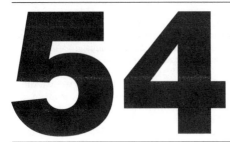

Burn Reconstruction

Keith G. Wolter

General Principles

I. **Goals**
   A. Maximize function.
   B. Minimize disfigurement.
   C. Restore appearance.
II. **Priorities for surgical procedures**
   A. **Urgent:** Required in the acute phase to preserve tissue and function. Examples: exposed ear cartilage and corneal exposure.
   B. **Essential:** Required to regain function. Examples: release of joint contractures; excision of functionally limiting heterotopic ossification.
   C. **Desirable:** Restore a more normal appearance. Examples: restoration of hair in the scalp or eyebrow.
III. **Timing**
   A. Most scars have matured reasonably by 6 to 12 months postburn.
   B. It is preferable to postpone surgical intervention until the scar fully matures, typically 18 to 24 months postburn.
   C. Tissue viability and functional concerns can override the desire to wait (e.g., proximal interphalangeal joint contracture).
   D. Waiting may be psychologically and/or occupationally debilitating. Selected patients may benefit from psychiatric consulation. Physical therapy should be instituted early.
   E. Exact timing of surgery is tailored to each patient's circumstances.
IV. **Hypertrophic scar and contracture**
   A. **Hypertrophic scar**
      1. Can begin to develop 3 weeks after wound closure.
      2. Typically is most pronounced at 2 to 3 months.
      3. Slowly regresses over 12 to 24 months.
      4. Most common in burns that are allowed to heal secondarily.
      5. Younger patients and those with darker skin are at greater risk.
      6. Major patient complaints include erythema, pruritus, and elevation of the scar.
   B. **Wound contracture**
      1. Occurs as collagen reorganizes.
      2. Fibroblasts and myofibroblasts lead to tissue contraction.
      3. **Extrinsic contracture:** Scarring of an adjacent area, pulling on nearby tissues; requires release. Example: ectropion from a cheek burn.
      4. **Intrinsic contracture:** Direct contracture of a region; requires reconstruction. Example: lower lid shortening from a lid burn.
      5. Always release extrinsic contractures first.
V. **Contracture prevention and nonoperative scar treatments**
   A. **Early and aggressive mobilization therapy** with active and passive range of motion (ROM).
   B. **Splints and/or garments** to prevent contracture formation
      1. May be combined with continuous passive motion devices.

      2. Customized splints are preferred over off-the-shelf models.
  C. External pressure dressings and/or devices
      1. Can decrease erythema, pruritus, and elevation of scar.
      2. 20 to 25 mm Hg of pressure is required to inhibit hypertrophic scar formation.
      3. Maintain use for up to 2 years while the scar matures.
      4. Must be worn nearly 24 hours per day, and be removed only for showering.
  D. Silicone gels and gel sheets
      1. The mode of action is unclear. Possible mechanisms include tissue hydration, localized cooling, into skin, and electrostatic effects.
      2. Often combined with pressure garments for increased benefit.
  E. Steroids: Topical creams, triamcinolone injections, and sustained-release topical tape.
  F. Dermabrasion: May avoid the need for excision in some areas.
VI. Surgery to minimize scar and contracture
  A. Better aesthetic and functional outcomes are typically realized with early burn wound excision and grafting. The face is a prime example.
  B. Only deep partial- and full-thickness burns need to be excised.
  C. Skin grafts
      1. Inhibit fibroblast proliferation and therefore contraction.
      2. Thicker grafts generally inhibit contraction more.
VII. Reconstructive options after excision
  A. Direct closure: Preferable if there is minimal tension across the wound.
  B. Adjacent tissue transfer (see Chapter 4, "Flaps"): Z-plasty, local advancement flaps, transposition flaps, and rotation flaps.
  C. Skin grafts (see Chapter 3, "Grafts")
      1. Secondary contraction of full-thickness skin grafts (FTSGs) is less compared with partial-thickness grafts due to the increased amount of dermis transferred.
      2. The donor site should be chosen for a good color and thickness match.
      3. Replace the entire aesthetic unit, if possible.
  D. Cultured epithelial autografts
      1. Can use if dermis is present, or if a dermal substitute is used.
      2. Costly, labor-intensive, and fragile.
  E. Tissue expansion (see Chapter 5, "Tissue Expansion")
      1. Minimizes the donor site deformity, but the complication rate is particularly high with burned tissues; therefore, patient selection is important.
      2. Expand one to three times per week, depending on location, goals, and patient tolerance.
      3. Optimal when the expander is placed directly over bone to allow for maximal outward expansion.
      4. The best results are achieved in the scalp, face, trunk, upper arm, and thigh.
         a. In expansion of neck tissues, tracheal compression must be avoided.
         b. It can be difficult to advance skin over the mandible.
         c. Complication rates are extremely high in the extremities.
  F. Serial excision: Requires multiple surgeries, but offers a less complicated solution than tissue expansion and therefore may be a better choice in poorly compliant patients and difficult areas.
  G. Flaps (see Chapter 4, "Flaps")
  H. Pretransfer expansion and free tissue transfer
      1. Expansion is followed by microvascular transfer.
      2. Provides large amount of vascularized tissue.
      3. The donor site can often be closed primarily.
      4. Surgical delay and dermal angiogenisis lead to robust flap tissue.
      5. Fat atrophy can make the skin more pliable.

Specific Anatomic Sites

I. Scalp
   A. **Acute coverage** is performed with skin grafts if the periosteum is intact. Otherwise, free tissue transfer is indicated. Scalp flaps are generally contraindicated in acute burn coverage.
   B. Treatment of the burned scalp differs from treatment of hereditary hair loss or male pattern baldness (the scalp is tight, thin, and less vascularized).
   C. **Rotational flaps** can be used to close small defects. However, hair follicle orientation is often incorrect.
   D. **Micrografting** of follicles is less successful in burned tissue.
   E. **Delayed tissue expansion** is the treatment of choice for scalp losses of less than 50%.
   F. **Free tissue transfer** (e.g., parascapular flap, radial forearm flap, omentum, and latissimus dorsi muscle) is the preferred option for scalp loss greater than 50%.

II. Face, forehead, and cheeks
   A. **Maintenance of aesthetic units** guides facial reconstruction; replacing only part of a unit can result in a quilt-like appearance.
   B. **Small burns** are excised and closed with primary closure or local flaps.
   C. **Larger burns** can be treated with tissue expansion in a delayed fashion, once primary wound closure has been accomplished.
   D. **For exposed bone**
      1. **A free flap**, such as a free parascapular flap, is optimal.
      2. **The "crane principle" flap:** The scalp is lifted and rotated into the defect, left in place for 2 to 3 weeks, and then returned to its native site, leaving behind a granulating base on the defect, which can be grafted.
   E. **Compression garments** are used to decrease hypertrophic scar.

III. Eyebrow
   A. For any of the hair restoration techniques, follicular alignment is key.
   B. **Aesthetic landmarks** are important; try to match the contralateral brow (make a template from the other side, if normal).
   C. **Vascularized island pedicle flaps from the temporal scalp** based on the anterior branch of the superficial temporal artery and tunneled under skin to the brow area can provide good results.
   D. **Micrografting** for hair restoration can be performed, but is tedious. This technique may give poor results for transfer into burned areas.
   E. **Scalp composite grafts:** Typically yield better results than micrografts.
   F. **Conservative management** options include tattooing or makeup.

IV. Eyelid
   A. **The first priority is to preserve vision.**
   B. **Indications for reconstruction:** Corneal exposure, ectropion, or canthal contracture.
   C. **Ectropion** is the most common cause of eyelid problems after burns. It may result from either intrinsic or extrinsic contracture.
      1. **Extrinsic contracture:** Address first.
         a. Releasing incisions are placed 1 to 2 mm away from the ciliary margin, extending 15 mm beyond the medial and lateral canthi.
         b. **Skin grafts** are used to fill the defect.
            (1) **Upper lid:** FTSG from the opposite side, avoiding the supratarsal fold.
            (2) **Lower lid:** FTSG from the retroauricular region.
         c. **Local flaps**
            (1) **Modified Trepier:** Upper eyelid skin and orbicularis oculi muscle, pedicled at the lateral canthal region, is used to resurface the lower eyelid.
            (2) **Fricke:** Forehead skin above the eyebrow, based laterally.
      2. **Intrinsic contracture:** Requires reconstruction of the entire eyelid thickness.

      a. Upper: If the ispilateral lower lid is intact, use Cutler-Beard or Hughes flaps.

      b. Lower: Mustarde cheek advancement. If no local tissue is available, then use a pedicled temporoparietal fascial flap.

      c. Consider a palatal mucosal graft for support of the middle lamella.

      d. Medial: Release bands of scar with Z-plasties.

      e. Lateral: Scar bands can be corrected by local transposition flap(s).

V. Nose

  A. Postburn scar contractures produce a foreshortened nose, elevated tip, and everted nostril.

  B. In more severe burns, nasal architecture is affected, with loss of skeletal support.

  C. Nostril stenosis may impair nasal breathing.

  D. Reconstruction must address all involved layers: mucosa, cartilage, and skin.

  E. For smaller burn scars affecting skin only, excise the aesthetic unit and cover with a full-thickness skin graft.

  F. Composite grafts from the ear work well for small (1 cm) burns of the alar rim.

  G. In larger burns, neighboring tissue is likely to also be affected and therefore not available for use. The paramedian forehead flap is effective in resurfacing most of the external nose in such cases.

  H. Distant donor sites include the Washio retroauricular flap and the radial forearm free flap, which can be prefabricated to include cartilaginous support.

VI. Ear

  A. Involved in 90% of facial burns.

  B. There is a high risk of suppurative chondritis caused by *Pseudomonas.* Sulfamylon antibiotic cream is used for prevention of infection and maintenance of a moist wound environment. Watch for acidosis.

  C. Symptoms of chondritis include severe pain, erythema, warmth, and swelling.

  D. Established infections require operative debridement.

  E. The reconstructive technique is dependent upon the amount of the ear that is affected.

    1. Small helical rim defects: The Antia-Buch advancement flap is optimal.

    2. Larger helical rim defects: Davis conchal transposition flap. A composite flap of skin and cartilage from the concha, pedicled at the crus helix, is transferred to the upper third of the ear. The donor site is closed with a skin graft.

    3. Extensive defects: A temporoparietal fascial flap is used to cover a cartilage framework.

  F. An osseointegrated prosthesis is an excellent option for total ear loss.

VII. Mouth

  A. Isolated oral commissure burns: Usually from children who have chewed on electric cords.

    1. Conservative management: Oral splint appliance, worn for 6 to 12 months.

    2. Surgical management: Gillies-Millard commissure repair, V-Y advancement, mucosal transposition flap, or tongue flaps.

    3. Be alert to the possibility of labial artery hemorrhage and instruct parents to apply digital pinch pressure.

    4. The lateral margin of the mouth is determined by measuring from the midline to the uninvolved side. Typically, this point is just below the pupil and the end of the nasolabial fold.

  B. Upper lip: This aesthetic unit includes the area bounded by the nasolabial folds laterally, the vermilion inferiorly, and the nasal sill and columellar base superiorly.

    1. Three subunits: Two lateral lip elements and the philtrum.

    2. Release burn ectropion by incising both nasolabial folds and the base of the nose to let the lip fall back into its native position.

    3. The columella can be lengthened with "fork flaps" from the upper lip.

    4. Some male patients desire hair. Use techniques for brow repair, which have the advantage of hiding scars.

    C. Lower lip: Responds well to aesthetic unit replacement.
      1. Soft tissue must be maintained on the pogonion for chin prominence.
      2. Scars can be set in the labiomental creases.
      3. Neck contractures must be released; otherwise, there will be secondary eversion of lower lip.

VIII. Neck and chin
    A. Neck scars are particularly prone to flexion contracture. They can produce extrinsic contracture of the lower face and mechanical disability of the mandible.
    B. Mentosternal synechiae are not uncommon. In children they may result in micrognathia.
    C. The most common error in management is inadequate scar release.
    D. Single or multiple Z-plasties can be utilized.
    E. Avoid injury to the marginal mandibular nerve.
    F. Large burn scars may require grafts, flaps, or both.
    G. FTSGs or split-thickness skin grafts (STSGs) can help limit contracture formation, but rescarring and contracture can occur. Hide graft margins under the jaw shadow, if possible.
    H. Tissue expansion is possible, although technically challenging due to the potential for tracheal compression.
      1. Placing infraclavicular expanders avoids tracheal compression.
      2. Multiple expanders often work well.
    I. Postoperative care: Neck immobilization, splinting, possible nasogastric feeding tube. Compression garments are used for 6 to 18 months to extend and contour the neck.
    J. Large burns may require sheet grafts, deltopectoral flaps, or free flaps.

IX. Breast: Treatment depends upon the age of the patient.
    A. Prepubuscent girls: Burn scars may hamper breast development.
      1. If the nipple-areolar complex (NAC) is burned, then progenitor cells for the breast bud may have been destroyed. If the NAC is intact, then breast tissue damage is less likely.
      2. Even if the breast bud is intact, skin contracture may impede normal development. Therefore, release scars before breast growth begins.
      3. An inframammary incision will release most contractures; the breast mound can then be resculpted and skin grafts used to fill in defects.
    B. Adult women burned as girls: Mammary development has often been impaired. A large amount of tissue replacement is usually needed.
      1. Tissue expansion
        a. Usually, the procedure of choice.
        b. Poor quality of scarred skin may increase the expansion time course.
        c. Ulceration, skin necrosis, and infection are more likely than with healthy skin.
      2. Autogenous tissue (e.g., TRAM and latissimus flaps)
    C. Adult women burned as adults: The reconstructive algorithm is based on the severity of the wound.
      1. If the breast parenchyma is intact, use scar releases with Z-plasties and full- or split-thickness skin grafts to correct asymmetries.
      2. If the breast parenchyma is burned, glandular volume must be restored.
        a. Similar to a postmastectomy defect, but the surrounding skin usually has poor quality. Therefore, flaps are often better than implants.
        b. Contralateral reduction is another option to equalize volume.

X. Abdomen
    A. Small defects: Closed with simple excision.
    B. Moderate defects: Use serial excisions.
    C. Large defects: Tissue expansion.

XI. Upper extremity
    A. Upper extremity contractures should be released in a proximal-to-distal fashion.
    B. Physical therapy and occupational therapy (OT) are as important, if not more important, than surgery.

C. Preoperative physical therapy loosens skin and joint contractures, and participation is an indicator of postoperative patient compliance. Maximal mobility of the joints via OT should be obtained prior to surgical release.

XII. Axilla

A. Adduction contractures can severely limit ROM. Contractures can be prevented or limited with early splinting and physical therapy.

1. **Three grades of axillary contractures**
   a. Type 1A: Involves anterior axillary fold
   b. Type 1B: Involves posterior axillary fold
   c. Type 2: Involves both axillary folds
   d. Type 3: Involves both folds and axillary dome

2. **Type 1 and 2 injuries are managed** with sequential release and resurfacing with thick STSGs or FTSGs.

3. **Type 3 injuries** require large amounts of skin. Composite flaps can be used, including parascapular and latissimus flaps.

B. Avoid displacing axillary hair and sweat glands out of axilla.

C. Scar release must continue through burn scar to normal tissue.

D. Splinting and physical therapy are critical postoperatively.

XIII. Elbow

A. If there is no exposed bone or nerve, use thick unmeshed STSGs.

B. If bone is exposed, then vascularized tissue is required. Consider a fasciocutaneous flap such as a reverse radial forearm flap.

C. A random local fasciocutaneous flap can be used, as long as the flap is based on the longitudinal axis to preserve circulation.

D. Consider a free flap if there is no available local tissue. However, muscle-containing flaps may be too bulky for use over joints because of interference with elbow flexion.

E. Heterotopic ossification, which occurs late after burn injury, may require excision to restore joint mobility.

XIV. Hand

A. It is easier to prevent contractures than to treat established ones.

1. Splinting and early mobilization are vital.
2. Aggressive and early tangential burn wound excision is key.

B. Postburn syndactyly is the most common secondary deformity. Most often, there is a web space contracture involving the dorsal skin of the web space. Treatment approaches include the following.

1. **Excision and/or release of the scar.**
2. **Local tissue rearrangements,** with a myriad of options, such as the following.
   a. "Jumping man plasty"
   b. V-M plasty
   c. Z-plasties
   d. Y-to-V plasty
   e. Tanzer rotation flaps
3. **Skin grafting**

C. Adduction contractures can involve muscle in addition to skin. The first web space is a common location. Treatment must include excision and/or release of contracted muscle tissue.

D. Palmar burns are less common. They typically occur in children who grasp hot objects (e.g., curling irons).

1. Release contractures.
2. FTSGs for palm resurfacing.

E. Claw hand deformity: From dorsal hand burn contractures. Patients have extended metacarpophalangeal (MP) joints, flexed interphalangeal (IP) joints, and a flexed wrist. Again, prevention is critical. If established, begin with aggressive OT, until maximized. MP joints and the wrist can be treated with capsulectomies. IP joint fusion may be required. Often, resurfacing with thin fascial or fasciocutaneous flaps is necessary.

F. **Shortage of skin** along joint creases results in contracture bands. Ensure joint mobility is maximized with OT prior to contracture release. K-wire fixation may be required to keep the joint in an optimal position during healing.

G. **Amputations**
   1. **Pollicization:** Used to restore thumb function.
   2. **Phalangization:** Shortened fingers can be relatively lengthened by deepening web spaces.
   3. **Toe transfer:** An option for severely burned hands.

H. **Nail bed:** Dorsal digital burns cause eponychial retraction and nail bed exposure. A single-stage bilateral transposition flap can be used to restore the nail fold.

XV. **Lower extremity**

A. **Early recognition of a potential compartment syndrome** can prevent limb loss.

B. **Joint contractures** are minimized with aggressive physical therapy, splints, compression garments, and early grafting.

C. **Scar release.**
   1. Narrow bands are lengthened with Z-plasties.
   2. Larger contractures require release and skin grafting.

D. **Long-term postoperative splinting**, particularly at night, can prevent recurrent contractures.

E. **Anterior knee:** Prone to unstable scars. Can be addressed with overgrafting.

F. **Achilles tendon contracture:** Can be covered with a temporoparietal fascial flap or reverse superficial sural artery flap.

G. **Pedicled or free flaps** are needed for exposed bone, nerves, vessels, cartilage, or tendons.

H. **Chronic lymphedema** is managed with custom-fit elastic compression garments.

XVI. **Perineum**

A. The severity of the burn will dictate whether contracture release or complete genital reconstruction is indicated.

B. **Extrinsic contractures** can be corrected with scar release and resurfacing.

C. **Complete reconstruction utilizes the techniques of gender surgery,** that is, a tubed pedicle flap or a radial forearm free flap for total phalloplasty or gracilis flaps for vaginal reconstruction.

Index